ELEMENTARY MEDICAL STATISTICS

DONALD MAINLAND

M.B., CH.B., D.SC., F.R.S.E., F.R.S.C., F.A.S.A.

PROFESSOR OF MEDICAL STATISTICS

NEW YORK UNIVERSITY MEDICAL CENTER

SECOND EDITION

W. B. SAUNDERS COMPANY

PHILADELPHIA AND LONDON   1963

PREFACE

The preface to the first edition of this book opened with the following paragraph:

"Those who have for many years stressed the importance of statistical thinking in medicine cannot be entirely happy to see statistics becoming established as a subject in the undergraduate curriculum, for it thereby becomes liable to the curse that is on all medical 'subjects': the emphasis on memorization, on techniques, and on preparation for board examinations which foster static pedagogy. If this is to be the fate of undergraduate statistical teaching it will indeed be regrettable, for modern statistics offers two things that are most obviously needed in medical education: a means of breaking down interdepartmental barriers, and a set of principles by which we can draw valid conclusions from experience."

During the succeeding decade more medical schools have introduced courses of statistics, and they are still sufficiently varied to prompt the hope that the day of rigid uniformity has been postponed. In too many of the courses, however, there is an overemphasis on statistical arithmetic, as evidenced by the nickname "Slide Rule Medicine" that is applied to some of them. The fault is not entirely that of the teachers, for even those teachers and textbook writers who have tried to show the meaning and limitations of the arithmetical tricks frequently meet people who have picked up and used the tricks without heeding the warnings against their misuse and misinterpretation.

During this same decade, however, a very encouraging phenomenon has been observed. The widespread acceptance of the controlled trial as the only way of testing most drugs and vaccines has shown that clinicians are by no means unwilling to apply statistical principles when they see their bearing on practical affairs. The writer of an elementary textbook can therefore use the properly conducted drug trial to illustrate an investigational standard recognized by medical workers; he could not easily do this ten years ago. He can show the difficulties of reaching this standard; he can even show that many laboratory experiments fall far short of it.

Even in discussing the vast area of medical research in which experiments in the strict sense are impossible, a writer can now use the controlled trial as a standard which, although not actually attainable in purely observational (survey) research, can be approached much more closely than was thought possible a few years ago.

This edition has been greatly influenced by these developments in the attitude of medical investigators. Its structure also has been greatly altered. In particular, the first ten chapters have been arranged in the form of questions that an investigator can ask himself regarding his projected, current or past research, and which a reader of journal articles can apply in the evaluation of others' work. Each question is taken as the text for an expository discussion.

This form of presentation originated in an effort to prepare questions that could be studied by members of the New York University Medical Center staff who came to the Department of Medical Statistics for consultation. Later, the questions were increased in number and discussion was added, for publication as a set of three articles in the American Heart Journal. Later still, a revised and expanded version was issued in mimeographed form to teachers and research workers in medicine and related fields, as part of a project entitled "Promotion of Biometrical Methods in Medical Research," which is supported by the National Institutes of Health, United States Public Health Service.* The method of presentation appears, therefore, to have been sufficiently well tested and received to justify changing the structure of this book in order to introduce ten groups of questions with greatly expanded discussions.

The emphasis in these discussions is upon statistical thinking rather than arithmetic, and an attempt is made to elucidate statistical jargon. In subsequent chapters (XI to XVI) specific methods of analysis are presented and discussed from the investigator's point of view, and the basis of the techniques is demonstrated by the results of randomization experiments. Nonparametric methods are particularly emphasized. Although attention is paid chiefly to those techniques that a small-scale investigator would be most likely to require, there is discussion, especially in Chapter XV, of mathematical developments, due largely to the use of electronic computers, that are now coming to the attention of medical workers — multivariate analysis, operations research in hospitals, and attempts at "machine diagnosis." Lines of critical evaluation of these developments are suggested.

For stimulating, informative and critical discussions that have contributed greatly to this revision, I owe a profound debt of gratitude to my present and former colleagues in medical statistics at New York University over the past twelve years — Miss Lee Herrera, Miss Claire Lingg, Miss Elisabeth Street and Miss M. I. Sutcliffe. I wish to thank Miss Hildegard Landsberger not only for typing the manuscript but for numerous constructive suggestions throughout that process.

New York University Medical Center   DONALD MAINLAND
550 First Avenue, New York 16, N. Y.

---

* This book has itself become part of that project, which is supported by Grant No. GM-06100 from the National Institute of General Medical Sciences, National Institutes of Health.

CONTENTS

CHAPTER III

THE POPULATION AND SAMPLING 29

CHAPTER IV

SUBDIVISION OF POPULATION AND SAMPLES 39

CHAPTER V

CHAPTER X

Table I. Limits of Binomial Population Percentages of X's Estimated from Random Samples—No. of X's in Sample: 0–50; Sample Sizes: 1–100, 358. Table II. Limits of Binomial Population Percentages of X's Estimated from Random Samples—Percentage of X's in Sample: 50–1; Sample Sizes: 100–1000, 362. Table III. Minimum Contrasts Required in Fourfold Contingency Tables to Insure a Type I Error of

Not More than 5 Per Cent (2.5 Per Cent in Each Tail), 364. Table IV. Minimum Contrasts Required in Fourfold Contingency Tables to Insure a Type I Error of Not More Than 1 Per Cent (0.5 Per Cent in Each Tail), 366. Table V. Percentages of Successful Experiments (%S) in Relation to Sample Sizes and to Percentages of X's in Populations A and B, 368. Table VI. Signed-ranks Test (Wilcoxon), 371. Table VII. The Gaussian Distribution—Frequency of Random Samples Lying Beyond Specified Multiples of the Standard Deviation Measured Above and Below the Mean, 372. Table VIII. Two-sample Ranks Test (Wilcoxon-White), 373.

CHAPTER I

QUESTIONS FOR USE IN PLANNING INVESTIGATIONS AND IN EVALUATING REPORTS

THE PURPOSE OF THE QUESTIONS

To many of us who indulge in medical research it often seems as if Nature, outside us and in ourselves (our desires, prejudices and stupidity), were laying traps on every hand to prevent us from approaching the truth. What we would like is a comprehensive, systematic and detailed scheme that would help us to detect and avoid Nature's traps. The same desire is felt even more keenly by many who are not research workers but who read journal articles and try to evaluate them. Such a scheme of warnings, detective devices and safety rules cannot, of course, create original research or critical insight, but it can help us to avoid mistakes in our own research and it can open our eyes to the good and bad features of others' work.

Any investigator could invent a scheme of this kind for himself through contact with a wide variety of research reports and research workers, if he paid attention to the planning and reasoning, rather than to results. Few research workers, however, have the time or inclination to obtain the necessary experience — to study "methodology." They can be helped by a scheme invented by someone who has had the experience; and it is just that kind of experience that a statistician accumulates if he immerses himself thoroughly in the investigations in which he is trying to give help. Indeed, I believe that the most useful role of a statistician in medical research at present is to apply such experience in a systematic way. The ten groups of questions, with accompanying discussions, that start in this chapter and are continued through Chapter X constitute such an effort by a research worker who gradually acquired the label "statistician."

With change of tense from future to past, the questions become a scheme for the basic "statistical" evaluation of research already performed, either one's own research or the reports of others' work. This is more fundamental statistics than are arithmetical tests; without it, the arithmetic is meaningless and dangerous. Only the investigator can properly perform this basic analysis of his own work, but the rest of us, by using such a series of questions as a check list, can help ourselves to form a balanced opinion of his work.

The scheme makes no claim to perfection or finality. Indeed, the best way for anyone to use it is to make it his own by changing it; but he would be well advised to retain in some form or other the topics dealt with in this scheme, even questions that appear insultingly elementary or unnecessary or repetitious. Repetition is particularly desirable, because if we do not score a hit by one question we may by another that repeats the same idea in another form or context.

The danger of such a scheme is, of course, that it may make research look like an industrial testing procedure which follows a plan from start to finish. Real research often starts from a hunch and it can have no detailed long-range plan, for it must be flexible in following leads as they appear. And yet even in acting on a hunch, thought before a leap is desirable, and this scheme of questions is intended to show the kinds of things that we ought to think about.

STATISTICS IN MEDICINE

The preceding paragraphs contain several references to "statistics," a word which has more than a hundred definitions (Kendall, 1952). Many of them are variants of the same idea, but some of them are distinct. In medicine the word has two common meanings:

1. Masses of figures, such as disease incidence and death rates — "statistics" as a plural noun.
2. Mathematical methods of treating such figures and also much smaller sets of figures collected in laboratory and clinical investigations — "statistics" as a singular noun.

Underlying these definitions and all the others, however, is the recognition of differences between individual things or events that bear the same label — between the heights, weights, heart sizes, arterial patterns and behavior of persons of the same race, sex and age; between many features in the same man at the age of 20 and at the age of 50; between different cases of measles in the same epidemic; between different heart attacks in the same person; between the physiologic reactions of animals at the beginning and end of a 3-hour laboratory period, even if the animals have not been experimented upon; between the numbers of patients who improve on a certain drug in two groups of fifty that are as alike as possible in the degree of severity of a particular disease; even between different specimens of the same "pure" chemical. All such differences are collectively called *variation,* and statistics as it is now practiced can be described as *the science and art of dealing with variation in such a way as to obtain reliable results.*

Any laboratory worker who finds the average of two buret readings or who selects litter mates for the comparison of two treatments is using a statistical method. So also is any clinician who judges that a patient's blood pressure is within the "normal" range, or who prescribes a certain treatment to a patient because he believes, from some evidence that he has observed or read, that it is likely to be more successful than a certain other treatment.

It is difficult to think of anything in medicine that does not, directly or indirectly, depend on counting or measurement. That is obvious in research, but it is true also in clinical practice. When a surgeon takes account of age and family history while investigating a lump in a woman's breast, he is using quantitative data, i.e., age incidence and family incidence of tumors. Even if he does not know the exact figures he is making a probability judgment, quantitative in nature although not expressed numerically. A physician does likewise when he tries to forecast, from a patient's history and present condition, the outcome of his disease.

In all counting and measurement whereby we argue from a sample to a larger group which the sample represents, or from a group to an individual, variation must be reckoned with, and therefore statistics is involved, although it is not always the statistics that we meet in textbooks bearing that title. Medical statistics is, in fact, coming to mean "the principles of quantitative medicine."

ABUSE AND MISUSE OF STATISTICS

Since variation is present everywhere in medicine, and since statistics is the science and art of dealing with variation, it may well be asked: "Why is there still antagonism to statistics among medical workers?"

One reason seems to be that, living in a world of variation and consequent uncertainty, we long for certainty, and much of our training in school, in college and even in medical school, panders to this desire by giving us the impression that there are yes-or-no answers to most questions.

A more obvious cause for skepticism regarding statistical evidence is that we are continually faced with conflicting, sometimes propagandist, interpretations of masses of figures in medicine, economics and other fields. It is therefore not surprising that some people still condemn all statistical activities by antiquated remarks such as, "Statistics can be made to prove anything" and "Lies, damn'd lies and statistics." Such critics are unaware of the development during the last 40 years of "experimenters' statistics." This has been created by statisticians working closely with laboratory and other investigators and by some of the investigators themselves, and it has now spread to every branch of pure and applied science.

The development of experimenters' statistics has done a great deal to clarify inductive inference, the process by which we learn from experience. It has improved the design of investigations, so that more reliable conclusions can be drawn. It has increased the *efficiency* of investigations; i.e., it has made it possible to draw conclusions with a known degree of precision from smaller sets of observations than were required to attain the same precision by the older methods — an economy in time, labor and money, and also a reduction in the numbers of animals and human subjects who have to suffer inconvenience or pain in research.

All these benefits have arisen from statistical thinking, but unfortunately they have been accompanied by a great evil, an epidemic of misapplied statistical tests. Many research reports are now peppered with statistical symbols — P and t, σ (sigma), χ^2 (chi-square) and others — which have numerical values attached to them, the results of statistical arithmetic, which is not the same as statistical thinking. Very often the tests are unnecessary, inappropriate or incorrectly interpreted.

In many published articles there seems to be a "negative correlation" between the amount of statistical testing and the soundness of the investigation. Poorly conceived experiments, carelessly performed on small samples of animals, human subjects or other material, can give "statistically significant" results and increase an investigator's annual publication rate, but they load the journals with unsound information. There is therefore no wonder that some laboratory workers utter dicta such as, "You cannot be a good biochemist and a biostatistician." Here again, however, the critics confuse statistical arithmetic with statistical thinking.

Most of us find arithmetic easier than thinking, and if the arithmetic seems to provide us with a "mathematical proof" of the validity of our results it is quite natural that we should pick up a test from one of the numerous statistical "cookbooks" and apply it to our data. The result has been a state of affairs that elicited a strong but hardly exaggerated statement from Lancelot Hogben, the experimental biologist who wrote the popular *Mathematics for the Million* and who later became a medical statistician. In 1950 he affirmed that "less than 1 per cent of research workers clearly apprehend the rationale of the statistical techniques they commonly invoke."

Whatever the exact percentage might have been in 1950, it has not increased greatly in medicine during the succeeding years, because the spread of techniques has been greater than the spread of understanding. More complicated techniques have come into use; these are not only arithmetical techniques but experimental designs devised by mathematicians, which most medical research workers find so mysterious that they have to trust that their consultant statisticians know what is really happening in the experiment and what the results mean when they emerge.

During that period, also, electronic computers, an inestimable boon when properly used, have spread a "virus" that may lead to another "epidemic." They have started to counteract the efforts of those clinicians and statisticians who were introducing the sound principles of careful laboratory research into the much more difficult field of clinical research.

The "virus" is the belief that if a clinician takes hundreds of patients' hospital records to a mathematician or engineer who is an expert at putting data through computers, much reliable and valuable information will come out. The computer experts do not (or should not) claim competence in the analysis of medical data or in the recognition of the numerous defects in hospital records, and the machines are not data-purifiers. They merely grind in the "dirt" and make it more difficult to detect.

The one hopeful feature in the present situation is that two kinds of people are disturbed by it — some investigators who are aware of the benefits and dangers of experimenters' statistics and some statisticians who have immersed themselves deeply in concrete research projects, as distinct from the theoretical development of techniques. These two kinds of people, who are not as distinct in their thinking or actions as their labels suggest, are coming to feel that statistics should be looked at from the inside of medicine, in order to separate what is useful from what is useless or dangerous. That is the attitude adopted in this book, and as a first step it is desirable to note the distinction between statistics and mathematics.

STATISTICS AND MATHEMATICS

A certain mathematician, who specialized in the mathematics of probability, stated that he knew an infallible way to prevent colds. When he felt a cold coming on he took a certain drug before going to bed, and he had no cold the next morning. His wife, however, declared that this was no proof, because he did not know whether he would have had a cold if he had not taken the drug. In contrast to her husband, she applied statistical judgment and illustrated a point that should be obvious from the foregoing discussion — statistics is not a branch of mathematics.

Like all other sciences, statistics uses tools made by mathematicians, but, as will be seen later, these tools, or their equivalents, could be developed experimentally. The experiments would take thousands of years, and the statistician who tests and uses the tools owes a great debt to the mathematicians who provide them. These mathematicians may be called "theoretical statisticians," and they may also become practical statisticians if they have an interest in research in the real world, if they work closely beside investigators and if they choose techniques of design and analysis because they are appropriate to the problem and not because of their theoretical interest.

THE RESEARCH WORKER AND STATISTICAL TECHNIQUES

In statistical techniques the mathematics is more obvious (more on the surface) than in many other techniques of science or everyday life, and this misleads many people. They feel that, because they cannot

understand in detail how formulae and tables are produced, their meaning in relation to the real world must remain a mystery, to be taken on
trust. They do not adopt the same attitude to other techniques, such as
driving an automobile, using a microscope or performing a surgical operation. No one feels it necessary, before turning on an electric light, to
know the mathematics by which an electric power plant is built and
operated. No competent laboratory worker, when choosing an instrument, takes the manufacturer's word regarding what it will accomplish.
He makes up his own mind, either from previous experience or by testing
the instrument.

To "apprehend the rationale" of a piece of statistical arithmetic is not
synonymous with understanding the mathematical proof of a formula,
i.e., the way in which it was invented. The mathematical proof is not a
proof that the formula is applicable in the real world. What we need to
know, before using any technique of analysis, can be described as follows:

1. We need to know what the results of the analysis will tell us in
terms of the subjects, material and events that we are investigating. We
can then decide whether this is the kind of information that we really
wish to obtain. We should, particularly, insist on finding out what
assumptions and approximations underlie the analysis.

2. Having selected the form of analysis that will tell us what we wish
to discover, we need to know what we must do at every point in the
investigation to make our data suitable for that analysis.

3. Whenever we plan to use a mathematical technique in analyzing
relationships, we must know in advance how we intend to test its safety
when it is applied to the real world.

An attempt to launch a man into orbit around the earth is based on
a vast complex of assumptions, many of them mathematical; but the
proof that the assumptions (plus some luck) are safe, is very direct. If
we propose to assume that a logarithmic relationship holds in a certain
chemical reaction, or that people's attitudes to the fluoridation of drinking
water can be expressed by an equation containing a number of social
variables, we ought first to ask ourselves: "What kind of 'launching test'
are we going to apply?"

In reporting the results of any statistical technique we ought to make
it clear that we possess these three items of necessary knowledge and that
we have acted accordingly throughout the investigation. If we do not
make this clear, a reader is justified in assuming that we belong to
Hogben's 99 per cent of research workers who do not really know what
they are doing when they apply such techniques. The reader does not
require to change that percentage if our report mentions a statistician in
the list of acknowledgments or even as co-author. We may not have
shown the report to the statistician. Or the statistician may have been
content to do the arithmetic after the investigation, saying that all the
rest is the investigator's responsibility. Or we may be working in an

institution where the statistician is subject to pressures of various kinds to induce him to coöperate with investigators on terms prescribed by them and approved by administrators who know nothing of the scientific, psychologic and even financial problems that a statistician meets when he tries to do clean work in some otherwise reputable medical schools.

The foregoing remarks lead to a question which many thousands of investigators must face if they wish to apply statistical techniques sensibly and safely: "What am I to do if I cannot find a statistician who is (1) suitable in experience and attitude, (2) willing to immerse himself in my project, and (3) sufficiently free from other duties to give me as much help as I really need – not merely the help that I think I need?"

In a sense, this whole book is an attempt to answer that question, but at this point it seems desirable to make a general statement about the ideas on which the answer is based.

No one should expect lectures or laboratory classes in statistics, or statistical textbooks, to make him able, without personal guidance, to apply safely to his own projects the techniques of design and analysis that he has learned. Such "do-it-yourself" ability is not expected in the individual sciences such as chemistry, physiology or any of the clinical research disciplines. Why should it be expected in what may be called the "general" science of statistics?

It should surely be no disgrace for an investigator to report on his work in the following terms: "This is what I did. These are the biases and other defects that I looked for. These are the doubts that still remain. This is my interpretation of the results and these are my reasons for that interpretation. I have little practical experience in statistical design or analysis, nor was there available anyone with such knowledge who could work with me throughout the investigation. Therefore tests of 'statistical significance' applied to these results might well lead to a false sense of security."

The ten sets of questions that are presented and discussed in this chapter and the succeeding nine chapters show the kinds of matters that we must attend to in research, whether we are going to apply a more technical analysis or not. Some of the discussions, however, show that statistical tests are very desirable, or even necessary, if we wish to avoid being overconfident or too hesitant in our conclusions. It should become obvious also that if we keep our plan of investigation very simple we can have confidence in our analyses, because we can see the connection between them and what we have done in the actual investigation. Chapters XI to XVI try to lay the foundation for such analyses.

SOURCES OF VARIATION

As we go through the ten groups of questions we should remember that the underlying theme is variation. Therefore in trying to see how each question applies to our particular project, or to a project that we are reading about, it is helpful to carry with us a simple scheme to remind us of the causes or sources of variation. Such a scheme is the familiar set of five questions that is employed to insure completeness of description of any event:

1. *Who?* The observer and all other persons who may influence the investigation.

2. *What?* The material, animate or inanimate, on which the investigation is to be performed.

3. *Where?* Variables associated with location, e.g., position of animal cages or hospital beds, different clinics in a multiclinic drug trial, right and left arms in subcutaneous injection.

4. *When?* Variables associated with time, from milliseconds to years. It will become obvious that the passage of time is the most subtle cause of mistakes.

5. *How?* Techniques, instruments and substances used in experimenting and in assessing effects by measurement or other methods.

THE TEN GROUPS OF QUESTIONS

The titles of the ten groups of questions are as follows:

    I.   The Nature of the Research and the Attitudes of the Researchers.
   II.   Purpose and General Method of Investigation.
  III.   The Population and Sampling.
   IV.   Subdivision of Population and Samples.
    V.   Skeleton Layouts for Results.
   VI.   Interpretation after an Experiment.
  VII.   Interpretation after a Survey.
 VIII.   Sample Sizes.
   IX.   Collecting, Recording and Examining the Data.
    X.   Lost Information.

For quick reference, all the questions are shown in the Contents, and for conciseness the questions are lettered and numbered — for example, "Q II – 2" is the second question in the second group. In order to make group numbers agree with chapter numbers we start here with Group I.

I. THE NATURE OF THE RESEARCH AND THE ATTITUDES OF THE RESEARCHERS

Q I – 1. Is our project actually research, or is it a demonstration or an educational program or provision of improved services?
Each of these objectives can be laudable, but we should not fool our-

selves by mistaking one for another. Someone who has developed a program of rehabilitation for persons with certain diseases or injuries may propose to evaluate it by analyzing his past or future records. Except for parts of his program that have failed to achieve their intended effect, he cannot really evaluate it, i.e., measure its value, without something to measure it against — a suitable "control" sample, which is commonly difficult or impossible to obtain. Therefore, such "evaluations" are usually demonstrations of apparent achievement.

A hint as to whether a piece of research is likely to be "real" research — an open-minded and systematic search for new knowledge — can sometimes be obtained from the statement of purpose. A statement such as, "I propose to prove that exercises of the mouth muscles prevent dental irregularities," or, "I am going to show that parental alcoholism is largely responsible for children's mental defects," is a warning signal. As one of my biologist friends remarked, the contrast between the scientific and unscientific approach can be expressed by saying that a scientist sets up a hypothesis and then tries to knock it down, whereas an unscientific worker sets up a hypothesis and then tries to keep it up.

Unscientific attitudes and assumptions may be well hidden, even from the research worker himself. Even if we start out with an open mind our ideas and results soon become our children. We defend them against criticism, and we are likely to be blind to their deformities. We may unconsciously move from research to a kind of demonstration in which our plans and actions are determined by a desire to show that our first results, or our interpretations of them, were correct. People who are aware of this risk, and wish to remain unbiased, seek methods of "blindfolding" themselves when they are examining specimens (e.g., x-ray films or tissues), animals and even human patients. Whenever possible they arrange for an independent observer to check their findings.

Q I – 2.   Are we going to turn a blind eye on some awkward bit of evidence?

Almost certainly we are, especially if it would mean retracting some of our previous statements; but we will perhaps do it less frequently if we remember this question.

Q I – 3.   Will we be hindered by our desire for a simple answer?

Perhaps we can reduce this danger by remembering the statement made by A. N. Whitehead, the mathematician and philosopher: "The aim of science is to seek the simplest explanation of complex facts. We are apt to fall into the error of thinking that the facts are simple because simplicity is the goal of our quest. The guiding motto in the life of every natural philosopher should be, Seek simplicity and distrust it" (Johnson).

Q I – 4.   If our research will entail experimentation on human beings, what will be its ethical justification?

If anyone should ask, "What has ethics to do with statistics?" he could be recommended to take two steps:

1. To place himself at the receiving end of data from a clinical drug trial in which the ethical problems have not been thought about, realistically and in detail, before the trial began.

2. To visit the clinical centers during the trial, see what is going on and discuss the trial informally with the doctors, nurses and all others who may have an influence on the results.

Perhaps some of the following remarks will obviate the need for such disturbing experiences.

Transition from Haphazard to Planned Experiments. Experimentation on human beings can be classified, in terms of its purpose, under two headings:

1. Procedures that are expected to add to medical knowledge but are not performed in order to help the individuals who are the subjects of the experiment. When the procedures may involve inconvenience or some risk, ethical (and also legal) problems arise.

2. Evaluation of a new method for the treatment or prevention of disease, or of a method already used but with apparently conflicting results.

Ethical problems in both groups can produce similar effects on data, and we will discuss here the second group. The very phrase "human experimentation" has such unsavory association that we speak of treatment evaluations as "clinical trials." And yet, whenever a doctor in routine practice administers a drug, even a well established drug, to see if it is followed by improvement, he is conducting an experiment. With many modern drugs, which are biologically powerful, the experiment is not without risk to the patient. From ancient times this has been the method by which we have accumulated knowledge, or beliefs, regarding the efficacy of treatments.

During the past 20 years, however, discontent with this method has grown rapidly. Indeed, anyone who has witnessed the changes in medical beliefs during the past few decades tends to be skeptical of the method. He thinks of the myriads of medications that have been enthusiastically advocated for a short time and then have dropped out of sight. He may think, for example, of the treatment of burns: The belief in Carron oil (linseed oil and lime water) was followed by the popularity of picric acid, which was dethroned by tannic acid, which was succeeded by gentian violet, which was again replaced by the use of oil, although with a different purpose and technique than formerly.

A glaring example of the way in which haphazard experiments can impede therapeutic progress was the history of the treatment of tuberculosis by gold compounds. During a period of more than 15 years, scores of reports were published, many of them with exaggerated claims for the efficacy of the treatment. A thorough search revealed only one trial in which controls (patients who did not receive gold) were compared with gold-treated patients, and this trial showed negative results (Medical Research Council, 1948). When we are trying to find out if a treatment is any good at all, a controlled trial requires that some patients must be deprived of the treatment under test, which we think might help them. Hence, the ethical problem.

Most of the main advances in therapy have been due to some method, such as penicillin treatment, which has been followed by phenomena strikingly different from previous experience and so rapid as to leave no reasonable doubt regarding the interpretation of cause and effect; but as soon as we start to explore the limitations of such a treatment, or to seek the best scheme of dosage, or to compare different treatments of the same type, planned experiments are necessary. Here ethical problems may arise because a clinician may feel that some particular patient would do better on drug B than on drug A, or better on a higher dose than on the dose assigned to him. The clinician may feel that his hands are tied because the assignment of patients is automatic, by a random system which is discussed in Chapter II.

Insight into Ethical Problems. During the past decade there has been a rapid spread of controlled drug trials in Great Britain and in the United States, and clinicians have developed clearer insight into the nature of the ethical problems. Among the general public also there has developed an appreciation of untreated controls for the evaluation of drugs and of preventive measures, as in the Salk poliomyelitis vaccine trial conducted in 1954, and in various prophylactic trials conducted by the Medical Research Council of Great Britain. The effects of this experience on many clinicians can be summarized as follows:

1. Clinicians have become better acquainted with what is required for convincing proof — the kind and amount of evidence. When they keep themselves in the dark as to whether individual patients are receiving the test drug or a "placebo" (an inert tablet, capsule or injection disguised to imitate the test drug*) they are impressed by the frequency of improvement among placebo-treated patients. They often see that what looks like evidence in favor of a drug (from their own previous impressions or other doctors' reports) is not evidence at all. Therefore they feel free to deprive half the patients of the treatment in order to make a valid test. Indeed, they may feel morally impelled to make such a test.

2. It has become clear that a sound experiment need not entail any more discomfort or risk to a patient than do the haphazard experiments

---

* In English writing a distinction is often made between a placebo and a "dummy" treatment. In *Medical Surveys and Clinical Trials* (Witts), Glaser distinguishes the two terms as follows: A placebo is given with the intention of producing a definite psychologic effect — to please the patient, and in clinical trials to prevent him from complaining about neglect. A dummy is given in order to prevent any differences between the psychologic effects of treatment and lack of treatment. In American usage, followed in this book, "placebo" is equivalent to "dummy" but it may not please the patient because whenever possible it has the disagreeable features of the drug that is being tested against it.

of routine practice. Indeed, patients in a controlled trial often receive more thorough attention than in routine practice.

3. Clinicians now know that a controlled trial does not deprive them of their right (and duty) to change a patient's therapy if they really believe that the trial therapy is affecting him adversely. Such a patient is taken out of the trial and counted as a "failure" against the agent (drug or placebo) that he received in the trial.

4. It is coming to be seen that the very existence of the ethical problem makes it desirable to test each new treatment, as soon as it appears, by methods that will provide a decisive answer as soon as possible, before the treatment acquires a reputation that will make clinicians hesitate to withhold it from patients.

Many responsible clinicians have given thought to these ethical problems. Recent noteworthy discussions are in articles by Hill and Witts in *Controlled Clinical Trials* (Council for International Organizations of Medical Sciences) and by Glaser and Knowelden in *Medical Surveys and Clinical Trials* (Witts). Probably most clinicians who conduct clinical trials would agree with Glaser's description of an ethical trial: "No patient should be worse off as a result of the trial than he might have been otherwise in the hands of a reasonable and competent medical man." They would probably concur also with his statement that in the majority of clinical trials it is possible to meet this condition. Nevertheless, ethical problems still exert a powerful effect on the data from some clinical trials.

Effects of Ethics on Data. These effects are most clearly seen in multi-clinic (multicenter) trials which are now rather extensively used because in many diseases no single center can provide a sufficient number of suitable patients within a reasonable period of time. The clinic chiefs, assembled to plan a trial, may decide that they really do not know whether any drug confers any real benefit on patients with a certain disease, and that therefore it is entirely ethical to administer a placebo to half of the patients while testing a new drug. But when they return to their clinics and face actual patients their feelings can change. They may then find various reasons for excluding from the trial certain patients who, according to the plan, are perfectly well qualified to enter.

The results of the trial will then apply to the type of patient described in the plan, *with the exception of* those who possessed a number of unspecified characteristics, physical, psychologic, social or economic, which prompted individual clinicians to exclude them — a very nebulous definition. But there are even more serious effects than ill-defined selection of patients:

1. Even when a clinician is in the dark regarding individual patients' therapies, he is tempted to remove patients from the trial as failures on more slender evidence than if he knew that neither of the agents was a placebo.

2. Because of the impulse to withhold patients, a trial can drag on far beyond its anticipated time limit. A trial that drags on loses interest, and the quality of the data deteriorates. New observers may be appointed who are unfamiliar with the system. Any clinical-trial coordinator who has tried to teach new observers in the middle of a trial, by correspondence, by long-distance telephone or even by a visit to the clinic, knows how unreliable the data from such a trial can be.

Unadjusted ethical conflicts have even greater force when some clinic chiefs during the planning sessions accept, against their own beliefs or feelings, the majority decision regarding the agents to be tested — drug against placebo, or two drugs one of which is disliked or feared by certain members of the group. The disturbing effects are probably most powerful when the clinic chiefs, having decided on a plan, depute the actual work of the trial to their assistants who have not shared in the planning and who differ from their chiefs in their opinion of the drugs under test or in their interpretation of the ethical situation.

In the most clinical trials nurses play as important a role as doctors. During their training nurses are rightly taught that they must give the best possible care to the individual patient. They are likely, therefore, to think that to do something to a patient — anything that might benefit him, and especially any standard procedure — is necessarily better than to avoid doing it. They are likely, therefore, to frown upon placebos. If they know that one is included in a trial and they think that a patient is going downhill, they may speculate, sometimes in front of the patient, regarding the possibility that this is one of the placebo cases.

Some years ago, when pediatricians began to suspect that oxygen administered to premature babies was a possible cause of retrolental fibroplasia and consequent blindness, a very carefully designed trial was organized in which half the babies received the usual (liberal) amounts of oxygen and the other half received restricted amounts. At the outset the nurses were horrified at the idea that any babies should be deprived of liberal oxygen, but as the trial continued and the suspicion that oxygen was dangerous increased in that clinic and elsewhere, the nurses changed sides completely and felt that it was criminal to give liberal oxygen to any babies.*

A nurse's work load may give rise to conflict between the care of patients and experimental treatments or observations that are not designed to benefit the patient. Clearly, care of the patient should come first, but the effect on the experiment and the resulting data may be devastating, and it is quite likely that neither the investigators nor a laborious statistician will ever find out.

Q I – 5. If we intend to conduct experiments on human beings how are we to insure that ethical conflicts will not vitiate our results?

The only way is to make sure that we have cleared up all the ethical

---

* I am indebted to Dr. J. T. Lanman for this example.

problems before we begin and thereafter keep close lookout for any that may arise. We need realistic thinking and frank discussion, involving all the personnel who will participate. If this includes nurses we must make sure, also, that there will be no conflict of duties owing to pressure of work. (Incidentally, clinicians could often learn from nurses a great deal about the actual day-to-day difficulties of conducting a sound experiment, including that very important factor, patients' psychology.)

A physician who pioneered in multicenter clinical trials wrote as follows: "Such trials are not easy to organize. They demand very careful planning; loose plans, loose methods give loose results, which are just as equivocal as the impressions of a single clinician and may be more misleading, since a semblance of scientific enquiry is presented" (Daniels). This statement applies to all components of clinical trials, at single as well as multiple centers.

A few years ago some experts in rehabilitation looked critically at the battery of treatments that had been developed at their institute for patients who had suffered paralysis due to vascular lesions in the brain. They realized that they had no real proof that the special treatments benefited the patients; therefore, they proposed to withhold these treatments from half the patients, and give them standard care instead. They found, however, that they could not carry out the plan because the resident staff rose in arms against it. One may lament the residents' dogmatic attitude, but their action did not promote pseudoscience, as would a pretended agreement with the plan, followed by secret sabotage. If ethical problems cannot be removed without coercion it is far better not to do a controlled trial at all.*

---

* To anyone who is concerned with the ethics of therapeutic trials, a recent article by Sir Austin Bradford Hill (Medical ethics and controlled trials. *Brit. Med. J.* 1: 1043, 1963) is highly recommended reading. The article points out that broad statements of principle are not enough, and that they may even be unrealistic and restrictive. Examples are given to show that each trial must be considered individually with regard to its ethical problems.

CHAPTER II

PURPOSE AND GENERAL METHOD
OF INVESTIGATION

Q II – 1. What is the immediate purpose of our investigation? What are the specific questions to be answered by it?

Q II – 2. What is the more remote (more general or ultimate) purpose of our investigation?

The formulation of purpose must usually proceed step by step, beginning with statements which, after further thought about our project, we will find very vague. Here are four examples of initial statements:

Ex. 1. Immediate question: Is cortisone preferable to aspirin in the treatment of rheumatoid arthritis? Ultimate purpose: Use of the preferable drug.

Ex. 2. Immediate question: Are persons who eat animal fats more liable to coronary heart disease than persons who eat vegetable fats? Ultimate purpose: Dietary recommendations.

Ex. 3. Immediate question: What is the "normal" structure of the human liver? Ultimate purpose: Elucidation of disease processes, or a diagnostic test (removal of a tiny fragment of a patient's liver for microscopic examination).

Ex. 4. Immediate question: What can be found by analysis of the records of patients with a particular disease (e.g., a certain type of kidney disease) treated by a certain physician during the past 10 years? The ultimate purposes here may be multiple:

a. To improve the physician's diagnostic skill. The survey will provide a rather precise picture of signs and symptoms, instead of recollected impressions. It may provide also a more reliable picture than do textbook descriptions — more up-to-date and more applicable to the physician's own patients, because textbook descriptions are often greatly influenced by advanced and hospitalized cases.

b. To improve the physician's prognostic (predictive) skill by showing the connection between the patients' condition on first examination and later developments in their disease.

15

c. To provide some clues to the cause of the disease.

d. To provide impressions of the value of various kinds of treatment, when systematic trials have not been done or are impossible.

These four examples refer to research on human beings, but analogous examples can easily be found in research on other organisms, individual organs, tissue extracts, inorganic material and organizations such as hospitals.

Specificity. The chairman of one of the grant-application reviewing committees of the National Institutes of Health (U. S. Public Health Service) once summed up the experience of many such committees by saying that the commonest and most fundamental defect in applications was lack of specificity. In trying to make a statement of purpose more specific we should say to ourselves, "What exactly do we mean by each word of that statement, and what do we not mean by it?" "How would we, or someone else, translate the statement into action?"

For instance, in *Ex. 1,* what do we mean by the "preferable" drug? Is it the drug that improves the patient's rheumatoid condition greatly but often produces other effects that are undesirable? Or is it the drug that causes less improvement, but more rarely produces undesirable effects? What do we mean by "improvement"? Do we mean the patient's statement that he feels better, or his greater capacity for work or other activities, or a lessened number of joints that are painful when pressed on, or lessened evidence of disease in an x-ray film, or any one of half a dozen other features that are commonly examined in rheumatoid patients? These various features do not commonly keep exactly in step when they change. Therefore, do we intend to measure improvement by an "index" produced by an arbitrary combination of some or all of them? Or will improvement in, say, three or more of these criteria be defined as "improvement in the patient's condition"? More fundamentally, do we mean relief of symptoms or actual lessening of the disease process?

Whatever arbitrary definition we adopt we can be sure that some other investigators will differ from us, and perhaps thereby reach a different conclusion when comparing the same drugs. The obvious solution of the problem is to report the change in each criterion separately.

The Two Classes of Variables. In spite of the unlimited variety of purposes in research, it appears that we are very often trying to find an association between one variable and another — between treatment and change of symptoms in arthritis, between diet and frequency of coronary disease, between liver function and liver structure, between blood pressures of patients when first seen and the subsequent progress of their kidney disease. In all of these instances we are trying to hang one variable on another variable, and it is convenient to call the variable that we start with — drug treatment, diet, liver function and blood pressure in the above examples — the "independent" variable, because we are not trying to hang it on to anything. The other variable, which we are trying to hang on to the independent variable — change of symptoms in arthritis, frequency of coronary disease, liver structure, progress of kidney disease — is the "dependent" variable.

These terms do not imply causal relationship. Indeed, at the outset they do not imply any relationship at all. They are operational terms, showing what we are trying to find out. For example, if we wish to compare the frequency of symptom X in patients with diseases A, B and C, the independent variable is disease, the dependent variable is the symptom (present or absent). If, however, we wish to find the frequency of diseases A, B and C in patients who come to us with symptom X, the independent variable is the symptom, the dependent variable is disease.

Q II – 3. Will the variables that we observe be the variables that we really wish to know about?

Indirect and Substitute Observations. In many of our observations in medicine something lies between what we would like to observe and what we actually observe. High blood pressure is often a clue to something wrong in the vascular system, now or in the future, but reading a blood pressure is not the same as direct examination of the vessels. If we come to think of high blood pressure itself as a disease, or if we equate it to arterial disease, we are playing what Dr. Yerushalmy, Professor of Biostatistics at the University of California, has called the "substitution game." We are substituting something that is easy to observe for something that is difficult to observe, and we have no right to do so unless we know the connection between the two things. We play the same game when we use the level of blood sugar as a direct measure of the severity or activity of diabetes and when we assume that treatment that lowers the blood sugar is attacking the disease.

Clinical observation is not the only field in which the substitution game is played. Animal experiments have helped human medicine so much that we have frequently forgotten the gap between the animal laboratory and the doctor's office. Textbooks of physiology for medical students and practitioners are transformed when they replace animal physiology by the most recently acquired knowledge of human physiology.

In the laboratory itself, illicit substitution of variables is not uncommon. As one of my colleagues in biochemistry remarked, to add a chemical to the fluid around a cell and assume that the results will be the same as if that chemical were produced within the cell is like assuming that gasoline poured over an automobile would produce the same results as gasoline poured into the tank.

The substitution game can continue beyond observation to inference. In *Ex. 2* under Q II – 1 and 2, we might answer the immediate question by finding that coronary heart disease is commoner in animal-fat consumers than in vegetable-fat consumers, but there is a very wide gap between this answer and the ultimate purpose, reduction of coronary disease by diet, apart altogether from the difficulty of controlling the diet. To answer the immediate question the independent variable would be a type of dietary fat, but to find the real cause of the difference in frequency of coronary disease between the animal-fat and vegetable-fat consumers, our independent variable perhaps ought to be something else associated with difference in type of fat consumed, such as the physiologic or psychologic make-up of the persons, their racial origin, upbringing, environment or socioeconomic status. Later in this series of questions we will describe the mistake as confusion of association and cause, but however we describe it we ought to ask ourselves, early in our planning: "What is the gap between the immediate question and the ultimate purpose of our study?"

Validity of Observations. If we prefer a more orthodox but less picturesque term than "substitution game" we can speak of the "validity" of our observations, in the sense that we speak of the "validity of evidence." It is worth noting that the word comes from the Latin *validus* (strong) and is related to "valiant." This conveys the concept of degrees of validity. External blood pressure has been shown to be, for ordinary purposes, a highly valid measure of intra-arterial pressure; but that does not mean that the relationship between the two pressures is the same in all persons, or in the same person at different times, or even at different phases of the heart cycle in the same person at the same time.

The "relativity of validity" may be illustrated by the story of the "rheumatoid factor," a protein (or more probably a group of related proteins) demonstrable in the blood of many patients with rheumatoid arthritis. At first it was thought to be a very valid indicator of that disease, but it has since been found in some of the patients who have other diseases in the same group as rheumatoid arthritis, i.e., the connective tissue diseases. Therefore it is a more valid indicator for the group than for rheumatoid arthritis itself. It is, however, not a very valid (or sensitive) indicator of the degree of severity of the patient's disease, as judged by clinical examination. Moreover, it is found in a small percentage of persons who have no other past or present evidence of connective tissue diseases, i.e., it is not a specific test for those diseases.

The terms "sensitivity" and "specificity" are looked at more closely in Chapter IX, in relation to diagnostic tests. Here we merely note that the validity of any method of observation has to be determined by some other independent method. Sometimes this can be very direct, such as the determination of blood pressures by sticking needles into arteries. More often it is indirect — for example, the diagnosis of a disease such as rheumatoid arthritis by a definition that has been established by physicians who have great experience of the disease.

If questions of validity appear difficult in the physical areas of medicine, they are much more difficult in psychologic and sociologic inquiries. In reading reports of such studies we should see whether the authors were aware of the difficulties and how they have met them.

Q II – 4. Will the investigation be an experiment in the strict sense, or a survey, or a mixture of the two?

Experiments.   The word "experiment" is often used so loosely that it forfeits much of its value. The distinctive feature of an experiment, in the strict sense, is that the investigator, wishing to compare the effects of two or more factors (independent variables) assigns them *himself* to the individuals (e.g., human beings, animals, or batches of a chemical substance) that comprise his test material.

Surveys.   A piece of nonexperimental research is best called a "survey," if we remember that a survey can be conducted on as few as half a dozen subjects. The amount of interference with, or manipulation of, our test material is not a criterion of experimentation. An investigator wished to compare the pressures inside blood vessels in cardiac and noncardiac diseases. He inserted needles into the arteries and veins of the patient; but, since he had not himself assigned the independent variable (disease) to the subjects, he conducted a survey, just as if he had compared male and female statures.

This apparently pedantic distinction lies at the root of modern science. Some people try to express it by the antithesis, "observation versus experiment"; but this is unsatisfactory because it suggests that an experimenter does not observe and that in a survey we do nothing to our subjects except look at them. "Survey" itself suggests the same idea, but it implies a systematic procedure. It will soon become apparent, also, that the other antithesis, between the statistical method and the experimental method, is out of date, because statistical thinking and techniques constitute a very important part of modern experimentation.

An Example from Drug Testing.   The essential features of an experiment, in the strict sense, can be seen by examining the method which during the past 15 years has become recognized as necessary to insure clear-cut answers in the testing of many drugs.

A physician wishes to compare the outcome after drug A with the outcome after drug B, using 50 patients for each drug. He chooses his 100 patients by certain criteria (perhaps sex, age range and severity of disease) which affect the behavior of the particular disease. He does this in order to reduce the differences in reaction between patients who are treated alike. He can expect the 50 A-treated patients to react somewhat similarly and the 50 B-treated patients to react somewhat similarly; and if there is a difference in the effects of A and B it ought to stand out as an intergroup difference.

However, the physician knows that "somewhat" is a very broad term. He knows that there are likely to be in each patient a different set of hidden factors tending to make some patients improve and others fail to improve, even if all patients were treated by the same drug. He knows also that, apart from the A and B treatments, many things may happen to different patients during the trial that may swing some toward a successful outcome and others toward failure. Therefore, if there is in reality no difference in the effects of A and B, but if a higher proportion of the "favorable" cases were allotted to drug A than to drug B, the verdict would seem to favor drug A, but the samples would be *biased.*

Bias. Bias can be defined as *something that makes a sample different from what it seems to be or purports to be* — something that causes *wrong labeling.* If the verdict in favor of drug A came about merely because more of the favorable cases had been allotted to that drug, the samples ought not to bear the labels "A" and "B" but "More Favorable" and "Less Favorable."

If at the end of the trial the A-treated patients show a much greater proportion of successes than the B-treated patients, the physician will wish to have little doubt that this was due to the difference between the drugs — that is, he will wish to have little risk of bias. He can achieve this by following two rules in performing the trial:

1. Assign the patients to the treatments by a strictly random method, i.e., randomize the treatments.

2. Permit no distinction between the treatment groups in the handling of the patients, i.e., in medical care, nursing, assessment of effects, or in any other way. This is equivalent to saying: Insure that the randomization alone is responsible for bias.

Randomization for Control of Bias.   "A strictly random process" means a method that is used in games of chance, such as card shuffling. Nowadays we customarily use a table of "random numbers" that have been obtained by card shuffling, spinning roulette wheels or by other such devices, and are equivalent to thousands of thoroughly shuffled cards. This is discussed in Chapter VI, but for simplicity we can speak of card shuffling here.

In order that the physician shall not know which of the two treatments any patient is to receive, he arranges for the randomization to be done by someone who will not be associated in any way with the care or assessment of the patients. In terms of playing cards, this person proceeds as follows. He takes 100 well made and uniform playing cards and marks on each card a number that will represent a particular patient, usually according to the order in which the patients will be started in the trial. He shuffles the cards thoroughly, puts them in one pile, and then takes the top 50 cards and calls them "A" to indicate the drug that these patients are to receive. The other 50 patients will receive drug B. He passes this information to someone who is going to dispense the drugs, e.g., bottles of tablets that look and taste alike, whether they are A or B. The dispenser, who, like the "randomizer," will have no other association with the trial, labels the appropriate bottles with the patients' numbers and removes any label or other mark that would identify the drugs. (For reasons that are discussed later he must not use identification symbols such as "A" and "B".) As each patient is admitted to the trial, his name is written on the bottles that bear his number.

This is the beginning of a "double-blind" trial — a trial in which neither (a) the patients nor (b) the physician and his associates know which treatment any particular patient is receiving. The "associates" include nurses, clinic secretaries and any other persons who might conceivably affect the outcome of the trial by influence on the patients or on the assessment of their condition. Even those who are to analyze the data must be kept "blindfold" until all problems in the data (e.g., omissions, ambiguities and obscurities) have been settled.

Bias from Leakage of Information. The bias-causing effect of apparently trivial actions may be very great, as in a drug trial recounted by Wilson (1952): "The experiment was very carefully designed with randomized controls, placebos, and precautions to keep the patients and examining physicians from knowing which were subjects and which controls. For several weeks the treatment showed excellent results, with very satisfying statistical significance. Then one day there was an obvious change, and thereafter only random fluctuations separated the subjects from the controls. The most searching examination failed to find the cause of this shift until finally it was learned that the receptionist on duty during the first weeks had started her vacation on the critical day. Further inquiry showed that she had known which of the patients had received the treatment. She thoroughly believed in it, with the result that her cheery greetings to the lucky subjects, 'How much better you look this morning, Mr. Smith,' had so brightened them up before they went in to be examined that the reports of the physicians were seriously biased."

How Randomization Acts. In a properly conducted double-blind trial the randomization not only determines how many initially "favorable" and "unfavorable" patients are assigned to each drug, but controls biases throughout the experiment. It was noted above that, in addition to receiving one or the other of the two drugs, individual patients may be affected during the trial by various events, unconnected with the drugs, which will push them into the "favorable" or "unfavorable" class. Some of the events that affect patients during a trial are due to the actions of doctors, nurses and others who come in contact with patients. Even a physician's self-conscious effort at neutrality can affect a patient. A completely double-blind trial insures that none of these actions on patients, physical or psychologic, shall occur simply because a person knows which treatment a particular patient is receiving. Therefore, unless there is a true causal connection between the drug and these actions, the actions will be like all the other events that are unconnected with the difference between the two drugs. The randomization then insures that it will be just a matter of chance whether an A-treated or a B-treated patient meets any one set of these events, which may render him "favorable" or "unfavorable," i.e., more (or less) likely to have a successful result.

Inferences after Randomization. From experience with card shuffling we know that the randomization will very likely push a few more of the "favorable" patients into the A-group than into the B-group, or vice versa — that is, randomization is almost certain to create a little bias. However, if we found after a properly conducted double-blind trial that all 50 A-treated patients were successes and all 50 B-treated patients were failures, we would not need to consult a statistician, or look up a table of "probabilities," or do any arithmetic before deciding that it was exceedingly unlikely that the randomization had created that much bias. Knowing that the experiment had closed other sources of bias, we would conclude that the drugs had differed in their effect.

When differences are less extreme a glance may not be enough to tell us that something more than randomization has probably caused the difference in outcome between the A's and the B's. Then we can use our centuries-old experience of games of chance to tell us how often randomization alone, without difference in drug effects, would cause such differences as we have observed in our particular experiment. How we do this is shown in Chapter XII; and Chapter XIV shows the analogous process in the handling of measurement data such as we would obtain if, instead of counting successes and failures, we compared the average fall in blood pressure in A-treated and B-treated patients.

The knowledge of how to control bias by randomization — how to make chance work for us, instead of worrying about it or trying in vain to eliminate it entirely — is one of the most important advances in scientific method made in the twentieth century. Examples of randomization in experiments on animals and on inanimate objects are given later.

Avoidance of Uncontrolled Bias. We are still sometimes told, even by experimenters, that the proper way to conduct an experiment is to "keep all factors constant except one" or "treat all individuals exactly alike except for the factor under test." As we will see, uniformity of treatment is a very important way to reduce variation in responses, but it is ridiculous to imagine that all individuals in an experiment will undergo exactly the same handling or other experiences, or that the most extreme efforts at uniformity will eliminate the risk of bias.

A properly conducted double-blind trial is an ideal way of insuring that the initial randomization will control biases throughout the experiment, but some drug trials, and many other kinds of experiments, cannot be double-blind. In such experiments the biases will be controlled by the randomization if we insure that knowledge of the treatment under test on a particular individual (subject or object) will not in any way influence the other experiences met by that individual in the experiment. Here, "experiences" is used in a very wide sense, to include what the investigator and others do to the individual, his location (e.g., hospital ward or cage position) during the experiment, the methods of assessing the outcome, and the times at which these assessments are made. The application of this rule often requires much forethought and vigilance.

Inferences after Surveys. After a properly conducted experiment the inference involves simply two alternatives: either the randomization alone or the randomization plus the factor under test. As a contrast, we recall the investigator who inserted needles into patients' arteries and veins in order to measure blood pressures. The independent variable, corresponding to the type of treatment in a drug trial, was the type of disease, cardiac versus noncardiac — rather heterogeneous classes, but suitable for this illustration. The investigator could not randomly assign these diseases to healthy subjects, but he could assume that "chance" had *to some extent* determined which individuals (with their blood pressures) came into his two samples, for we are all, throughout our lives, subject to some random shuffling by the events that happen to us.

The investigator could also seek for, and remove, certain possible causes of bias, such as sex and age, which are known to influence blood pressures; but he could never be sure that all undetectable biases had been controlled by random shuffling. In fact, the safest assumption would be that some hidden biases had not been so controlled, because many observations that have looked bias-free on the surface have revealed bias on deeper digging.

In surveys of this kind it is impossible to obtain final answers to such questions as the following: "What else in these patients, besides the type of disease, may have made the cardiacs differ from (or resemble) the noncardiacs in blood pressure?" "What nonrandom factors may have brought a certain type of cardiac patient to me, and what different factors may have brought the noncardiacs?" "Could these factors be in any way connected with blood pressure differences?" "How do I know that, in blood pressures, my two samples were equally representative of cardiac and noncardiac patients outside my clinic?" "How do I know that many of the cardiacs (or noncardiacs) with unduly high pressure did not die or go to another clinic, instead of coming to me?"

As will be seen later, every kind of survey raises questions of biased selection, and some of the questions in each survey are unanswerable. Therefore, when we find a difference between two samples in a survey, the causal inference does not take the simple "either-or" form. In a survey there are three possible explanations of such a difference: (1) the independent variable (or variables) that we are studying, (2) randomization effects, and (3) hidden biases not controlled by the randomization effects.

This might discourage us from all surveys, but that would eliminate the greater part of the research that is done on patients and on healthy persons. What we must do, therefore, is try to bring surveys as near to good experiments in quality as we can, but we must always remember the doubt attached to inferences based solely on surveys.

Students' "Experiments." Many college graduates, and even many medical graduates, may find the foregoing description of an experiment, and the distinction between an experiment and a survey, rather unfamiliar. One reason is that most of the so-called "experiments" conducted in college and medical school laboratories are really not experiments, but exercises designed to familiarize students with facts and techniques. Another reason is the slow penetration, among academic laboratory workers, of the ideas of experimentation that were introduced into agriculture and animal husbandry a quarter of a century ago, and that have since then spread widely in other applied sciences.

Q II – 5. If the investigation is a survey, will it be anecdotal or evaluational?

Anecdotal surveys, merely recounting experiences and impressions, are not to be despised, any more than are the oral anecdotes of an experienced physician. We benefit by knowing what can happen, even though we do not know how often it happens, or why it happens — for example: the survival for more than 57 years of three persons with a congenital heart defect that usually kills its victims when very young; unusual autopsy findings after a certain treatment of a disease; a surgeon's difficulties in performing a certain kind of operation.

In evaluational surveys, sometimes called "statistical" surveys, we compare groups of subjects by percentage frequencies (e.g., alive or dead) or by average measurements (e.g., weights, blood pressures), trying to find associations between different phenomena and clues to possible causes. Many surveys that aim at being evaluational but are inadequate in methods and data would have value as anecdotal surveys, if they would avoid statistical tests, causal explanations and attempts at generalization. The mere fact that we may have on punch cards the records of thousands of patients and can obtain money for card sorting or even for electronic computer service in no way affects this statement. What is meant by "inadequate methods and data" appears in subsequent discussions.

Q II – 6. If the investigation is a survey, will it be retrospective, prospective or instantaneous (cross-sectional)?

Retrospective Surveys. In a typical retrospective (backward-going) survey we start with a group of subjects in whom some event, X, such as a coronary heart attack has already happened. Then we find another group that is like the first in certain respects, such as sex, age and occupation, but has no history of the event under study — the not-X's. We seek in both groups, X and not-X, for some feature which we suspect may be a cause of X, such as the consumption of animal fats (A) in contrast to the consumption of vegetable fats (B), before the event occurred in the X's and during the corresponding period in the not-X's.

Prospective Surveys. In a typical prospective (forward-going) survey we start with two groups of subjects in whom the event, X, has not happened, and who are alike in many respects but differ in the feature under study (A versus B). Then we follow all the subjects forward for a certain period and compare the frequency of occurrence of X in the two groups, A and B.

A prospective survey can, of course, start at some point of time in the past and stop at the present time or be continued into the future. A common example is a physician's "follow-up" study (see *Ex. 4* under Q II – 1 and 2 at the beginning of this chapter).

Instantaneous (Cross-sectional) Surveys. In these surveys we examine subjects as they are at the moment, or during the time that it takes to make the survey — for example, to ascertain blood chemistry levels in healthy persons, or to seek for an association between two diseases, or an association between a disease, X, and some other characteristic present at the same time, by comparing the frequency of X in two groups, A and B. These "snapshot" surveys are called "cross-sectional" in contrast to "longitudinal" surveys, which may be either prospective or retrospective. When instantaneous studies entail comparison of the frequency of X's in A's and B's, they look somewhat like prospective surveys, but they are more akin to retrospective surveys, in that the events have already occurred at the time of the survey, and their various biases are like those of retrospective surveys.

Many cross-sectional surveys are essentially bookkeeping operations, but if their lack of depth is recognized they can be very useful, for example, to an administrator who wishes to know the state of affairs in his organization at a particular time. The notification of births, deaths and infectious diseases provides public health authorities with a kind of series of cross-sectional surveys. Insofar as such data are valid and complete they can provide a basis for administrative action, such as an attempt to stop an epidemic in its early stages. Such data also indicate where a more scientific study of a health problem may be desirable. The largest human cross-sectional survey is, of course, the national census.

Some Defects of Large Surveys. Retrospective surveys can be so laden with hidden biases that the method has been stigmatized as "backward in two senses"; but prospective surveys are by no means free from danger of bias. Some of the dangers in both types emerge in later questions (especially in Chapter VII).

As compared with retrospective and instantaneous surveys, the primary disadvantage of a prospective study, starting with healthy persons, is its size. This leads to great expense in time, labor and money. For example, if one death from a certain disease occurs per thousand persons each year, in order to obtain records of 1000 such deaths we have to follow 200,000 persons for 5 years or a million persons for 1 year. With such multitudes to be studied, we may have to employ inadequately trained workers. Every year, also, more of the subjects originally in the study will be lost sight of. Therefore the other two survey methods, in spite of their defects, may be desirable at the outset, because they may give hints that seem to justify further search by a prospective study or by some kind of experimental approach, or they may dispel an impression that has arisen from casual observation, and thus prevent us from being drawn by flimsy evidence into a costly prospective study.

The difficulties and defects of clinical follow-up studies become clear in later chapters. Two of the most serious defects are:

1. The records, made for clinical purposes, are seldom suitable for any profound analytical study.
2. Many patients are commonly lost sight of.

Q II – 7. If the investigation is a survey, what is the imaginary experiment which, if it were possible, we would perform instead of the survey?

Of all the questions in the ten groups, this is the one that I have found most generally useful in trying to find defects in surveys. Some defects can be spotted easily, but the spotting method has often left me wondering whether I have not missed some even more serious defect. An imaginary experiment helps to remove this doubt, and we should use it when thinking about all the questions on surveys in these ten groups. It is the best way of bringing to light the difficulties and uncertainties inherent in survey research, and it shows what we should try to achieve, as far as possible, by our survey methods. Often a broad and simple outline of an experiment is sufficient, such as the drug trial discussed under Q II – 4.

We should note three cardinal features of a good experiment:

1. "Controls" (contrast-groups).
2. Randomization.
3. Complete follow-up. We account for all individuals at the end of the experiment.

Q II – 8. What will be our contrast-groups? How comparable will they be initially?

The word "control" is a rather inconvenient term because it is used in several senses, for example, when we speak of control of bias by randomization or of quality control in industry. Moreover, when we are comparing treatments A and B, each treatment group is in a sense a "control" for the other. Therefore the term "comparison group" or "contrast-group" is preferable.

It is difficult to see how one can draw any conclusions about anything without having something to compare it with. In all four examples of investigational purposes given at the beginning of this chapter under Q II – 1 and 2, the need for comparison was implied. Even the search for the "normal" structure of the liver would require considerable knowledge of the differences between livers in healthy and diseased subjects and between livers at different ages.

The reference to contrast-groups gives us an opportunity to summarize what has been said before regarding the difference between an experiment and a survey. In both methods of investigation the contrast-groups differ from each other, not only in the independent variable that is to be studied, but in other variables, and many of these may be entirely unknown. We can visualize each individual as carrying a particular net (or resultant) effect of these variables. In a properly conducted experiment these net effects are randomly assigned to the variables (treatments) that are to be compared, and our knowledge of games of chance enables us to make allowance for them at the end of the experiment. In a survey we cannot do this. Therefore, we must put much thought into our efforts to make the samples comparable, and be very cautious in our interpretation of the results. Questions in later chapters show the dangers that we must try to avoid.

Q II – 9. Are we trying to answer too many questions by one piece of research?

This is a very common tendency. When conducting a clinical trial on adults, if a few child patients are available it appears to be wasteful not to include them. Actually, unless we know that children with the disease in question react like adults it is usually a waste of effort to use them in the trial. Rarely will they give a definite verdict by themselves. If they seem to have reacted in the trial like the adults we have still no right to pool the two groups and strengthen the evidence, because the similarity may have been a result of chance.

The number of observations proposed for each subject in a survey may be very unrealistic. For example, a certain dermatologic clinic had a large number of patients with a wide variety of skin diseases. The head of the clinic decided that henceforth there should be recorded as much information as possible about each patient in certain of the disease categories, so that after 5 or 10 years numerous relationships could be studied. He called in a statistician to scrutinize his proposed record form.

Faced with such a problem, the statistician may sympathize with the clinician's motives, but if he has suffered the frustration of trying to draw conclusions from even better-than-average clinic records he will be very skeptical about the usefulness of the plan. He will see many possible future hypotheses, but few or none that are now definite enough to show what specific form of data would be needed to test them. He will visualize a succession of different persons filling in the record sheets hurriedly and interpreting the questions differently. He will visualize the record sheets themselves being altered from time to time, as the clinic chief or someone else thinks of ways of improving them, and, consequently, out of 10 years' data there may be only 2 consecutive years of comparable information. Finally, being aware of the changes of knowledge, interest and fashion in medicine, he will be inclined to wager that some of the salient questions 10 years hence will find no answer in the vast mass of accumulated data.

Even in a short survey or clinical trial the making of a multitude of observations on subordinate features often distracts the observer's attention from more important features. In any study there are usually some observers who believe that more phenomena should be recorded than the data sheets call for. Sometimes they add this information but fail to answer an important question that is actually in the data sheets, or they may even answer this question incorrectly.

When we are tempted to ask additional subordinate questions in any kind of study we should remember that very seldom does any one study give the last and complete verdict on any subject.

Unless we see clearly that we are not too ambitious in our plans, the best way to make ourselves face realities is to conduct a pilot study.

Q II – 10.   Do we intend to conduct a pilot study before starting our definitive investigation?

If we are not very familiar with the subject matter of the proposed research, the methods and the magnitude and complexities of the intended investigation, it is very desirable to conduct a pilot study, i.e., a small preliminary study that is as nearly like the intended study, in every detail, as we can make it — a full dress rehearsal. We should then review our experiences in the pilot study very critically, looking for defects in our plan, our methods and our recorded observations.

Q II – 11.   Have the questions that our research is intended to answer been already answered by someone else?

This does not imply that we ought not to repeat an investigation that someone else has done; but it means that we ought to find out what has been done that is relevant to our work. If our particular question has not been answered, similar questions may have been attempted or answered, perhaps on other material.

A proposal was made for certain modifications in the handling of children in a pediatric clinic and for a study of the effects of the changes. The investigators felt that they had to devise the methods of study *de novo* because they had found only one reference to such research in pediatric literature. If, however, they had searched the literature pertaining to adults they would have found reports of many such studies. In another research proposal the responses of cardiac patients to certain changes in clinic conditions was looked upon as an unmapped area of study; but the proposers might have obtained useful leads from a publication on tuberculosis patients' behavior under similar conditions.

Q II – 12.   Is this research outside our accustomed field?

It is sometimes very valuable for research workers to enter fields that are not their own; but there is such an abundance of information and complex techniques in most fields that one who steps across a boundary should be very cautious. A specialist in immunization against infectious diseases may propose to study the behavioral characteristics of patients in the clinic. He may have a thorough grasp of experimental principles, but he is likely to be an amateur in the application of them to psycho-social problems. Many family-incidence studies by medical workers are found to be meaningless and misleading when examined by a *human* geneticist, because many necessary data have not been obtained and environmental factors have been neglected.

If we wish to cross boundaries we should sink our pride and seek expert guidance, but sometimes we do not know which expert we need. It is desirable, therefore, to discuss our proposed research with persons of diverse interests. Even if they cannot help us directly, they may know the kind of help that we should seek.

CHAPTER III

THE POPULATION AND SAMPLING

Q III – 1.   What is the initial definition of our population – the kind of subject or material which is to be studied, and to which our conclusions will be applicable?

Nearly all research is aimed at generalization from a sample to subjects or material *of like kind*. Even if we examined every member of an existing population – all persons with a particular disease in a certain country, or even in the whole world at a certain time, or all animals, now living, of a certain species and strain – we would have only a sample, restricted by time or place or both, of the "material of like kind" to which we would want to apply the results of our investigation.

Obviously, therefore, we must define our population, and that really means describing our sample. Our initial definition will be supplemented and modified by our answers to subsequent questions regarding selection of subjects, methods and times of observation, and other features or phenomena that have an influence on the outcome of our investigation. Indeed, to define our population as adequately as we can we must wait until the end of our investigation, because the statement of what was done to or occurred in the sample, besides the factors under test, is part of the required description.

The term "population" is, of course, a carry-over from the beginning of statistics, the counting of persons, and its modern application often seems far-fetched; but it is useful because it reminds us that our material, and therefore our sample, must be composed of "individuals," whether these are different persons each providing a blood count, or drops of blood from the same person, or pipetfuls of fluid from the same solution, or animal cages, each cage containing a group of animals. The "individuals" that compose the sample are the *sampling units*.

Q III – 2.   Is the initial definition of the population adequate for the selection of subjects?

To test the adequacy of the definition we can ask two questions:

1. Would everyone applying this definition make the same decision as to whether a subject is or is not qualified for the study?

2. Is the definition appropriate to the purpose of the study? For example, the purpose of a clinical drug trial is the application of the resulting information to patients diagnosed by certain specified methods during life. If some patients who were in the trial die and an autopsy is performed, the postmortem diagnosis is irrelevant, although it may help us to improve our clinical diagnostic criteria in the future.

Q III – 3.   What other populations are excluded by the definition of our population?

Whenever we define, we separate something from something else, and we should ask: "What kinds are we excluding?" Unless we do so, we run the risk of "illicit generalization" and tend to form inflated notions of the universality of our discoveries. If we developed the habit of more detailed description and of making more modest, qualified and tentative inferences, we would run much less risk of having our conclusions "refuted" by other people who have studied somewhat different populations. The differences, subtle and perhaps unrecorded, may lie in the events that led to the selection of the sample, or in the experimental methods, or in the criteria of assessment.

Volunteer Subjects. The way in which we obtain our subjects may introduce an important but ill-defined restriction on our population. People who volunteer for a study are very likely to differ in various ways from those who refuse to participate. Some may be excessively interested in their condition or, in the case of healthy volunteers, interested because a certain disease has been common in their relatives. On the other hand, some sick persons may be extremely indifferent to their condition but willing to cooperate. Some people enjoy being the center of attention. Some are even masochistic.

Restriction by Previous Therapy. We ought to scrutinize every item in the definition of our population, although we are sometimes disturbed by what we find. Let us suppose that we plan to test for 6 months a new drug (B) against an older and widely used drug (A) in patients suffering from a chronic disease, such as rheumatoid arthritis. If we decide to exclude patients who have ever received drug A, our population will be largely restricted to early cases, with perhaps some patients whose disease has been of longer duration but so mild that they have never received drug A, and possibly some patients who have been treated by a physician who seldom uses drug A.

If, then, we decide to admit to the trial patients who have been previously treated by drug A, the question will arise: "Suppose that a patient has been treated unsuccessfully with drug A. Is it fair to expose him to a 1:1 chance of being treated by it again for 6 months? If the randomization assigns him to that drug could we not count him immediately as a failure before even putting him on the drug?" The answer is: "If we do so, we will no longer have a proper experiment, because we have no right to assume that at this time, and under the conditions of this trial, he would behave as he did previously." Physicians who know the unpredictable behavior of rheumatoid arthritis would very likely adopt this point of view and enter the patient in the trial. On the other hand, in the treatment of a rapidly progressing and often fatal disease there might be much more hesitation.

Even in a disease that is neither rapidly progressing nor fatal, a difficult question can arise: "Are we going to risk admitting patients to a trial who have already had undesirable symptoms when treated with drug A?" The answer will depend on the nature of the symptoms. Sometimes it will be: "Admit them to the trial and, as usual, watch all patients carefully; then remove those who exhibit undesirable symptoms." Sometimes it is unethical to admit such patients at all, but then our definition of the population must be appropriately changed. Moreover, we will not be able to compare the A-treated and B-treated patients in the trial with respect to frequencies of undesirable symptoms.

We should visualize, as fully and realistically as we can, all such contingencies that may arise in a proposed trial. Even if we discover that we cannot with clear conscience start the trial at all, this is better than agreeing to a plan at a conference table and then breaking the agreement, secretly or openly, when we face actual patients, instead of the abstract "cases" discussed in a planning session.

Q III – 4. Will the definition of the population be strictly observed throughout the study?

If we are to obtain any clear-cut and usable answer from a study it is important that we adhere to the rules that we have set up for definition of the population, methods of observation and all other features. If we find that the rules really do not work we should drop the study and start afresh. In clinical trials in which patients are scarce, the temptation to relax the admission rules is very strong, and the question may arise: "Why did we make this restrictive rule?" It is therefore desirable at the outset to write down the reasons for all the rules regarding selection of subjects.

Q III – 5. How may the study itself affect the definition of the population?

It is still sometimes forgotten that laboratory animals are in unnatural conditions. We may not "murder to dissect," but we often have to distort in order to study. Those of us who loathe questionnaires may be as abnormal as laboratory animals when we are compelled to answer them.

In a time-study of interns' activities it was proposed to have each intern continuously accompanied by an observer throughout his hours on duty, the observer being provided with a bed in the intern's room. The definition of the intern population so sampled would have to include (1) willingness (or inducement or compulsion) to undergo constant surveillance, and (2) performance under those conditions. What these supplementary definitions would do to the original definition "interns on such and such a service," is not clear, but physicians who have been interns and have worked with interns might hazard a guess.

It requires great insight and ingenuity to devise ways of measuring and reducing the biasing influence of study methods. Many of us who are medically trained, including even psychiatrists, are naïve regarding the psychologic and sociologic aspects of research on man and animals; and it is often not easy to find a suitable (i.e., experimentally minded) psychologist or sociologist to help us.

In drug trials it is often considered necessary to take patients out of the experiment when they display certain undesirable symptoms. It might then be considered perfectly valid to define the population to which the therapeutic results of the trial would apply by a phrase such as: "Patients who did not require removal from the trial." Sometimes, however, it is possible to discover the following kind of note in a case history: "Patient had side effects and was not benefiting; therefore, was taken out of trial." The implication is that if the patient had appeared to be benefiting he might not have been removed from the trial, in spite of the occurrence of side effects. Moreover, in other records, in which such notes are not found, the same double motive may have led to removal of patients with side effects. It is doubtful if any workable rules could be set up that would stipulate the kind, number and degree of undesirable symptoms that would determine whether a patient should be kept on, or taken off, the trial therapy. The only safe rule is to count patients who were taken off therapy, ostensibly because of side effects, as failures for the therapy that they were receiving.

Q III – 6. By what technique will we obtain our samples?

Since we wish to argue from a sample to its parent population, we should obviously try to obtain the sample by a reliable method. By this we do not mean a method that guarantees that the sample will exactly represent the population in the variables under study, e.g., the percentages of X's and not-X's or the mean value of some measurement. No method guarantees this, unless we possess certain kinds of knowledge of the population or material under study beyond what the sample provides. Extreme examples of such knowledge occur in physics and chemistry. For instance, if it is found that a very highly purified sample of a certain chemical, under certain specified conditions, crystallizes in a certain form, although this is the only such sample in existence the chemist can feel confident that a population of such samples would crystallize in the same form.

We seldom have such basic general knowledge when we sample in medical research. In this area, when numerous samples are taken from a large population and then compared with the population as a whole, it is found that relatively few samples show exactly the population value (e.g., percentage of X's) compared with the numbers of samples that give values above or below it. Therefore, by a "reliable" method of sampling we mean one that enables us to estimate how far the population value may be above or below the observed sample value. The only method is some form of strictly random sampling.

Strictly Random Sampling. Perhaps the simplest introduction to random sampling in medicine is by an example that seems rather remote from clinical and laboratory research. Let us suppose that there is a population of 20,000 persons in a certain industry, and we wish to find what percentage of them possess a certain characteristic (X) — some anatomic, physiologic, biochemical, psychologic or pathologic feature. Owing to lack of time and money we can examine only 200 individuals (a 1 per cent sample), but we wish to select those 200 in such a way that we can estimate the possible difference between our sample percentage of X's and the "true" (population) percentage. That is, we wish to estimate our possible error, because no numerical estimate of any kind means anything unless it is accompanied by an estimate of error.

In an actual investigation of this kind we would probably divide the population by sex, age group, and probably by type of job within the industry, and then we would take a sample from each subpopulation; but for simplicity we describe the taking of one sample of 200 from the total 20,000.

In essence, the sampling method is the same as was used by the "randomizer" in the drug trial described under Q II – 4. After shuffling the cards, when he took the top 50 and called them "A" he had a strictly random sample of the total 100 cards; but in the drug trial the other (random) sample of 50 cards would also be used, to indicate what patients would receive drug B, whereas in our industry survey we would use only the sample of 200. Obviously, the shuffling of 20,000 cards would not be a practical way of obtaining the sample, and random numbers are now commonly used; but the essential process is best revealed by a method that is still employed in various sampling experiments — disk sampling.

To obtain a random sample from our population of 20,000 we would take 20,000 plastic disks, say one inch in diameter and precision-made to insure uniform shape, size and texture. On each disk we would mark one person's employment serial number or other identification symbol. We would shuffle the disks very thoroughly in a barrel and then, without looking at the marks on the disks, we would take a sample of 200 — the persons to be examined.

Arguing from Samples to Populations. If we found that 16 of our sample of 200 persons (8 per cent) were X's, we could then state that the population percentage was unlikely to be as low as 4 per cent X's or as high as 13 per cent X's. How we arrive at such figures is shown in Chapter XI. At present the essential point to note is that they are based on our knowledge of random processes, as in games of chance and in experiments of the disk-sampling type. From this experience we know that if the population value were 4 per cent X's or less, and we did a large number of disk-sampling experiments (say 1000) taking 200 disks in each experiment (and replacing each sample after we had counted its X's), we would rarely find samples containing as many as 16 X's. By "rarely" we mean in this instance "in fewer than 2.5 per cent of random sampling experiments." Similarly, if the population value were 13 per cent X's or greater, we would rarely find samples of 200 containing as *few* as 16 X's.

Therefore, if we adopt this definition of "rarity" in all our random samplings, our risk of error, i.e., the frequency with which we will be wrong in such statements as "not as high as 13 per cent X's," will be less than 2.5 per cent. In the present example, our conclusion would be that the population value lay somewhere between 5 per cent and 12 per cent X's. If we assumed that it was any closer to the sample value (8 per cent X's) our risk of being wrong would be greater than 2.5 per cent.* As will be seen later, we can set this risk at any level that we wish; for example, at 1 per cent.

Equal Opportunity of Selection. In our description of disk sampling an important item was omitted. If we wrote on the disks the serial numbers from 1 to 20,000 we would be altering the surfaces of the disks unequally — changing their frictional properties to different degrees. In the shuffling some disks might move less easily over their neighbors than others, and the sample might contain an unduly large proportion of the higher (or lower) numbers; it would be a biased sample. That this is not fanciful was revealed in an actual sampling experiment in which counters (disks) of different colors were used. The population percentages were known and in the sampling "there emerged a persistent bias against counters of one particular colour. After careful investigation the only explanation seemed to be that these particular counters were slightly more greasy than the others, owing to pecularities of the pigment, and hence slipped through the sampler's fingers" (Yule and Kendall, 1949, sect. 18.22).

Readers of this book will presumably use random numbers, and not disks or playing cards, in randomization; but the anecdote is worth remembering because (1) it shows how little it takes to create bias, and (2) it illustrates a basic requirement in random sampling: Each individual unit must start with an equal opportunity of appearing in the sample and must retain that equality, except insofar as the random process itself pushes it toward or away from the sample.

Q III – 7. What is the danger of haphazard selection?

"Experience has shown that the human being is an extremely poor instrument for the conduct of a random selection. Wherever there is any scope for personal choice or judgment on the part of the observer, bias is almost certain to creep in. Nor is this a quality that can be removed by conscious effort or training. Nearly every human being has, as part of his psychological make-up, a tendency away from true randomness in his choices" (Yule and Kendall, 1949, sect. 18.21).

---

* Although the population in this example is finite, it is so large relative to the sample that the "infinite population limit" method of Chapter XI is applicable; and for greater safety the limits found in tables (Mainland, Herrera and Sutcliffe) have been expressed as integers: 4.70 as 4 per cent, and 12.61 as 13 per cent.

An experienced investigator, Dr. G. W. Corner, reported an instructive example of bias in the choice of experimental animals. He and W. M. Allen were trying to extract from the corpora lutea of sows' ovaries the hormone (progesterone) which causes proliferation of the uterine mucosa in early pregnancy. To test the extracts, they injected them into female rabbits. They had been so successful that they were writing a paper on their methods, but decided to see whether a less skillful chemist than Mr. Allen could follow their directions.

Dr. Corner therefore carried through the whole procedure himself, but failed repeatedly. Greatly perturbed, the investigators spent much time and labor trying to find errors in the method of extraction. They even blacked out Dr. Corner's laboratory because they thought that the bright sunlight might have spoiled his extracts. Finally, they made a batch together and divided it into two lots. Each of them tested one lot. Mr. Allen's worked, but Dr. Corner's did not. The reason may be given in Dr. Corner's own words:

"The explanation will seem so silly that I almost hesitate to admit what it was. The fact is that rabbits do not respond well to progesterone until they are about 8 weeks old and weigh about 800 grams. We did not know this, and our rabbits ranged from 600 to 1200 grams. When we went to the cages to inject them, Willard Allen's idea of what constitutes a nice rabbit led him to choose the larger ones, while I must have had a subconscious preference for the infants. My extracts had been as good as his all the while, but my rabbits were insensitive. It is staggering to think how often the success or failure of research may hang upon an unimaginable contingency" (G. W. Corner).

Strictly random sampling from the stock of rabbits throughout the experiments would have resulted in some successes and some failures in the hands of both investigators, even with the same batch of extract. A search for causes of failure would have led them quickly to notice the association with differences in weight.

"Random," standing alone, is a dangerous word, for it has the colloquial meaning of "haphazard" or "without conscious bias." The only safe way to distinguish the technical use of the word is by a phrase such as "strictly random" or, better still, by naming the instrument or method (e.g., random numbers). Without such information, unless we know an investigator's practice the safest assumption is that his samples were not random in the technical sense. For example, the shuffling of bits of paper in a hat may prevent psychologic bias, but it is unlikely to remove physical bias, due to the order in which the papers were numbered and placed in the hat.

Q III – 8. What is the danger of a purely systematic selection method?

As was noted in the sampling of industrial employees, we can systematically divide the total population into subpopulations by sex, age group, type of job and so forth, and then take a random sample from each group; but here we are to consider systematic sampling without random selection at any point. If we select, say, every fifth, tenth or nth name in a list, and then use our sample for population estimates as if it were a random sample, we are faced with the difficult, often impossible, task of showing that it is, for our purposes, equivalent to a strictly random sample.

Every nth Name.   A medical school in a large city proposed to institute a television program for the postgraduate education of physicians in their own homes. It wished to discover physicians' opinions of the proposal, and therefore sent a letter to every fifth physician in the directory, an alphabetical list of names. Such a list is clearly nonrandom. It contains clusters arising from racial origin, from blood relationship, and even from marriage, when husband and wife both practice under the same last name. Therefore it was impossible to make a reliable estimate of the responses of the total population of physicians.

If we read about an "every nth name" sample, even if we know that the investigator is well acquainted with the principles and techniques of sampling, we ought to scrutinize carefully his justification, looking for evidence that the method was actually safe with his material.

"Representative" Samples.   Persons who are not well acquainted with the principles of sampling choose this systematic method not only because it is easy, but because they think that it spreads the choice more evenly among the population and so provides a more "representative" sample than does random selection. For instance, in the taking of a 20 per cent sample from a large collection of hospital records the admission numbers ending in 0 and 5 may be chosen because it is not supposed that the terminal digits would be associated with any particular characteristic of the patients, and that, if more patients are admitted in one season (or in one month) than in another, correspondingly more 0's and 5's will be found; whereas a random sample might take in too many June patients and too few December patients, or vice versa.

The trouble with this systematic method is that we do not know exactly how representative it is — how evenly or unevenly it spreads its net in relation to the multitude of variables, such as time (seasons, months, or time of day), sex, age, disease, and so on, which may create clusters of various sizes. We cannot use it like a random sample to provide a reliable estimate of population values, and it gives no other basis for such estimates.

Q III – 9.   If our samples are not strictly random, how can we generalize, i.e., argue from them to their populations?

Medical Samples Seldom Random.   In contrast to the sampling from finite and known populations, such as the employees in a particular industrial company, let us now consider two much commoner types of sampling in medical research. Let us think of patients with a certain disease who come to a particular physician, clinic or hospital. They often have much in common, and differ as a group from patients who go to other physicians or clinics or hospitals. They may be selected by such features as area of residence, economic and social conditions, and even the partiality to a particular physician. Let us visualize also the differences between physicians (and clinics) in diagnostic customs and standards, in methods of assessing the severity and progress of a patient's condition, and in general patient care. When we think about these things we see very good reasons to conclude that no group of patients investigated by an individual physician, or in a clinic or in a hospital, is likely to be equivalent to a strictly random sample of the population which, by diagnostic label, it purports to represent. This will still be true even if we divide the group into samples with more detailed labels to indicate sex, age range, severity of condition, duration of disease and type of previous therapy. It will still be true if we take a dozen clinics and pool their contributions, whether they are equal or unequal in numbers.

Next, let us visualize the circumstances and practices in the farms or institutes where laboratory animals are bred — the factors that determine which animals shall be delivered to a particular laboratory on a particular day. The animals are born in litters and are grouped in cages, and the breeder or handyman, in picking the type desired to fill an order, does not do anything equivalent to the disk mixing that we have described. Our sample consisting of clusters and parts of clusters, is not even a strictly random sample of the breeder's own population of the specified type, and even if we insist on pairs of litter mates, these pairs are not randomly selected pairs. Indeed, even if the breeder went to great trouble to obtain a random sample of his animals of a particular species, strain, sex, age and weight range, we could not assume that it was equivalent to a strictly random sample of all the animals to which those labels could be applied, for it is known that two lots of animals of the same "pure" strain, bred at different institutions, come to differ from each other.

It is true that in the production of our samples of patients and animals random processes are at work, i.e., forces, independent of each other, pushing individuals this way and that, like the forces set in motion by our hands in a disk-sampling experiment. The point to remember is that Nature does not *try* to randomize. Strict randomization requires special precautions, such as uniform disks, well made playing cards, or thoroughly tested roulette wheels; it requires also much labor and much time.

The Path of Generalization.   And so, after learning that strictly random sampling is nearly always essential if we are to make a reliable estimate of the possible error in our conclusions, we learn that most of the samples that come to us are not strictly random samples of the populations to which we wish to generalize. After we have spent 6 months or a year on a clinical trial, with random assignment of drugs, double-blind techniques and all other precautions, and have proved beyond reasonable doubt that drug A was more effective than drug B on the patients in the trial, it is very discouraging to be told that, because we had not a strictly random sample of all present and future patients of like kind, our results do not necessarily apply to other patients elsewhere or to our own future patients. We must admit the same uncertainty regarding much of our laboratory research, and we seem to be driven to scientific nihilism — to a confession that in most of our research we cannot generalize from what we have observed.

And yet the knowledge that has given man the power to control his environment is the product of inductive inference — arguments from samples to populations. Our situation in research is in fact no more discouraging than in many other activities of life. In all the generalizations on which we base our actions we are doing something akin to what mathematicians call "extrapolating," i.e., carrying a line on a graph beyond the observed points. In doing so we are trusting to a uniformity or consistency in Nature and our trust is often justified, not only in the physical sciences but in biology and medicine.

Such justification is progressive. As our experience and the experience of others increases, if we find no contradictory evidence under widely varying conditions we gain more and more confidence in our generalization. Moreover, if we penetrate more deeply and can *explain* the facts that we have discovered — by seeing how they fit into a system of other facts or by discovering underlying mechanisms — our confidence increases still more. Even in this process of enlarging our experience, however, we must beware of bias. Uninteresting "negative" results, and results that run strongly counter to current beliefs, are less likely to be published than are exciting "positive" results or results that are fashionable.

Because generalization is stepwise, it behooves each of us to make his particular step as sound as he can, not only by care in the investigation but by a detailed description of what was done.

Value of Detailed Descriptions. To help others, either in applying our results or in studying them for further research, we must reveal as best we can the possible extent and limits of generalization, by telling what we know about the parent population of our sample. We can do this only by describing our sample, how we selected it, and what factors beyond our control may have influenced its composition, and trying to include all the information which, according to current knowledge or opinion, is relevant to the problem. Overall statements, such as age range, numbers of males and females and numbers in different stages of the disease when treatment started, are not very helpful. There is an old saying that one table of raw data is worth more than half a dozen tables of figures derived from the raw data; and it is amazing how much information on each patient, animal or other unit can, with the help of abbreviations, be packed into a fine-print one-page table. It may even be possible to include in the same table the chief observations (e.g., responses to tests or to therapy) made on each unit. Incidentally, such tables furnish an answer to a common criticism of "statistics" — that it deals only with groups and averages, and ignores the individual.

CHAPTER IV

SUBDIVISION OF POPULATION AND SAMPLES

Q IV – 1.   Do we intend to subdivide our original population in order (a) to study a sample from each class separately, or (b) to confine our study to one class? If so, why?

In a trial of drugs for the treatment of rheumatic fever (Medical Research Council of Great Britain and American Heart Association), the patients were divided by age (0 to 15 years; 16 years and over) and by duration from onset of attack to start of therapy (14 days or less; 15 to 42 days; 43 days and over). The division provided six subgroups for the comparison of drugs A, B and C within each subgroup. This procedure is so characteristic of experimentation of all kinds, and of all good surveys, that discussion might seem superfluous; but before deciding whether to subdivide in any investigation, and how far to subdivide, we should recall why we subdivide.

The term "stratification" is now rather widely used for this subdivision of populations. It suggests division into layers lying on top of one another, as do geologic strata, and it is appropriate enough for age groups, or duration-of-disease groups, which can be arranged in ascending or descending numerical order, but if the differences are qualitative the term is less suitable. Stratification by sex, for instance, hardly seems fitting, at least in a statistical sense. The term should imply, also, that we intend to take a sample from each of the classes (strata), but we often take only one class for investigation, and the division is then equivalent simply to a restriction of the definition of the population to be sampled.

Reduction of Variation. Subdivision of populations is our primary weapon for attacking variation — the differences that exist between things that bear the same name. For example, rheumatic fever patients, like sufferers from all other diseases, vary from each other in response to treatment; but the clinical-trial investigators had good reason to believe that, if they studied children and adults separately, they would find less variation in response to treatment within each of these two age classes than among the total patients, adults and children combined.

Similarly, in children (or in adults) they expected less variation in response to treatment in any one of the duration-from-onset groups than in all the children (or adults) considered as one group. In some diseases the early cases are more amenable to treatment, and in other diseases the patients tend to improve after a certain length of time, with little or no treatment; but whatever the natural history of the disease, it is often desirable to subdivide by duration.

As these examples show, the total undivided population contains more variation than do its subclasses, i.e., it is more heterogeneous; and we can express this by a kind of equation:

Intraclass variation + Interclass variation = Total variation.

The purposes of subdivision of the population can be described as: (1) Increase of specificity, (2) Reduction of bias, and (3) Increase of sensitivity.

Increase of Specificity. If drug A is more effective than drug B in advanced cases of a certain disease, whereas B is as effective as A in early cases, it may be very useful to know this difference, especially if A is a more hazardous drug, because we can avoid using it with early cases. In general, the more we know about the specific characteristics and behavior of the various subclasses of any material — their similarities and differences — the nearer we are likely to come to underlying principles.

Reduction of Bias. In an experiment, however heterogeneous a group of subjects may be, random assignment of the factors under test will control the bias in such a way that we can state our risk of falsely concluding that the factor under test has caused the observed results (Chapter II, under Q II – 4). In a survey our situation is different. Let us suppose that in the rheumatic fever study the investigators had not been comparing drugs but had wished to find out whether males or females fared better when all were treated by the same drug. Let us suppose, further, that sex difference itself had no influence on the outcome, but that patients treated earlier in the disease did better than those who started treatment later.

Obviously, if there were a higher proportion of early cases among the males and we simply compared males and females without division by duration before treatment, we would obtain a biased verdict in favor of the males. To avoid such risks we would have to compare the outcome in the two sexes in each duration-before-treatment class separately, and we would have to do likewise with other independent variables such as age — a sex contrast of outcome in each age-duration subclass.

Increase of Sensitivity. In an experiment, although randomization will control the effects of bias in a heterogeneous group, it will not correct another effect of the excessive variation, and this effect is present in surveys also. Let us suppose that we had tested two treatments, A and B, with the following results:

Out of 100 A-treated patients, 65 improved
Out of 100 B-treated patients, 50 improved
Difference = 15 per cent

Scrutinizing the data however, we make the following tabulation:

	Treatment A	Treatment B
Early cases	45 out of 60 improved	45 out of 60 improved
Late cases	20 out of 40 improved	5 out of 40 improved

In the early cases, A and B were equally effective (or ineffective), but the difference in the late cases = 50 minus 12.5 = 37.5 per cent.

For simplicity we have supposed that the randomization had assigned exactly equal numbers of early cases to the two treatment groups, and also exactly equal numbers of late cases — that is, it had entirely prevented bias due to differences in duration of disease — but the mixing of early and late cases in the first analysis partially masked or damped the contrast between the effect of the two treatments.

Damping Effects. If we remember damping effects we may save ourselves much waste of effort. Thus, if we were testing a possible preventive of colds, we ought not to load our samples with persons who seldom or never have colds. In testing anti-inflammatory drugs in rheumatoid arthritis it is customary to exclude two types of patients: (1) those whose symptoms have been present for only a few months, because they often improve greatly with little or no treatment, and (2) the "burnt-out" cases, in which the disease shows no inflammatory activity but marked anatomic deformities which cannot be reduced by drugs.

"Placebo-reactors." In testing headache remedies it may be worth while to begin by administering a placebo to all subjects and then to eliminate from the trial all those who report relief — the "placebo-reactors" (Jellinek). This does not imply, however, that we can omit a contrast-group in the trial itself. A person who had not obtained relief in the all-placebo test might, for some reason or other, obtain relief while on placebo during the trial.

The "Hawthorne Effect." This phenomenon is analogous to the placebo effect. It obtained its nickname from the Western Electric Company's Hawthorne plant in Chicago, where during the 1920's many investigations were conducted on the working conditions of the employees (Roethlisberger and Dickson). In one experiment a control group worked under a more or less constant illumination throughout. The test group worked at different times under three different levels of illumination: (1) approximately the same as that of the control group, (2) twice, (3) three times that of the control group. The result was a very appreciable production increase in both groups, with no appreciable intergroup difference in its magnitude.

In another experiment the controls worked under a constant level of 10 foot-candles. In the test group the levels were decreased from 10 to 3 foot-candles by one foot-candle at a time. During this period the efficiency of both groups increased slowly and steadily; and it was only when the illumination for the test group reached 3 foot-candles and the operatives could hardly see what they were doing that their production rate decreased.

Whether we call this phenomenon "placebo effect" or "Hawthorne effect" or the effect of an "associated agent" we must remember it whenever we plan to do anything to a human being and measure its effect.

Damping in Measurement Data. To show the damping effect of interclass variation in measurement data, let the measurement scale be 1, 2, 3, and so on, and let each individual in two samples of 8 subjects be represented by the letter "x":

Treatment A	x	x	x	x	x	x	x	x				
Treatment B					x	x	x	x	x	x	x	x
Measurement scale	1	2	3	4	5	6	7	8	9	10	11	12

The B-treated subjects have a higher total (or average) reading than the A-treated subjects; but there is considerable overlap of the two samples. Looking at the data, we discover that children (c) and adults (a) are in both samples, and adults give higher readings than children under the same treatment:

Treatment A	c	c	c	c	a	a	a	a				
Treatment B					c	c	c	c	a	a	a	a
Measurement scale	1	2	3	4	5	6	7	8	9	10	11	12

When we separate the children and adults in both treatment groups, the treatment differences stand out clearly.

Q IV – 2. Apart from the factor under test, what are the variables that are associated with differences in the phenomena to be observed?

Categories for Subdivision of the Population. When we wish to decide whether a person is "underweight" or not, we select the part of our weight tables appropriate to the person's sex, age (adult or child), and stature. We ought to choose, also, a table suitable to racial stock, unless it has been shown that allowance for stature corrects sufficiently for interracial differences in weight. The construction of weight tables, therefore, provides a simple example of population division and also exemplifies three categories that are used in many kinds of research: (1) stock, species or kind; (2) sex; (3) age. Subdivision by stature illustrates a fourth category or group of categories — features relevant to the particular problem.

Stock, Species or Kind. "Racial stock" is very difficult to define, and when used in medicine it should seldom be taken to mean more than the country or region in which a person's ancestors lived for many generations. However, even our rather vague and superficial classification (Anglo-Saxon, North European, South European, Negro, Japanese, and so on) reminds us of differences *associated with* racial stock — anatomic, physiologic and psychologic differences, also differences in liability to certain diseases.

The term "associated with" is desirably noncommital, for in many instances the differences are probably not hereditary but environmental. Different food habits can produce differences in nutritional status. Differences in economic and social conditions of different racial groups can produce different hygienic conditions, different attitudes to disease, to doctors and to people who pester them with questionnaires. The grouping of members of the same stock in the same area can promote the spread of a particular disease among the group.

The term "stock" reminds us also of differences between strains of the same animal species and interfamily differences. "Species" means "kind," and reminds us of the differences between different kinds of the same thing. Muscle contraction time is not necessarily the same in a frog's gastrocnemius and a toad's gastrocnemius, or in a frog's gastrocnemius and a frog's sartorius.

Every disease contains "species" and "subspecies," because a "disease" is simply a label for a group of phenomena which either (a) spring from a common cause, such as a particular microorganism, or (b) frequently occur together and are suspected to have a common cause. The chief value in the label is therapeutic — to enable us to prescribe what is, currently, considered an appropriate treatment — and the label can mislead us in our search for the real nature of disease. When people talk about the cause and cure of "cancer," it is well to remind them that in bygone days "fever" was considered a disease. Increase of knowledge has led us to the separate labeling of innumerable conditions, all of which have fever as one manifestation. On the other hand, increase of knowledge can lead to grouping of conditions — for example, the discovery of the tubercle bacillus justified the application of a common label to phenomena in the lungs, kidneys, lymph nodes, joints, skin and other organs, which appeared to be different diseases.

Sex. As a rule we allow for sex differences that have been already recognized, e.g., in statures, body weights, blood counts, emotional characteristics and the predilection for certain diseases; but recent discoveries suggest that this may not be enough. To most investigators a kidney was a kidney, histologically, whether male or female, until there was discovered a sex difference in the shape of certain cells which could easily be mistaken for the results of experiment or disease (Crabtree). During many decades millions of cells of all kinds had been examined before there was reported in 1950 a small body that looked like a "satellite" of the nucleolus in the nuclei of female cats' nerve cells (Barr, Bertram and Lindsay). Thereafter the same kind of particle was readily seen by other workers in a wide variety of female cells (including women's leukocytes) stained by routine techniques.

Age. We still know little about the phenomena of aging in adults, especially the distinction between disease and "healthy" aging, but we know enough to have it serve as a warning. For example, various chemical blood tests appeared to be very successful in detecting the presence of cancer, until it was discovered that the healthy control subjects were those most easily available to the inventor of the test, such as nurses, laboratory technicians and hospital interns — all much younger than the majority of the cancer patients. The tests have, therefore, merely "diagnosed" middle age or old age, and, in some instances, debility in the cancer patients.

Other Relevant Features. Every investigation has its own set of features that could affect the outcome, in addition to the independent variables under study. In research on patients, whether treatment trials or surveys (e.g., of blood pressure or blood chemistry) there is seldom difficulty in finding a dozen or more such features — for example: total duration of disease; age at initial onset; duration between present attack and treatment; severity; manifestations of present attack; accompanying diseased conditions (complications); occupation; social and economic condition; previous treatments of the disorder; diet; recent emotional disturbances; conditions under which treatment will be carried out; and various other treatments, supplementary to those under test.

The five questions mentioned in Chapter I — *Who? What? Where? When? How?* — can help to remind us of categories for subdivision and for exclusion of subgroups. We ought not to complete our list of categories before answering the questions in Chapter IX (Collecting, Recording and Examining the Data). Differences in the conditions under which observations are made, and in the methods employed, can create different subpopulations of the total material about which we are trying to learn.

Q IV – 3. Which of the variables listed in answer to Question IV – 2 will we use as a basis for subdivision of the population? Why not the other variables?

Q IV – 4. If we choose a measured variable (e.g., age) as a basis for classification, how will we decide on the coarseness or fineness of the subdivision?

"In expositions of the scientific use of experimentation it is frequent to find an excessive stress laid on the importance of varying the essential conditions only one at a time. . . . This ideal doctrine seems to be more nearly related to expositions of elementary physical theory than to laboratory practice in any branch of research" (Fisher, *The Design of Experiments,* sect. 37). Although this was written more than a quarter of a century ago, we have noted (under Q II – 4) that some investigators still tell us that the proper way to conduct an experiment is to hold all relevant features constant, or as constant as possible, except the factors under test. If we tried to follow this injunction literally we would confine our animal experiments to litter mates from highly inbred strains, our human investigations to uniovular twins. More likely, we would never begin an investigation at all, because there would always be some relevant (or conceivably relevant) features, in the environment, in our experimental techniques and in our observational methods, that we could make more uniform if we tried to do so.

Guidelines for Division of Population.   What we have to decide before every investigation is where to draw the line between desirable and excessive uniformity of material, conditions and methods; that is the reason for Questions IV – 3 and IV – 4. Decisions regarding the selection of material for investigation, categories of subdivision, numbers of subclasses, uniformity of conditions, standardization of equipment, and experimental and observational methods should be based chiefly on five considerations:

1. Simplicity, clarity and objectivity of definitions, such as the dividing lines between classes.
2. Relative weights of the variables under consideration — their ability to produce differences in outcome, and thus to lower sensitivity.
3. Feasibility and convenience.
4. Usefulness in application of results.
5. Relative costs of increased uniformity and increased sample size.

Several of these topics require further discussion.

Simplicity, Clarity and Objectivity of Definitions.   Potential users of our results should be able to classify our material exactly as we have done, and to reproduce our techniques very closely. Classes should be both mutually exclusive and complete, i.e., there should be a niche for every individual that may be met in the population that we wish to sample. Difficulties and defects of classification can be illustrated by schemes that have been devised for the descriptions of stages (progression) of a disease, its activity and severity.

Stages in a Disease.   A classification that is based on objective observations may be widely used for a decade or more, and clinicians may think that they are therefore using a reliable common language; and yet when it is critically examined it may be found unworkable. A scheme that represents the general or "typical" progress of a disease in successive steps, ABCD, breaks down when it meets a patient whose pattern is ACBD. If each of these letters contains information from different tissues, organs or functions, or a mixture of x-ray and clinical observations, we can be sure that the scheme will often break down.

The best way to demonstrate the quality of a scheme is to have the observers examine a wide variety of individuals and record the presence or absence of each of the features that the scheme utilizes, and then make the classification themselves. In the testing of one scheme 153 such records and classifications were made. The observations were on bones, joints and neighboring soft tissues. If the scheme had been workable, anyone (for example, an office clerk) ought to have been able, by following the rules for classification, to arrive at the same result as anyone else who used the same data. This could not be done because in 59 instances (38.6 per cent) classification was impossible. This was not due to incomplete or self-contradictory observations but to the combination of features, present in the several tissues, that disqualified the case from each of the four classes, and did not even permit labeling it as transitional between one class and the next.

And yet in each of these instances a class had been assigned by the observers. Presumably they had supplied a mental correction term to the prescribed scheme. It can be taken for granted that different observers will differ in their mental correction terms, and the scheme cannot, therefore, be a common language.

If a multiple-criteria system of classification is desired, the only dependable method is by a hierarchy of classes and subclasses, along the lines: X_1 present or absent, X_2 present or absent, X_3 present or absent. (When measured variables are used, one can, of course, substitute for "present-absent" a dividing line, such as X_1 above or below a certain level.)

At the other extreme but equally ambiguous are systems that permit subjects to be placed in more than one category. A good example is given by Fletcher and Oldham in *Medical Surveys and Clinical Trials* (Witts). In a survey of a group of persons to determine the prevalence of chronic bronchitis, the diagnostic scheme permitted three different interpretations and, depending on which interpretation was used, the same group was found to have three different frequencies of the disease: 12.5, 16.5 and 39 per cent. The chief source of the confusion was that in order to "strengthen the diagnosis in cases of doubt," yellowness of sputum, colds going to the chest, and time off work due to chest trouble were used as supplementary evidence. In classification the rule should be: Apply all criteria to all cases.

Feasibility and Convenience.   The investigators in the rheumatic fever trial, mentioned under Q IV – 1, could have divided the total group of patients into numerous subclasses by various combinations of the manifestations of the disease present on admission to the trial, such as the presence or absence of chorea, the severity of heart involvement, and the degree of fever. They could have divided ages by single years, and duration of treatment by 3-day intervals. Such schemes would not only have been difficult to operate; they would have broken down because there would seldom have been found three patients (for treatments A, B and C) sufficiently alike in all particulars to go into any one subclass.

Usefulness in Application of Results.   Before beginning any investigation, we should ask: "By whom, for what purpose, and under what circumstances, will our results probably be used?" Extreme refinement of conditions may be desirable if an experiment is one of a series to be conducted in our own laboratory, but if we wish to offer a generalization to others we should remember that restriction of conditions narrows the basis of generalization.

For example, in order to increase the sensitivity of a drug trial we may restrict the criteria of admission so severely that our patients are far from typical of the general run of patients to whom we wish to apply the results of the trial. Similarly, pure-line strains of animals may be useful for a first experiment, but this should often be followed by experiments on more typical examples of the same species.

Relative Costs of Increased Uniformity and Increased Sample Size. Increase of uniformity of material and conditions is not the only way to increase the sensitivity of an experiment. As will be seen later, we can achieve this also by increasing our sample sizes, provided that by spreading our net we do not catch still more heterogeneous material, or by prolonging our experiment we do not introduce more variation in technique. In choosing between these two methods, we must compare the costs in time, labor, money and in human or animal suffering.

In summary, subdivision of the population and other methods of increasing uniformity of material and conditions should be carried, *not as far as possible,* but as far as *convenient* and *useful;* and often a balance must be struck between these two requirements.

Subdivision in a Survey. The foregoing remarks are designed chiefly for experimental investigations. In a survey, subdivision of the population (i.e., of our available sample) is our principal method of reducing bias, because we cannot control it by randomization. Let us suppose that a physician is surveying his case records of a particular disease in order to see whether there appears to be a relationship between the outcome of therapy and the duration of the disease when first treated, so that he can appropriately modify his therapy in type and dosage. If he uses what may be called "analysis *en masse*" he may be grossly misled. For example, if he merely divides all his data into duration-before-treatment classes he may find (or fail to find) a difference in outcome solely because of different sex ratios in the different duration classes. If he tries to explore the sex difference by pooling the duration classes again and dividing the whole series by sex, he may be misled by another variable such as age, or by the duration variable itself.

There is, of course, no possibility of removing bias due to unknown variables, but we can go a long way toward reducing the bias due to variables that we can identify. To do so, we adopt to a large extent the traditional experimenters' prescription, trying to make all things as uniform as we can, except the variable under test. That is, we try to match individuals, or groups of individuals, on all variables except the one that we are studying — duration before treatment in the physician's series. This procedure will often leave many unmatched individuals, but that will bring home to us the fact that many collections of data do not contain nearly so much usable information as their gross bulk would suggest.

It should be mentioned that "analysis *en masse*" is defended by some people who believe that, after we have divided the total data by reference to one variable or perhaps two variables (e.g., sex and age), the residual (intraclass) variation is due to so many variables, many of which are independent of each other, that we have practically the equivalent of random assignment of individuals with respect to all other variables except the one that we are studying. An experimentally minded worker is not inclined to trust such an argument. He looks with caution also on mass analyses that employ much more elaborate mathematical techniques mentioned in Chapter XV.

Q IV – 5. If our research is an experiment in the strict sense, are we going to make paired comparisons within the same subject or between matched subjects? If so, why?

Advantages of Paired Comparisons. We have already noted the usefulness of matching in an attempt to reduce bias-causing variation in surveys. Here we are concerned with the reduction of variation in experiments. The advantage of using a patient as his own yardstick or "control," and of using litter mates in animal experiments, can be illustrated by a simplified and exaggerated example. Of 20 animals, not litter mates, 10 have received treatment A and 10 have received treatment B. A baseline reading of a certain variable was taken before treatment, and the increases in the values of the variable after treatment are as follows:

Treatment A	3 7 4 1 8 10 2 9 6 5	Average = 5.5 units
Treatment B	6 2 10 7 8 10 5 11 3 9	Average = 7.1 units

There is a difference of 1.6 units between the averages, but there is so much intersubject variation within each treatment group, and so much overlap of the two groups, that it would require a vast increase of sample sizes and a persistence of this contrast (B greater than A) to convince us that the treatment difference had anything to do with the difference in readings.

If, however, we had used 10 pairs of litter mates, applying treatment A to one member of each pair and treatment B to the other, and if we had then obtained exactly the same figures as above, but in the following arrangement, we would have been considerably impressed.

Litter	*a*	*b*	*c*	*d*	*e*	*f*	*g*	*h*	*i*	*j*
Treatment A	3	7	4	1	8	10	2	9	6	5
Treatment B	5	10	6	2	9	11	3	10	7	8
Difference (B−A)	+2	+3	+2	+1	+1	+1	+1	+1	+1	+3

The average difference is, of course, the same as the previous difference between the averages, +1.6 units; but every one of the ten differences is positive, and this would very rarely be produced by the coin tossing or other randomization by which we would have assigned A and B in each pair. The matched-pair comparison has produced evidence that would have required a much greater number of animals in an intergroup comparison; and it has done so by eliminating the interanimal variation in the readings themselves. All we need look at is the interlitter variation in the *differences* (B minus A), and this variation has not been great enough to obscure the tendency to produce positive differences.

Q IV – 6.   What are the risks of paired comparisons in an experiment?

Just as very restricted selection of human subjects or pure-line strains of animals may mislead us in generalization, so may human twins and litter mates. We should remember also that if we lose one member of a pair during the experiment its mate will be of little use to us, because our conclusions depend on intrapair differences. In addition, when the matched observations are from the same individual (intrasubject comparisons) we should beware of the following three risks: (1) the confounding of time and treatment, (2) interference of treatments with each other and (3) doubling the duration of the experiment.

Confounding of Time and Treatment.   "The subject as his own control" is a misleading phrase, for it has caused people to embark on trials of therapy, or of diets, with statements such as: "The patients will be their own controls; hence a control group will be unnecessary." Let us suppose that we give drug A to certain patients for a certain length of time and then drug B to the same patients for the same length of time. If the group of patients appears to respond differently, or in the same way, to the two drugs, how can we safely attribute this finding to the drug? We cannot do so, unless we know that if the patients had been kept on drug A, instead of receiving B, during the second (B) period, they would have reacted in the same way, and to the same degree, as they did during the first (A) period. We are very seldom justified in believing this, and we run a serious risk of bias, because the proper label for the contrast is not "drug A versus drug B" but "A-period versus B-period." We have *confounded* time and treatment, i.e., we have mixed them together or confused them.

To avoid the risk of confounding we must use a cross-over (switch-back) design — two groups, one with the AB sequence and the other with the BA sequence, and we must assign patients to these two groups strictly at random. Then we may be able to show that in both groups, A was associated with a greater degree (or greater frequency) of improvement than B.

Interference of Treatments with Each Other.   In an intrasubject drug comparison, when we pass from A to B (or from B to A) the phenomena in the second period may be due partly, and sometimes largely, to one or other of three phenomena: (1) a carry-over of effects from the first drug, (2) a violent rebound of symptoms due to withdrawal of the first drug, and occasionally (3) a benefit from withdrawal of the first drug.

To minimize such risks is difficult, especially with an unfamiliar drug. If we try to separate one effective drug from another by a period on placebo we invite a breakdown of the trial. Even if the patient stays with us and even if we know that cessation of treatment for two weeks will do him no permanent harm, it is not easy to withstand his entreaties to give him something that will make him feel as well as he did last week.

Doubling the Duration of the Experiment.   If we are testing each treatment for 48 hours, the cross-over design requires only 4 days' study of each subject; but if the period of treatment by each agent under test is 6 months, each subject requires a year's observation, and then the risks, especially in clinical trials, are great: loss of interest by the observers, change of observers and other personnel because they move to other appointments, and losses of patients, commonly called "drop-outs."

Because of the numerous disadvantages, we ought to be very sure that any proposed paired comparison has compensating advantages, and these advantages exist only when members of a pair, treated alike, react very similarly. In general, litter mates do so, but it is well known that patients who show good response to a certain treatment at one time may show little or no response to it another time, even when the interval is short. Often there is not enough information to prove that an intrasubject comparison will effect a great economy in sample size.

Individuals versus Groups.   There still seems to linger in many minds the notion that an intrasubject comparison, even with only one trial of each treatment per patient, tells us something about the relative effects of the treatments in each individual patient. Obviously, to obtain that kind of information we would require several separate trials of each treatment in the same patient. All that we can learn from a single cross-over design is a group effect — that drug A was followed by a certain effect more frequently (or in greater degree) than was drug B. If this difference is too great to be wholly attributable to the randomization, we expect to find the same overall direction of differences in similar patients, but even if we used the same patients over again the first experiment would give us no *legitimate* assurance that the *individuals* would behave as they did before. Therefore, the only advantage of such an intrasubject comparison is reduction of sample size. If we increased our sample (often by only 25 per cent or thereabouts) we could obtain as reliable information from two equal groups, each on a different treatment.

If we wish to know whether an individual patient benefits more by one treatment than by another, we must consider that patient as able to provide a "population" of observation periods, and then we must apply each treatment in several of the periods. This is what we attempt to obtain in clinical practice and in everyday life by the "on-and-off" method of observation. "Whenever Mrs. Smith is on drug A she does better than when she is on drug B." "Whenever Johnny eats strawberries he gets a rash." In practice, even if we can obtain no better evidence than this, we nevertheless feel justified in giving Mrs. Smith drug A instead of drug B, and in telling Johnny to avoid strawberries for a season. But if we wished to design an experiment that would give sounder evidence we would start by asking such questions as: "How often is 'whenever'?" "How long was Mrs. Smith on drug B on each occasion? When we tried it again did we take her off it quickly because it had failed on the first occasion?" "Does Johnny develop the rash because he knows that he has eaten strawberries?"

Our experiment would aim at obtaining reliable information regarding A versus B in Mrs. Smith, or strawberries versus no strawberries in Johnny — the kind of information, regarding individuals, that clinicians desire, but which they cannot obtain from clinical trials conducted on groups. Such information, especially relating to fine distinctions between the effects of drugs, is not easy to obtain. A skin test might give some objective confirmatory evidence of Johnny's sensitivity to strawberries; but Mrs. Smith would have to be subjected to a series of A and B treatments involving a combination of systematic and random assignments, the details of which are beyond the scope of this discussion.

Q IV – 7.   If our research is a survey, what will be the advantages and risks of a matched comparison?

We have already seen how, in the analysis of data already accumulated, a series of matched comparisons can help to reduce the risks of bias. Matching is used also in the collection of new data. If we wish to find out whether a disease (X) is associated with exposure to a certain noxious influence such as radiation, we can take each X-patient and match him against a not-X of the same sex, age, place of birth, occupation and other attributes.

Proper matching is often difficult and there are complicated risks of biased selection in this method, but in addition there is a risk of too close matching. If we are looking for a causal factor, A versus not-A, we may choose X's and not-X's who are alike in possessing attributes B, C, D and E. If, unknown to us, the presence (or absence) of X is associated in some manner with the presence of one of these attributes we may fail entirely to find the association of X with A.

Q IV – 8.   If our research is an experiment, do we wish to increase its efficiency by utilizing a rather more complicated design than the two-group or paired comparison? If so, what are the advantages and risks?

Advantages of Balanced Designs.   Of the designs referred to, the three commonest bear the names "randomized blocks," "the factorial design" and "Latin squares." They were primarily developed in agriculture but are now widely used in many branches of science. Essentially they are an outcome of the matched-pair (including intrasubject) comparisons, but they enable us to compare more than two treatments or other factors in the same experiment.

The factorial design, in particular, allows us to test any number of factors simultaneously on the same subjects. For example, in a study of x-ray bone density measured by a photoelectric densitometer, an experiment was set up to test on cadaver bones the effects of seven of the procedures in x-raying and processing the films (Mainland, 1956). Two levels or variants of each factor were contrasted: a higher versus a lower kilovoltage, two positions of the bones on the films, two positions of the films during processing, two strengths of developer, two fixation periods, two washing periods, and drying at room temperature versus exposure to warm circulating air in a film dryer.

The number of different combinations of seven factors each with two variants (or "levels" or "doses") is $2^7 = 128$. Therefore 128 films were exposed in random order, 64 of them at the higher kilovoltage and 64 at the lower. Both groups had equal numbers of two bone positions, film positions during processing, and so on. In fact the whole series was completely balanced (symmetrical) with respect to all seven factors. Therefore it was possible to compare variants (1) and (2) (or higher and lower levels) of each factor in turn by dividing the total group into two samples of 64 in seven different ways. If the "one factor at a time" method had been used it would have required 128 films to compare variants (1) and (2) of the kilovoltage with other factors set at variant (1). Then, in order to measure the bone-position contrast with all other factors set at variant (1) it would have required an additional 64 films with the bone-position factor at variant (2). The testing of each factor, with all other factors at variant (1) would have required a total of 512 films. Then another 1344 films would have been required for the next series of questions that were answered by the same 128 films — questions on the "interactions" of two factors, such as: "Was the high-low kilovoltage contrast in bone density different when the fixation period was different?"

This example illustrates the superiority of the factorial design over the old-fashioned method not only in the tremendous economy that it provides, but in its closer kinship to natural working conditions in which many factors vary simultaneously.

When one has become thoroughly accustomed to the standards required in the simpler experiments it is very desirable to become acquainted with these somewhat complicated designs. Good introductory discussions in relation to clinical research are given by Truelove in *Medical Surveys and Clinical Trials* (Witts) and by Reid and Doll in *Controlled Clinical Trials* (Council for International Organizations of Medical Sciences). For more extensive and detailed description, Finney's *Experimental Design and Its Statistical Basis* is highly recommended.

Some Risks of Balanced Designs. The various balanced designs are extremely valuable in experiments on inanimate material, but I am not so optimistic as I used to be regarding their potentialities in clinical research or even in experiments on laboratory animals. Designs that depend for their success on balanced numbers and symmetry can easily be ruined by mishaps like infections among animals, drop-outs of human subjects and omissions of items from clinical records. It is true that on certain assumptions it is possible to fill "holes" in the data by estimation from the figures that remain; but the safest assumption for a clinical investigator is that a missing piece of information indicates bias and therefore cannot be estimated with confidence.

Another drawback of these designs in clinical research is that the methods are chiefly applicable when the data are to be measurements rather than frequencies.

Q IV – 9.   What two effects of variation should we remember at every point in an investigation?

This is a review question which summarizes much that has been said in this and previous chapters and much that will be said in subsequent chapters. The answer is of course (1) bias, and (2) the lowering of sensitivity or precision. Whenever we consider any characteristic of our investigational material, or anything that has already affected it or anything that occurs during the investigation, and whenever we make any decision while planning or conducting the study, we should consider whether the risk of bias will be thereby increased and whether the sensitivity (precision) will be reduced. In a sense this is the one basic question, and our ten groups of questions merely develop its implications.

CHAPTER V

SKELETON LAYOUTS FOR RESULTS

Q V – 1. What skeleton layout must we prepare to receive our results?

This is really an extension of Question I – 1 – What are the specific questions to be answered by the investigation? If at the beginning we cannot visualize our skeleton layout, e.g., the headings of our tables of results, there is little prospect that at the end we will have the proper information — the tissues required to fill and clothe the skeleton. We are not concerned here with rules for constructing tables and graphs, but with the types of information that should go into them. If the layout is not written down it should at least be clear in our minds.

Basic Types of Data. In face of the variety of arithmetical displays that we meet in medical literature, it is helpful to remember that most of the questions that are asked in medical research, and the numerical data that are required to answer them, can be classified in a rather simple fashion. Thus, we can ask either, "How many?" or "How much?" — and these questions often give a clue to the method of presenting and analyzing the data.

The question, "How many?" leads to frequency data (enumeration data) — counts of individuals in various classes. Often the classes denote qualitative features (attributes or events) such as sex, drug treatments, diseases, death or survival, and location of residence. However, even if we have taken measurements of a variable we may choose to group the measurements into two or more classes, e.g., diastolic blood pressure above 90 mm. mercury, at or below 90 mm.

Sometimes frequencies are expressed as percentages, and it is curious that some writers still fail to appreciate the difference, in weight of evidence, between 20 per cent of 5 cases and 20 per cent of 50 cases. *Percentage frequencies without the denominator (the total number of cases or events) are essentially meaningless.*

The question, "How much?" leads to measurement data (mensuration data), often expressed as an average measurement, such as the arithmetic mean. We should never forget that *an average, without a statement of the variation between the individual component measurements, tells us almost nothing.*

There is no absolute division between enumeration data and measurement data. Thus, the class headings of a table of frequency data may be measurements, such as statures, ages, blood pressures or doses of a certain drug.

Although some variables cannot be precisely measured on a scale with equally spaced marks, they can often be arranged in order of rank. For example, although we cannot measure on an absolute scale the functional capacity of patients with rheumatoid arthritis, we can rank them (1, 2, 3, 4) in ascending order of incapacity, from patients who can perform their previous activities with hardly any inconvenience, to those who are completely bedridden. Severity of pain in various diseases can be ranked by the potency of the pain-relieving drug that is required to give relief, from pain that is relieved by aspirin to pain that the most powerful opiates cannot relieve.

Estimates and Comparisons. The form of our results will depend on the numerical purpose of our investigation. Sometimes this purpose is to obtain an estimate of a particular population value, such as the proportion of patients, treated by a certain method, who show improvement at the end of 6 months from the start of treatment (Chapter XI); or the average and intersubject variation of the concentration of a certain substance in the blood of healthy women within a certain age range (Chapter XIII). More often our purpose is a search for relationships by comparison of frequencies (Chapter XII) or of measurements (Chapter XIV). The data are infinitely diverse, but the types of layout that we commonly need are remarkably few and simple. Both in frequency comparisons and in measurement comparisons we may compare groups that have different attributes (or have been treated differently) or we may make matched-pair comparisons (including intrasubject comparisons).

Intergroup Frequency Comparisons. Two examples:

1. Two hundred men with cancer of the prostate gland were randomly assigned in equal numbers to a certain drug (A) and to a placebo (B) and were classified at the end of four weeks' treatment as "improved" (X) or "not improved" (not-X). In a subsequent trial on the same patients, A was a daily dose of 5 mg. of a certain drug, and B was a daily dose of 500 mg. of the same drug.

2. A number of prospective surveys of the following type are now being undertaken. Men within a certain age range who have no history or signs of coronary heart disease are classified according to their diastolic blood pressure: above 90 mm. mercury (A), 90 mm. or below (B). They are followed for 5 years in order to compare, in the A's and B's, the proportions who develop coronary disease (X) and who do not develop it (not-X).

Frequency comparisons are best displayed in a table containing the actual numbers of individuals:

Independent Variable	Dependent Variable		Total
	X	Not-X	
A			
B			
Total			

This is an *association table,* to show an AB difference and an accompanying X–not-X difference. The four spaces within the table, excluding the totals, are commonly called "cells."

As will be emphasized later, an association by itself does not prove a causal relationship. The table is called also a *contingency table* because it displays the joint occurrence of two sets of events or attributes, the AB set and the X–not-X set (cf. "contact," from the same Latin root as "contingency"). The table shown here, the fourfold table (AB; X–not-X), is the one most commonly seen; but there can be any number of rows (A, B, C, and so forth) and any number of columns (X, Y, Z, and so forth). More than two drugs can be tested at once; diastolic blood pressures can be divided at other levels, in addition to the 90 mm. division; patients can be classified as "improved," "no change," "worse."

Matched-pair Frequency Comparisons. In a litter-mate experiment, injection A may be a certain chemical, while injection B may be another chemical or the medium in which chemical A was dissolved or suspended. X may be death, while not-X is survival. In a human drug trial, A and B may be different drugs administered during different periods to the same patients; X and not-X may be "improved" and "not-improved." For all such comparisons, the general form is as follows:

Outcome	No. of Pairs
(1) A X, B X	
(2) A X, B not-X	
(3) A not-X, B X	
(4) A not-X, B not-X	
Total	

The first outcome (A X, B X) and the fourth are "tied pairs," and, as is shown in Chapter XII, our main interest is in the untied pairs. If the difference in numbers of pairs between (2) and (3) would rarely occur as the result of random assignment of the treatments, we feel justified in concluding that there is a difference in the effect of A and B, even if the tied pairs are numerous.

If we were to put such data into a contingency table and analyze them accordingly (Chapter XII) we would be breaking a fundamental rule: *The method of analysis must spring from the design of the investigation.* If, for example, we had 20 pairs of observations and put them into a contingency table, with row headings A and B and column headings X and Not-X, we would in effect be pretending that we had 20 pieces of information regarding the outcome after treatment A, independent of the 20 pieces of information regarding the outcome after B; and the contingency table analysis would give us an answer in accordance with our pretence. We would also throw away the very information that we wished to discover — whether there was any difference in outcome after A and B when both were measured by the same (or a very similar) yardstick.

Intergroup Measurement Comparisons. Two examples:

1. A common type of comparison is met in attempts to establish "norms." For example, healthy males and females in a certain age range are compared with regard to the average level and intersubject variation of blood constituents. Even if the constituent is counted (e.g., so many thousand white blood cells per cubic mm. of blood), the data are essentially measurement data, just like pulse rates.

2. In a 3-month clinical trial on 76 rheumatoid arthritics approximately half received the drug under test (A) and half received placebo tablets (B), but no patient was deprived of treatment because all patients were allowed to take as much aspirin as they wished. One method of assessment in rheumatoid arthritis is to record the strength of hand grip when a patient squeezes a rubber bag connected to a mercury manometer. Therefore the A and B groups were compared with respect to the average change in grip between beginning and end of therapy. Another type of assessment was the intergroup difference in the average change in the numbers of joints that were painful when squeezed by the examining physician. As in blood examination, although the joints were counted, the numbers were essentially measurement data.

As with frequency comparisons, we are not confined to a comparison of two classes, A and B. We can compare average changes after three or more drugs, and the average blood pressures of men in any number of different occupations (A, B, C, and so on).

Matched-pair Measurement Comparisons. As with matched-pair frequency comparisons, our presentation and analysis must conform to our experiment design. That is, we are concerned with the average of the AB differences and with the variation between these differences, not with a comparison of the A average and the B average, or with the variation among the readings that contribute to these averages (see example under Q IV – 5).

Concomitant Variation and Trends. In the examples of frequency comparisons we classified both the dependent and independent variables by qualitative differences or coarse measurement differences (A, B, and so on; X, not-X, and so on). When we used actual measurements instead of X and not-X, we passed to a method that is more precise and more sensitive than merely "counting heads." If we can also substitute measurements for the classes A, B, and so on, we have a still more sensitive method of detecting relationships and differences.

For example, if we record blood pressures in healthy males of different ages, we can plot them as a dot diagram (one dot for each individual) with age on the horizontal axis and blood pressure on the vertical axis. If we find the percentage mortality in batches of mice subjected to six different dose levels of cocaine (20 animals at each dose), we can graph the six dots, with dose on the horizontal axis and mortality on the vertical axis, to obtain a suggestion regarding the nature of the relationship between the two variables. Some further discussion of this very big subject, concomitant variation and trends, is given in Chapter XV.

Q V – 2.   Are measurements to be presented and analyzed as measurement data or as frequency data? What will determine the choice?

Some of the rheumatic fever drug trial data (Q IV – 1), such as temperature, pulse rate, and heart size on x-ray films, were measurements, and therefore could have been used to compare the treatment groups in terms of average changes and time trends of measurements. Instead, the report presented measurement data as frequency data. For example, it displayed the percentage of children, in each treatment group, who showed changes in the transverse cardiac diameter of 0.6 cm. or more, between the start of treatment and the end of the third week. Thus, the report deliberately sacrificed some of the information that the measurements had offered.

Before doing this in any investigation we should (1) see clearly what the analysis by measurement-data methods would tell us, and (2) decide whether we desire that information. For example, the average change in heart diameter might have differed between the treatment groups owing to various causes, such as small changes in the same direction in many children in one of the groups, or large changes in a few children. Apparently the rheumatic fever investigators did not consider an *average* difference, by itself, of practical importance. They wished to know whether a *greater proportion* of children showed a change of over half a centimeter in one treatment group than in another.

By contrast, in a trial of drugs in tumor-bearing animals, the arrest, or even slight delay, of tumor growth might provide a useful suggestion to chemists for the preparation of a related compound that might be more powerful. The extraction of full information, by analysis of actual measurements, would therefore be desirable. In human cancer patients the precision of measurement appears to be seldom great enough to justify this effort.

Q V – 3. If we intend to present measurements as frequency data, when will we select the dividing lines between the classes?

When we put measurement data into a contingency table it is very important that we set up the dividing lines — for example, 0.6 cm. change in heart diameter; with fever, without fever; slow pulse, normal pulse, rapid pulse — before we inspect the data. Otherwise, we may draw the lines in such a way that they will emphasize or obscure a contrast according to our desires. Or we may be so anxious to avoid such a bias that we may create a bias in the opposite direction.

Q V – 4. Will our sampling units be independent of each other, except insofar as randomization brings them together?

In a drug trial the sampling units are individual patients, and the randomization assigns them independently to the treatments, in the sense that cards in thorough shuffling have freedom to locate themselves independently. This requirement is fairly obvious, but many research workers are rather vague about their sampling units and the need for their independence.

Wrong Sampling Units. Let us suppose that a dentist, having attended to the teeth of two boys, instructs one of them to use toothpaste A and the other to use toothpaste B, and insures by parental cooperation that his instructions are carried out. After a certain length of time he finds that the boy who used toothpaste A has 8 carious teeth, whereas the other boy has no caries. In terms of numbers of teeth, this looks like an impressive difference, but we need no profound knowledge of dentistry or of statistics to realize that it provides no adequate evidence that the difference in toothpaste was responsible. Persons differ in their tendency to develop caries; therefore the individual teeth in any mouth do not provide independent pieces of information about the effect of a toothpaste. It is boys, not teeth, that are the sampling units, and there is only one sampling unit in each of the A and B samples — no true *replicates*, i.e., sampling units that receive the same test treatment but are otherwise independent.

In this simple case the point is obvious, but it was not obvious to a distinguished worker in nutrition and dentistry who reported on the caries in 36,196 teeth in the mouths of 1870 children. By examining about 20 teeth per child the investigator had measured over and over again the same tendency (or resistance) to caries, but in the analysis each tooth was counted as if it gave an independent piece of information. This error — the error of wrong sampling units — can be called also "spurious enlargement of samples," "spurious replication," or "counting the same thing over again."

In the large dental caries study the proper sampling units were children, and one way to express the information would be by the numbers of children with, and without, caries (and this was done in another part of the report). A finer measure would be the number of carious teeth per child, with some form of adjustment for the number of filled and missing teeth.

Animals and Cages.   Scientific research workers in animal husbandry have known for at least a couple of decades that a pen of pigs fed on diet A and another pen of pigs fed on diet B are analogous to the two boys in our imaginary toothpaste experiment. The pigs in any one pen are subjected to the same influences, from outside the pen and also from inside the pen, including their pen mates (feeding and excretion, behavior, parasites and other influences). There would therefore be no replicates in the comparison of diets; diet differences would be *confounded* with pen differences.

In contrast to research workers in animal husbandry and agriculture, some prominent laboratory experimenters still believe that if they put 20 control animals in one cage and 20 treated animals in another cage, they have two samples, each containing 20 sampling units. Enlightenment, however, seems to be coming from high places, as in a government-sponsored experiment on mice exposed to the radiation effects of an atomic bomb explosion (the "Greenhouse" experiment). This experiment involved approximately 5000 mice, and each mouse was placed in an individual cage during irradiation and during subsequent observation in a laboratory.*

Group Therapy and Social Experiments.   In some chronic diseases, such as certain kinds of heart disease, the progress of a patient who is no longer hospitalized depends considerably on his attitude toward the conditions and problems that meet him in everyday life. Some social workers believe that such patients can be helped by discussing their problems in a group of similar patients under the guidance of social workers, psychologists and physicians. An experiment to test the efficacy of such group therapy presents many difficulties. One of them is the risk of spurious replication. A single treatment group and a single control group, even after strictly random assignment of patients, constitute only two sampling units, each treated differently, i.e., there are no true replicates. The chief factor affecting all members of the treatment group may have been the chance assignment to it of one or two dominant and optimistic (or pessimistic) persons who spread a "contagion."

Groups as Sampling Units.   In a certain mental institution it was

---

* I am indebted to Drs. Jacob Furth, A. W. Kimball and Jack Moshman for information on this experiment, which is no longer restricted (classified) material. To me, the most encouraging feature of the story, as recounted by a very senior experimental pathologist who had participated in the research, was the pathologist's own attitude. Unlike many other senior medical laboratory scientists, he understood, and expressed admiration for, the statistician's insistence on (1) a separate cage for each mouse, (2) randomization of cage positions in the laboratory, and (3) the location of the statistician himself adjacent to the laboratory, so that he would be continuously aware of what went on.

decided to test the effect of a certain drug on amebiasis, an infection caused when the protozoan *Entamoeba histolytica* inhabits the intestine. The test of efficacy was absence of the organism from the patients' stools for a period of four months after treatment ceased. It would have been legitimate to assign the drug and no treatment (or placebo) by a random process to equal numbers of all who suffered from the infection in any one building, and to have considered the patients as sampling units in the analysis of the results, but this method was not used, because the benefit of the drug might easily have been obscured by reinfection from untreated patients, an occurrence that is more difficult to prevent in mental institutions than in other hospitals. The only simple solution of the problem was to treat all patients in any one building alike, and use other buildings and other institutions as replicates.

An analogous difficulty arises in research on vaccines, such as the testing of a vaccine that is claimed to prevent colds. Half the workers in an organization, such as a factory or office, may be given the vaccine, the other half a placebo; but if the vaccine is effective it will reduce the spread of colds to the unvaccinated subjects. The ultimate comparison between the two groups may then reveal no greater difference in the incidence of colds than could easily be attributed to the initial randomization. Even in large-scale prophylactic trials, as of poliomyelitis vaccine, this phenomenon could occur. Whether the phenomenon is a spread of infection or a spread of protection, it can be called a "contagion."

The question might now be asked: "Even when individuals have been assigned independently at random to the treatments, if contagion can occur are the individuals true replicates — independent sampling units?" If we answered "No" we would have to apply the same ruling to many controlled drug trials, because there is often the risk of psychologic and sometimes physical contagion. Replication in an experiment implies random assignment of individuals not only to the treatments but to subsequent events. If in one building of the mental institution both drug and no-drug treatment had been used, the randomization would have determined whether any particular set of circumstances, involving risk of infection, would be met by a drug-treated or control patient. In that sense the sampling units (the patients) would have been independent. The randomization would, as always, have fulfilled its purpose: the control of the risk of a verdict that the treatments differed in their effects when in fact they did not differ. Randomization does not guard against the risk of a false "no difference" verdict. If there is risk of contagion we must systematically design the experiment in such a way as to reduce that risk.

Q V – 5. Are we going to mix the sampling units?

Perhaps the best way to answer that question is to ask ourselves: "Of what population do we desire an estimate?"

Mixed Sampling Units in a Clinical Survey. A diagnostic procedure that entails some risk to patients is the injection into arteries of fluids that are opaque to x-rays, in order to discover by roentgenography whether the arteries are dilated or otherwise abnormal. One physician reported that he had performed this injection 86 times without mishap. This may impress us, but it does not give us an estimate of the risk run by *patients* who are subjected to the technique. We can obtain such an estimate by noting that the 86 injections were performed in 18 patients, the numbers of injections ranging from 2 per patient to 10 (in one patient). We can, therefore, assert that in 18 patients, each injected twice, no harm was done, and we could make similar statements, regarding fewer patients who received more injections.

If we are tempted to argue that the injection is the sampling unit, we should remember that this implies that the risk of harm is quite unrelated to the patient and his vascular system, and we should ask ourselves: "If the injection had been performed 86 times in only one patient, would we be as confident about the lack of risk as we would be if the injection had been performed once in each of 86 patients?"

Mixed Sampling Units in the Laboratory. This mixing is not uncommon in medical research. If we obtain a total of 69 readings, of any kind, from 11 dogs, and then calculate the average of the 69 readings and their variation from each other, we have a mixture of sampling units, i.e., readings and dogs — a mixture of interanimal and intra-animal variation. The same would be true if we obtained an equal number of readings from each dog, e.g., 6 readings per dog, and treated the 66 readings in the same way. We would be implying that dogs did not differ in their average readings — that we would be quite happy if we could obtain all 66 readings from one dog. To anyone with a biological upbringing this must be a fantastic concept, unless he has been hoodwinked by an elementary statistics book that has led him to believe that, if he has found no "statistically significant" difference between the averages for the various dogs, he is at liberty to pool the readings of all the dogs.

In order to clarify our thinking about sampling units in measurement as in counting, we should ask ourselves the following kinds of questions: "Of what population (or populations) do we desire estimates? Is it a population of *readings* from the same animal, or is it a population of *animals,* each investigated in the same way and to the same extent?" "To the same extent" implies the same number of readings per animal — one reading, the average of two readings, the average of three readings, and so on. If we take more than one reading per animal we can obtain both intra- and interanimal estimates, but we must not mix them up in presentation or analysis.

Mixed Sampling Units in Reports. If a report makes a statement regarding an average or frequency obtained from M readings (or "experiments" or "trials" or "episodes" such as epileptic fits or coronary attacks) in a total of N subjects (M being greater than N), we can infer a mixing of sampling units. Moreover, if the numbers of readings differ in different subjects, even if there is no mixture of sampling units, we should become very suspicious. We should ask: "Why did the investigator stop short in some subjects? Was it because something went wrong — something that may have introduced bias, even in the readings that were taken? Did the investigator reject some readings that did not seem in line with the others, or with his notion of what the readings ought to be?"

Bilateral organs such as limbs and kidneys, if right or left side is not specified, easily lead one to count the same thing twice (the same subject's tendency to have an abnormality for instance); and they lead to confusion in other ways also. We may read about some peculiarity that occurred 30 times in 100 sciatic nerves from 50 cadavers, but we do not know whether it occurred on both sides in 15 cadavers, or on one side in 30 cadavers, or sometimes on one side and sometimes on both sides.

Q V – 6. Will the denominators be correct?

Wrong Denominators. The following example, published in one of the best medical journals, dates from World War II, and it is to be hoped that most readers will be insulted by the kindergarten lesson that it contains; but it was several years after medical graduation when I first learned the lesson, and some very recent graduates appear to be in a similar plight.

In 139 out of 2312 British Air Force women there was delay in menstruation (temporary amenorrhea). To show the relationship of this to occupation, the 139 women were classified as follows:

Clerks	52 (37.4%)	Equipment assistants	8 (5.8%)
Cooks	20 (14.4%)	Batwomen	7 (5.0%)
Drivers	16 (11.5%)	Flight mechanics	4 (2.9%)
Unskilled workers	9 (6.5%)	Waitresses	3 (2.2%)
Telephone operators	9 (6.5%)	Spark plug tester	1 (0.7%)

Administrative staff, safety equipment workers, radio operators, tailoresses, and instrument repairers   2 each (1.4%)

The conclusion was: "The greatest number of cases therefore occur in those with sedentary occupations."

The percentages were obtained by dividing the number in each occupational class (52, 20, and so on) by the total number of cases, 139. The clerks seem to be thirteen times as likely to have amenorrhea as the flight mechanics, but this would be the ratio that we would expect if there were, in the 2312 women, thirteen times as many clerks as flight mechanics, without there being any relationship between occupation and amenorrhea. (Note that, to find the 13 to 1 ratio, percentages need not have been calculated at all.)

A simple imaginary experiment provides a model for this survey. If we were comparing treatments A, B, C, and so on, each applied to a different group of subjects, to discover whether the treatments differed in the frequencies with which they produced an undesirable symptom

(X), we would ask: "What proportion of A-treated subjects developed X?" "What proportion of B-treated subjects did so?"—and so on.

Similarly, to compare the frequencies of amenorrhea in the different occupational classes there ought to have been calculated for each class a percentage such as:

$$\frac{\text{No. of clerks with amenorrhea} \times 100}{\text{Total number of clerks}} = \text{per cent of clerks with amenorrhea}$$

This uses the proper denominator, the particular group exposed to risk. (The phrase "population at risk" is more traditional, but it suggests a distinction between populations and samples, and that is not the present issue.) The report on the Air Force women stated nothing about the sizes of the groups exposed to risk, i.e., the numbers in the various occupational classes.

"*Sex Incidence.*" Perhaps few editors or medical journal readers would nowadays be misled by such a blatant case of wrong denominator; but many of us are apt to be led astray when we read that, in a series of patients with a certain disease, one sex greatly outnumbered the other. Probably we are, almost unconsciously, applying as denominators the approximate one-to-one sex ratio in the general population, as did the skin specialists who believed that acne was much commoner in girls than in boys, until a survey of schoolchildren revealed that the percentage frequency was equal in the two sexes. The explanation of the error was, of course, that girls were more concerned than boys about their appearance and sought the skin specialists' help. An even more striking distortion of sex difference in frequency was the impression, formed by physicians in an oriental country, that breast cancer (which is predominantly a disease of women in Western countries) was commoner among the native men that among the native women. Then it was discovered that modesty commonly deterred women from going to a doctor for breast examination.

Q V – 7. What will be the groups exposed to risk?

The above examples should warn us to look closely at the meaning of "the group exposed to risk." Let X be an individual with a certain attribute, or the subject of a certain event, such as death or a rise in blood pressure. Then the relative frequency of X's is their frequency expressed in relation to the group exposed to risk, often as a percentage:

$$\frac{\text{No. of X's} \times 100}{\text{No. of X's} + \text{No. of not-X's}}$$

In order that the denominator shall be the true group at risk, the not-X's must be the individuals who, if they had been X's, ought to have been in the numerator. (When X is rare, the expression "per thousand" or "per hundred thousand" is often useful, in order to avoid many decimal figures.)

Importance of the Not-X's.   In a report on hospital patients suffering from ulcers of the stomach or duodenum, the observers presented a chart of "age incidence" showing the numbers of patients in each age group. The conclusion was: "This shows the maximum incidence for gastric ulcer between 40 and 60, but duodenal ulcer has an earlier peak at 35 to 39." In a subsequent issue of the same journal a critic wrote: "Surely it is time to insist that clinicians use the term 'incidence' as used in vital statistics to signify the ratio of observed cases to the appropriate population at risk."

The observers might have defended their presentation along these lines: "Granted that we cannot define our population at risk (our potential patients), surely we can assume that over a short period of time our populations at ages 35 to 39 and at ages 40 to 60 will remain almost constant. These two populations will not be of the same size, but this is irrelevant when we are comparing the ratios of gastric to duodenal ulcers in the two populations."

Unfortunately this would be too simple a concept. It would overlook the complex forces that determine whether a patient with a certain condition comes for medical attention, or enters a particular hospital — not only the effect of symptoms on patients' decisions, but socioeconomic and psychologic forces. The population ratio of gastric to duodenal ulcers might be one-to-one in both age groups; but if the resultants of these forces differed in the two groups with respect to the two types of ulcer, the hospital ratios could be vastly different. That is one reason why it was stipulated above that the denominator for relative frequency should include the subjects who, if they were X's, *ought* to have been (not would have been) in the numerator. There are many unknown forces that may keep them out.

All such examples lead to a generalization: To discover how often X (a disease or anything else) occurs in a population (or in a subgroup of the population) we must investigate the population (or subgroup), not the persons who come to our notice because they have X.

"Age Incidence."   Prominent investigators still sometimes use wrong denominators in so-called "age incidence" data. They present a graph that shows age on the horizontal axis and, on the vertical axis, the number of patients who had a certain disease (or the percentage frequency, with the total number of those patients as the denominator). Often the graph line rises at the earlier ages and falls again at the later ages, and the investigator will state, or imply, that the peak indicates the age at which the disease is most likely to occur. He seems to forget that a decline with increase of age is what he should expect, even if the incidence of the disease were the same at all ages, because in the later decades there are progressively fewer persons left alive. (The incidence of any disease at the age of 200 years is zero!) Even the earlier rise may be partly an artifact, because the investigator may have relatively few child patients.

Such a graph might be said to show the "incidence of ages" in the sample. It does not show the incidence of the disease at different ages, even in a segment of the population that would contribute all its "X's" to the investigator's collection. For that purpose he would require to know the size of each age group in the segment.

"*Average Age.*" Wrong denominators can be hidden in statements like, "The average age of male patients admitted with coronary heart diseases was Y years," and, "The average age of female patients was higher than that of male patients." To exaggerate and simplify, we let the incidence of disease X be 10 per cent in both sexes at age 50 and also at age 60, and we invent the following figures:

Females	Age 50	Age 60
Exposed to risk	100	100
Number of female patients	10	10

Average age of female patients with disease $X = 55$ years.

Males	Age 50	Age 60
Exposed to risk	100	20
Number of male patients	10	2

Average age of male patients =
$(50 \times 10 + 60 \times 2)/12 = 620/12 = 51.7$ years.

The "average age of death" still traps some workers. From autopsy or hospital records, or by following their patients for a number of years, they find the average (arithmetic mean) age at death *for the patients who have died.* Obviously, we cannot find the mean age at death for a group of patients with a certain disease, unless we wait until all of them are dead. We might seem to be on safer ground in comparing the mean ages at death in two groups (e.g., with different diseases); but we have no right to imagine that the error (of underestimation) will be the same in both groups.

What we are usually trying to discover by an average age at death in sufferers from a certain disease is the life-shortening effect of that disease, and a little thought makes us doubt whether the age at death, even if derived from all patients, would be a satisfactory answer, because it depends not only on the duration between onset and death but on the age at onset — compare, for example, the average age at death in (1) a disease that attacks and kills children and (2) a disease that attacks and kills old people.

If, however, we ask about the duration of life after we have first diagnosed the disease, and if the disease kills some patients before any patients are lost to follow-up, we can obtain at least a partial answer to our question. For instance, we can say: "By the end of three years P per cent had died of the disease, Q per cent had died from other causes, and R per cent were still alive."

Alternatively, if we can follow all patients in the group under study until half of them have died, this will give us (in years) the median (midpoint) duration from diagnosis to death. Even then, we have not fully answered our question unless we have made allowance for the mortality among a similar group not afflicted by the disease that we are studying, and it is by no means easy to find suitable groups for comparison. Official statistics of mortality, either national or local, commonly cover too broad categories of persons to be dependable for this purpose.

"Condition When Last Seen." In a follow-up study a clinician may survey 20 years' experience of a certain disease and report the data for the whole group in terms of the patients' condition when last seen. The interval between the first visit and the last may range from 1 year to 20 years, and the question arises: What does the condition on the last visit really tell us? The information is analogous to what we would obtain from an animal experiment in which we made observations on some animals half an hour after the experiment began, on other animals the next day, on still other animals a month later, and then pooled all the observations to give an average reading or a percentage frequency of the phenomena under study.

If we are about to conduct any kind of survey on a group of patients or their records, probably the best way to make ourselves face reality is to imagine that we are going to apply our findings for predictive purposes to a new patient in the same category. A clinician could imagine himself saying to the new patient: "If the figures from my survey apply to you, the chances are X out of 100 that you will be in such and such a condition when you make your last visit to me (or my successor); but I cannot tell whether this is a prophecy of your condition next year or 20 years hence."

Such a statement would surely lead the clinician to an analysis that would permit him to make the following type of assertion: "If the figures from my survey apply to you, the chances (out of 100) regarding your position 5 years hence will be as follows: X_1 that I will not know how you are, because you will not be coming to me any more; X_2 that you will be dead and I will know it; X_3 that you will be alive and I will know that you are in such and such a condition . . . " and so on. Unless X_1 in the survey were very small, the data would not be very informative. Perhaps, also, it would be found unwise to combine, say, the 1936-1940 figures with the 1956-1960 figures; but the denominator, i.e., the group at risk (patients studied for 5 years) would at least permit an intelligible prediction, in contrast to the previous version — the condition when last seen.

Q V – 8. Will the difference between "incidence" and "prevalence" mislead us?

In the foregoing paragraphs the word "incidence" has been used rather loosely. We must now look at a strict definition, and at the distinction between "incidence" and "prevalence." These are both expressions of relative frequency and have the same general formula, but the *preva-*

lence of X is the relative frequency of X *at a certain time,* whereas the *incidence* of X is the relative frequency of occurrence of X *during a certain period.* Prevalence answers the question: "How common?" Incidence answers the question: "How often?"

This distinction is made chiefly by specialists in "vital statistics," which are large masses of population data on the major events in life, such as births, deaths and diseases. The rest of us use "incidence" to cover both kinds of frequency, and we can defend ourselves on the grounds of custom, if we take care not to deceive ourselves and others. The term "attack rate" has sometimes a clearer meaning than "incidence"; and even if we intend to use any of the more technical terms it is often best to start out by using percentage frequency (or frequency per thousand or per hundred thousand), specifying whether we are referring to one particular time or to a span of time.

Deceptive Prevalence Figures. In an experiment or in a forward-going survey we compare the incidence of X in two or more groups, A, B, and so on, between times T_0 and T_1. In a cross-sectional survey we do not know when time T_0 was, but we compare the prevalence of X in two or more groups at time T_1. Let us suppose that the incidence of X (some disease or disability) was higher in the A's than in the B's, that X was also more severe in the A's, and that therefore a higher percentage of the AX's have been removed (e.g., by death, change of occupation or locale) than of the BX's. This is not an unreasonable supposition, because greater susceptibility to disease often manifests itself not only by greater frequency but by greater severity. Such an occurrence can make prevalence figures very misleading (Neyman, 1955), as can be shown thus:

At time T_0 there are 100 A's and 100 B's.

Between T_0 and T_1 the incidence of X in the A's is 50 per cent, leaving 50 A's who are not-X's. Of the 50 AX's, 90 per cent disappear before T_1, leaving only 5.

Between T_0 and T_1 the incidence of X in the B's is 20 per cent, leaving 80 B's who are not-X's. Of the 20 BX's, only 10 per cent disappear, leaving 18.

We make our cross-sectional survey at T_1 and find the following figures:

	X	Not-X	Total
A	5	50	55
B	18	80	98

Prevalence of X in A's = 9.1 per cent.
Prevalence of X in B's = 18.4 per cent.

The contrast in prevalence is the reverse of the contrast in incidence, and we have a *spurious association* — an association that is not present in the population. With certain other figures for incidence and for the disappearance of X's, this reversal does not occur, but the amount of the difference in prevalence is no safe guide to the amount of the difference in incidence.

A record of prevalence can also mask a real association. If a survey of men aged 60 years revealed the same average and range of blood pressure in heavy smokers as in nonsmokers, several explanations would be possible, one of them being that smoking had killed many of those whose pressure it had raised, while many of those whose pressure was raised by other factors had survived.

To avoid the prevalence-incidence fallacy we must, before starting a survey, visualize a period that stretches back for years, and ask ourselves: "Is it at all possible that the X:not-X ratio has changed through the years? If so, is it possible that the change was different in the A's and B's? What information can we seek to reassure ourselves on this problem?"

The Time Factor in Incidence and Prevalence. It is time, the father of so many biases, that produces the prevalence-incidence confusion; but time can mislead us in either of those estimates taken by itself. Let us suppose that a physician's population contains equal numbers of persons with disease X and with disease Y. Both diseases have periods of quiescence followed by periods of activity, but in X the recurrences are more frequent than in Y. For simplicity, we suppose that all patients with either disease go to the same physician when their diseases are active. If the physician counts the number of patients who have come to him during a particular span of time, he will find more X's than Y's.

We should always remember that prevalence, although measured in the present, depends on the past. It is the resultant of competing forces: incidence (attack rate), recovery rate, and rate of loss by death or other events.

Q V – 9. What do we expect to be the order of magnitude of the frequencies and measurements that we observe, and of quantities that we calculate during the analysis?

Such information has several uses, for example:

1. We need it before we can make any estimate of necessary sample sizes, or of the likelihood of success in our search for differences, if real differences exist (Chapter VIII).

2. Whenever we are doing any calculation, we should continually scrutinize our figures, to see if they "make sense." Otherwise, we may make some fantastic blunders.

3. When we are reading a report, if we have some knowledge of the magnitudes of frequencies or measurements to be expected under the conditions described, we should see if the reported figures appear reasonable. If they do not, we should try to find out why. If, in the report itself, there are inconsistencies of numerical values in different batches of data, we should again try to discover the cause.

CHAPTER VI

INTERPRETATION AFTER
AN EXPERIMENT

In order to see how we will be able to interpret our results, we must look closely at the questions that our experiment is to ask, and how we are going to conduct it, with special attention to problems of variation and risks of bias. At this stage we are not concerned with "interpretation" in the sense of a profound explanation of the observed phenomena, and we will use "causal" in the everyday (nonmetaphysical) sense of the term.

This chapter contains much discussion of "statistical significance tests," and one might well ask: "Why not describe the tests first and talk about them afterward?" The reasons for not adopting that sequence are threefold:

1. Underlying all tests of statistical "significance" and all estimation of population values from samples, there are certain principles, derived from our experience of random processes ("chance" in the strict technical sense of the word). Unless we grasp these principles, and unless we know what the tests and estimates can and cannot tell us about the real world, the techniques are dangerous.

Before becoming involved with the special features and arithmetic of any particular technique we can, without great difficulty, start to grasp the principles by reference to such phenomena as card shuffling and the sampling of disks in a barrel. Such phenomena are not only our chief sources of knowledge of chance, but are used in modern experimentation in the real world. By starting in this way we can avoid the need for repetition of principles, and of warning against dangers, with each individual technique.

2. Many of us, having learned a few techniques, illustrated by simple examples in a textbook or classroom, have applied them to complex data, or to bits of such data, without knowing what fools we were making of ourselves. If we had known more about the tests in general, we would have had a better notion of what kind of test to seek for and what to avoid. Often, we might have decided not to use a test at all. Indeed,

if this chapter helped to reduce the "incidence" of tests, but promoted simpler, more thoughtful and more systematic investigation, followed by more cautious interpretation, I would be very happy. At all events, it may help to reduce the incidence of reader-deception by tests that will doubtless continue to appear in medical journals.

3. Individual statistical tests may come and go, but random processes in Nature will always be with us, mixed with trends, systematic differences and other sources of bias. They will even remain with those workers who seem to think that they can shut out chance by closing their laboratory doors. Even if we do not contemplate applying any of the tests that the statisticians have devised, the principles underlying those tests provide a groundwork for a kind of thinking that we must do when we are planning, performing and interpreting any investigation.

Q VI – 1.   What exactly is the hypothesis that we wish to test by our experiment?

This is a more specific question than Q II – 1 — What is the immediate purpose of our investigation? Let us suppose that our hypothesis is that drug A, administered to a certain type of patient under certain specified conditions, causes improvement in a higher proportion of patients than does drug B administered to the same type of patient under the same conditions. Obviously, our hypothesis would not be proved true merely by showing that in the A-patients a higher proportion had improved than in the B-patients. We must show that the observed difference would rarely occur unless A was more effective than B. That is why we arrange that the random assignment of drugs to patients shall be the only difference-causing factor besides the possible difference in drug effects. We know how often the randomization itself causes differences of various magnitudes, and if the observed difference is rare according to the standard that we have chosen, we accept it as proof of our hypothesis regarding the drugs.

The Null Hypothesis. In reality the hypothesis that we are testing — the one that gives us numerical values (numbers improved and not improved) by which we judge our observed values — is the hypothesis that there is no difference between the drug effects. Such a "no-difference" hypothesis, involving either frequencies or measurements, is commonly called a "null" hypothesis. By disproving (rejecting) the null hypothesis we prove (accept) the original hypothesis; but it is important to note that we can never prove that the null hypothesis is true. Treatments may really differ in their effects, but not enough to create in the experiment a difference that is any greater than what is often produced by randomization alone.

Null hypotheses are often illustrated by comparisons of two or more treatments or other independent variables (A, B, and so on), the dependent variable (X) being a frequency or a measurement. However, null hypotheses are equally basic in the study of relationships between measured variables, such as different amounts of a certain dietary supplement (A_1, A_2, A_3, and so on) and the amounts of growth (X_1, X_2,

X₃, and so on) in different children or groups of children during a certain period. After the experiment, we draw a dot diagram, with the A's on the horizontal axis, the X's on the vertical axis, and a dot for each child. If the null hypothesis (no AX relationship) were true, and there were no other source of variation (individual differences in amounts of growth) the dots would lie along a horizontal line; but of course such dots are always scattered, and there may be a suggestion of trend. A glance may suffice to tell us that this suggestion would be often produced by the randomization that assigned the amounts (doses) of supplement to the individual children; but for greater assurance we may perform a numerical test.

Hypotheses in General. The aura of dignity and importance that often surrounds the word "hypothesis" would be removed if we remembered that it is merely the Greek form of the Latin *suppositio*. It is a supposition that we express in such a form that we can test it. Hence, three general requirements should be obvious:

1. The hypothesis must be clearly defined. This often necessitates the breaking down of a complicated hypothesis into its components.
2. The consequences of the hypothesis must be fully worked out — what would happen and what would not happen, if the hypothesis were (a) true and (b) false.
3. The experiment must be so designed that its outcome can be placed alongside the deductions obtained in (2).

"Hypothesis" when loosely used can be very misleading. When a person who is not familiar with research decides to conduct an investigation he may use the word "hypothesis" as equivalent to "premise" or "axiom" or "belief"—something that he takes for granted, not something to be tested by the investigation.

Q VI – 2. By what rules are we going to insure that the causal interpretation after the experiment will take the form: "Either the randomization or the factor under test"?

The two rules given in the drug trial example under Q II – 4 can now be repeated in more general terms:

1. Assign the sampling units to the variants of the factor under test by a strictly random method.
2. During the experiment permit nothing to interfere with the effects of the randomization except the factor under test; that is, insure that the randomization is solely responsible for the biases throughout the experiment.

The main purpose of this chapter is to amplify those rules.

Q VI – 3. Is randomization necessary if we are not going to apply a statistical test?

Probably the best way to answer that question is to consider what a good experimenter does after an experiment. Even if he is going to apply an arithmetical test later, he looks at the results and tries to decide whether the numerical differences, which appear to be associated with treatment differences, could easily have been caused by something else, such as intersubject variation or measurement error or biases that he could not control. In so doing he actually applies a statistical test — the "eye test." Of course, the eye cannot detect a hidden bias, but neither can arithmetic. As Wilson (1952) has remarked, "fifty pages of higher mathematics will not salvage an experiment with a hidden bias."

The purpose of randomization is to control the biases that may result from the variability of our material, our procedures and other circumstances affecting the experiment. Therefore the question about the need for randomization is best put in another form.

Q VI – 4.   What is the risk in trusting to our pre-existing knowledge of variability and to our way of conducting the experiment, instead of using randomization?

To an increasing number of experimenters this would be a pointless question. They would say: "Randomization is an integral part of our experiments." However, the question needs consideration because this attitude is by no means universal in medical laboratories.

Randomization as a Routine Procedure. In medicine we could learn from industrial laboratories an appreciation of the value of routine randomization, as in the following incident reported by Wilson (1952).

In the manufacture of a certain plastic object, hot plastic was introduced into a mold and pressed into shape. In order to ascertain the effect of duration of pressure upon the strength of the object, six batches of plastic were pressed in the same mold, the first batch for 10 seconds, the second for 20 seconds, and so on. When the strength of each object (Y) was plotted against the duration of pressure (X) the six points formed a smooth ascending curve, which was interpreted as showing a strong dependence of strength on duration of pressure.

However, the research supervisor objected to the experiment because the durations of pressure had not been arranged in random order. When the experiment was repeated with the sequence of the six durations randomized, there was no suggestion of a relationship between duration and strength. The source of the error in the first experiment was easily discovered. As successive batches of plastic were introduced, the mold became hotter, and the higher temperature was the cause of the greater strength of the objects. Time and treatment had been confounded.

Incidentally, as Wilson pointed out, even when randomization is used it is important to keep accurate records of the order in which tests are made. When the data from the second experiment were plotted with strength as Y and order as X, the same kind of relationship was found as in the first experiment, and this gave the clue to the cause.

Reasons and Excuses for Not Randomizing. It is desirable to look at three of the reasons expressed or implied by medical laboratory workers who do not see why they should use randomization.

1. "The reasoning after my type of experiment is not statistical. I reduce my experimental error to a very small quantity and then accept as 'real' only those measurement differences that are of a different order of magnitude from my error." In certain lines of medical research akin to "pure" chemistry and "pure" physics this attitude is certainly tenable, but the statement suggests a confusion between statistical tests and statistical thinking. Many workers who claim that they do not use statistics do not feel comfortable unless they have repeated an experiment at least once, on the "off chance" that something "unusual" happened the first time.

2. "I am so well acquainted with the variability of my material and with my experimental error that any hidden bias will be unimportant. If I suspect a more serious bias I do another experiment designed so as to avoid it." This argument may be legitimate for certain workers in certain of their studies, and when they are observing by measurement rather than enumeration, but when it is adduced as a general defense of individual judgment it prompts the following three reflections:

a. It appears to imply that an experimenter knows everything important about an experimental situation except the factor that he is testing. It would seem, therefore, more appropriate to routine industrial testing than to original research, which is a probing into the vast unknown. And yet randomization has come to be recognized as vital in industrial testing, perhaps because mistakes and wastage can be measured there in dollars.

b. The dependence on previous experience prompts the question: "How can we be sure that the new situation was like the previous situation, qualitatively and quantitatively, in all relevant respects?" This does not imply that we should ignore past experience in setting up an experiment and evaluating its outcome. What we are asking is that the experiment shall itself give us information by which we can evaluate what it seems to tell us.

c. Estimates of experimental error are often not nearly as reliable as they are supposed to be. Useful but sometimes embarrassing questions are: "What exactly do you mean by the statement that your experimental error is ± 2 per cent?" "How often would you expect that value to be exceeded in a hundred experiments?" "How many observations, under what conditions, provided your estimate of error?" It would often take several hundred observations to justify the confidence that many experimenters place in an error estimate derived from a dozen or twenty observations. Even an extensive special study of error leaves unanswered the question: "Will the conditions in the experiment in which we are going to use this estimate be exactly the same as in the study that produced it?"

3. "The biases that we have not eliminated by the design and conduct of the experiment are due to chance and can therefore be allowed for by a statistical test." This still rather common faith in statistical arithmetic seems to reflect a confusion between the colloquial and technical use of

the word "chance." Experimenters are not entirely to blame, because the confusion can be traced not only to statistical "cookbooks" but to some of the fundamental writings that introduced modern statistics to experimenters (Mainland, 1960).

Randomization in Medical Laboratories.   Unlike the industrial laboratory worker who tested the plastic mold, distinguished professors in the medical sciences do not have research supervisors who will tell them to do an experiment over again, introducing randomization. It would perhaps help such professors if they would open-mindedly share the experience of a biological statistician who has been called in to perform an "autopsy" on a long series of experiments. He often finds traces of havoc caused by failure to randomize when he compares data from animals "treated alike," and close together in time, with data from animals that were also "treated alike" but farther apart in time. He can seldom do more than raise doubts which may cause a wise experimenter to discard the results of months of work. The reader of a journal article is of course much less able to detect such faults than is a person who can talk to the experimenter.

Perhaps the best advertisement for randomization is the feeling that it confers on the experimenter—a freedom from worry about bias. However carefully we set up and conduct an experiment, unforeseen and unpreventable things are almost certain to occur. An instrument may break down. We repair it or replace it by another of the same kind. We may be able to apply a correction term to all readings taken by the new instrument, trying to make them equivalent to those from the first instrument; but we cannot be sure that the corrected readings are close enough to those that the first instrument would have given so that we will have no hidden bias. Even when an instrument functions as well as possible throughout an experiment it may fluctuate or drift, and although we repeatedly check it and apply correction terms we can never be quite sure that they are adequate.

The animals or other material on which we are experimenting may be different, perceptibly or imperceptibly, at different times in an experiment. The experimenter may unwittingly alter certain methods of procedure, observation or assessment during the course of the experiment.

We ought not to be careless about these and many other possibilities or fail to correct for disturbances when we can do so, because any increase of variation reduces the sensitivity of our experiment. But if we have placed our sampling units in random relationship to such events we know that we can make proper allowance for the bias that they may have introduced.

Q VI – 5. What are the risks in using the method of "alternates" instead of true randomization?

From time to time this question is still asked, because this method seems to be such an easy "unbiased" way of assigning treatments to patients in their order of admission to a clinical trial or to animals in the order in which they are taken out of a cage—treatment A to Nos. 1, 3, 5, and so on; treatment B to Nos. 2, 4, 6, and so on. The objections to the method can be described as logical and psychological.

Logical Objections to Alternate-subject Assignment. A clinician, talking to a statistician, said: "In a drug trial I arranged that the clinic attendant would hand out the A and B drugs to alternate patients as they left the clinic. What was wrong with that as a method of randomization?" An appropriate answer would have been: "How did you prove that it was right?" As in the selection of every nth subject from a sample (Q III – 8), whenever anyone proposes to substitute a systematic selection method for a strictly random method the onus is on him to prove that the substitute is sufficiently equivalent to the random method for his purpose.

When numbers are taken from a roulette wheel for the construction of a table of random numbers, it requires an enormous exploration, with thousands of digits, to prove that the wheel is sufficiently unbiased. In an experiment containing a few score subjects such a proof would be impossible, even for the characteristics of the subjects that we can observe and record; and we know, moreover, that there are likely to be undetectable characteristics that will have great bearing on the subjects' reactions in the experiment.

We can distinguish two ways in which the alternate-subject assignment can interfere with the logical structure of an experiment: (1) by introducing bias, and (2) by automatic matching.

Bias Due to Alternate-subject Assignment. During an outbreak of infectious disease the severity of successive cases may in general increase during the earlier stages of an outbreak and decrease during the later stages. If during the later stages we apply treatments A and B to equal numbers of patients in the order ABAB, the B's will on the average be less severe cases than the A's.

When we reach haphazardly to take animals from cages, our selection is far from random. The lively ones that pop up may be the ones we take first, or it may be easier to catch the sluggish ones. In fact, weight trends have been demonstrated in more than one series of animals so selected. The ABAB design applied to such series invites bias. Similarly, if during a 6-hour laboratory period 6 animals are subjected to one or other of two operations, A and B, in the order ABABAB, the B's will have been subjected for an hour longer than the A's to whatever influences the waiting period under laboratory conditions may exert on them, and these influences are often far from negligible.

A grossly simplified picture, fictitious but based on an actual investigation, will help to show how unsuspected and probably undetectable rhythms may cause bias. A surgeon wished to find out whether a certain seasickness remedy would reduce the incidence or severity of postoperative vomiting. In order to avoid biased selection, he administered the drug to alternate patients.

Let us suppose that there are two surgical operating days, Mondays and Fridays, and that there is some factor that tends to make the incidence or severity of vomiting greater on one of the days than on the other. Such a factor might be one of the following: the relationship of the operating day to a weekend or to a hospital visiting day, which often disturbs patients; different nurses or different attitude of the nurses; the surgeon's other activities; difference in preoperative preparation, such as maintenance of body fluid balance. Let there be on each day some most common number (modal number) of the operations used in the study: 5 on Mondays, 3 on Fridays. For simplicity we imagine these numbers constant. Allocating the drug (D) and no-drug (N) to alternate patients, we have in each week:

Monday, DNDND; Friday, NDN.

There are equal numbers of D's and N's, but if Monday tends to be the "more favorable" day the drug will be favored. In practice there might be other biases that would counteract this bias, but we have no right to assume so. More complicated rhythms, within any time period from a day to a year, can be similarly conceived.

Automatic Matching by Alternate-subject Assignment. If two subjects, taken at the same time or close together in time, are more alike than those taken farther apart, the ABAB sequence will create a series of more or less matched pairs. This could occur in the examples given above —the trend of increasing (or decreasing) severity in an outbreak of disease, and the selection of animals from cages. It could conceivably have occurred in the drug trial in which the attendant handed out drugs A and B to alternate patients as they left the clinic. Junior physicians may deal with the less difficult or less serious cases and dismiss them early in the clinic period, whereas the more complicated and more serious cases will be retained for consultation with the clinic chief, perhaps with other specialists and perhaps to receive special advice or treatment.

Now if we have in reality a series of matched pairs and then analyze the data as if we had randomly assigned the treatments through the whole group (e.g., by contingency table analysis) we are applying an inappropriate method of analysis. Each member of the A-sample will have its mate in the B-sample, and the outcome in the two samples may be much more alike than if we had created the samples by overall randomization. When we allow for this larger variation before being willing to accept the proof of an A-B difference, we are making an unnecessarily large allowance and we may miss a difference that actually exists.

The alternate-subject method of assignment does not in fact lead to any valid analysis. There is always the risk of confounding sequence and treatment. If we wish to use matched pairs in spite of their drawbacks (see under Q IV – 6) we must assign A and B within each pair strictly at random and then set up the results for analysis in terms of pairs.

Psychological Objections to Alternate-subject Assignment. One of the most notable instances of vast labor wasted by a systematic assignment of therapy is described by Truelove in *Medical Surveys and Clinical*

Trials (Witts). In a trial of anticoagulant therapy in coronary heart disease it was arranged that patients admitted to the participating hospitals on odd-numbered days of the month would receive the test treatment and those admitted on even-numbered days would not. After the trial was over it was found that there were 580 treated patients and 442 controls. This was far too big a difference to be accounted for by the slight excess of odd-numbered days in a year. It was then reported that some patients had been put into the treatment group at the request of their relatives and private physicians, and it is impossible to determine how many others may have been steered into it by arranging for their admission on the odd-numbered days. Consequently, no one can say what the results of this very large trial really mean.

When I hear a clinician's proposal to assign treatments according to whether the patient's hospital admission number is odd or even (because he cannot see how this assignment could be selectively manipulated), I am surprised at his lack of faith in man's ingenuity.

The psychological danger of the alternate-subject and similar methods of assignment lies not only in the risk of purposive steering of patients to one or the other treatment. When a conscientious physician is deciding whether a patient qualifies for admission to a trial, he is afraid of being biased by knowing which treatment will be administered. In his effort to avoid bias he may come to a different decision regarding admission from the decision he would have reached without that knowledge.

Q VI – 6. What instrument are we going to use for randomization?

Tables of Random Numbers. These tables provide the easiest and most dependable method of randomization, and they are now readily available to research workers. They can be looked upon as equivalent to thousands of thoroughly shuffled playing cards, each card bearing one digit from 0 through 9. The digits, when originally recorded in random order (by methods to be mentioned) are, as it were, in one long line, but are broken up into columns, rows and blocks to facilitate reading. The following is a small portion of Fisher and Yates' (1938-1957) six-page table which contains 15,000 digits:

26	72	39	27	67
43	00	65	98	50
16	06	10	89	20
09	65	90	77	47
65	39	07	16	29

To use the table, we select a digit anywhere in it without previously inspecting the numbers themselves, e.g., by opening at a page and placing on it anywhere a pointer such as the corner of an index card. We start at the digit touched by the pointer and proceed by consecutive digits up or down or to right or left, passing from block to block without interruption. Having come to the end of a row or column we can start at the next one on either side and proceed in the same or reverse direction.

If we are performing a series of investigations that will be connected with each other we must avoid using the same sequence of digits on two occasions. Therefore it is desirable to keep a note of the part of the table that we have used.

Examples of the Use of Random Numbers. A few simple small-sample illustrations will indicate the principles. (For complex experiment designs or very large samples, special methods published with the various sets of tables are desirable in order to prevent one's using up too many digits.) The examples can be expressed as instructions to the randomizer, who should check each step very carefully before he goes on to the next one.

Ex. 1. Assignment of treatments A and B, each treatment to 5 patients.*
Take ten index cards ($5'' \times 3''$) and write on each card a number representing one of the patients (e.g., the order in which he will be admitted to the trial). Suppose that the pointer has landed on the zero of "10" in the middle of the above table. Write on the first card "10," on the second card "89," on the third card "20," on the fourth card "09," and so on. Arrange the cards in a pile in ascending (or descending) order of the random numbers and then take off the top five cards and mark them "A"; mark the remainder "B." The systematic arrangement of the random numbers has transferred the random order to the patients.

	Random No.	Patient No.
A	09	4
	10	1
	20	3
	39	10
	47	8
B	65	9
	65	5
	77	7
	89	2
	90	6

The duplicates (two 65's) cause no disturbance because both of them have led to the assignment of treatment B. If, however, one 65 had been the fifth item and the other the sixth item it would have been necessary to decide whether patient No. 5 or patient No. 9 should receive drug A. This could have been decided by picking up two random numbers somewhere else in the table and letting their ascending order of magnitude determine the relative positions of the cards with duplicate numbers. We can do likewise with triplicates and other ties; but it is

---

* As Herrera (1955) has pointed out, a method that was prescribed in the first edition of this book for separation of subjects into two or more groups by random numbers did not entirely remove the risk of bias.

often best to reduce the number of such problems by using four-digit numbers for the randomization.

To resume the procedure, make a list of patients and their assigned treatments:

Patient No.	Treatment	
1	A	
2		B
3	A	
4	A	
5		B
6		B
7		B
8	A	
9		B
10	A	

It is useful to arrange the A's and B's in separate columns, to prevent misreading of letters, and in case carbon copies of the list should become smudged.

If the trial is to be double-blind, a copy of this list can be sent to the drug dispenser who will put the patient's numbers on the proper bottles or other containers and remove all clues to the identification of drugs. If the trial is not to be double-blind the physician and all others concerned with the patient can be kept in the dark, until treatment is actually to begin, by preparing an envelope for each patient with his number on the outside. Inside is placed a card with the patient's number and also the assigned treatment, along with paper or cards to prevent anyone from being tempted to hold the envelope up to a bright light. The envelopes are sealed and delivered to the physician or other responsible person.

NOTE. — If the number of available patients were odd, say 11, the top five (or six) cards could be marked "A" and the remainder "B"; no uncontrolled bias would result.

Ex. 2. Treatments A and B are to be applied to 10 pairs of litter mates, one treatment to each animal. Write down an identification number or letter for one member of each pair. Assign to these animals the treatments by single-digit random numbers, letting even numbers (including 0) represent treatment A and odd numbers treatment B. The other member of each pair will receive the other treatment.

Ex. 3. Ten tubes in a laboratory (or 100 x-ray films or 50 histopathologic slides) are to be arranged in random order. Write the serial number or other identification of each tube (or film or slide) on an index card and proceed as in Ex. 1, stopping short of division into A and B groups.

Ex. 4. There are 234 animals in stock and a random sample of 40 is required. First, identify each animal. If they are not in single-animal cages, a temporary or permanent mark can be made on each of them. On each of 234 cards write the identification of a particular animal. Write a four-digit random number on each card, arrange the cards in ascending order of random numbers and take the first 40 cards to indicate which animals shall comprise the sample.

Ex. 5. An intersubject comparison of treatments A and B has to be completed within a certain number of months. It is difficult to predict how many subjects will become available during the period. It would be permissible to assume a certain total and randomly assign A and B to equal numbers. Even if the assumed total was not reached by the end of the period, and even if the numbers in the treatment classes were unequal, the randomization would still control the bias. However, more than the anticipated number of subjects might arrive, and the combination of two sets of observations, each randomized within itself, presents some problems. The best solution seems to be random assignment of the treatments to each subject at the very beginning of the experiment, using odd numbers for A and even numbers for B, without trying to make the samples equal in size. One can assign treatments to more than the anticipated numbers of subjects, but if one runs short of the assignments before the end of the experiment, one can supplement them by the same process.

Manufacture and Testing of Random Numbers. At present there are in common use three large sets of random numbers:

1. The table of Fisher and Yates (1938–1957) already mentioned. It was derived from the 15th to 19th digits in a twenty-figure logarithm table, the selection and arrangements of the digits being determined by two sets of playing cards.

2. The tables of Kendall and Babington-Smith (1939, 1946), containing 100,000 digits. This was produced by the use of a disk with digits 0 to 9 equally spaced around it. The disk was rotated at uniform speed in the dark, and was illuminated at irregular intervals by flashes of light from a lamp controlled by an operator working a telegraph key. Each digit thus rendered visible was recorded. (It is recommended that these tables be read horizontally because they were more thoroughly tested in that direction than vertically.)

3. *A Million Random Digits* produced by the Rand Corporation (1955) by an equipment constructed and operated on the principle of a roulette-wheel but employing an electronic random frequency pulse.

For many small investigations a sufficient supply of random numbers is to be found in *Tables for Statisticians* by Arkin and Colton (1950–1959), which reproduces the first 8000 digits of the Kendall and Babington-Smith tables.

All these tables were thoroughly tested by the application of our knowledge of what happens in random processes — for instance, the approximately equal frequencies of the digits 0 to 9, the extent to which departures from equality occur, the intervals between digits of the same value, and various other relationships analogous to those found in card games (e.g., one of the tests applied to random numbers is called the "poker" test).

"Pure chance" — a completely random arrangement or sequence — is of course an ideal, a limit which natural phenomena and man-made instruments (like tables of random numbers) can approach but can never reach. The tables doubtless contain spots of nonrandomness, but they are the best instruments for randomization available to the experimenter, and have been far more thoroughly tested than many of his other instruments.

Q VI – 7. What sources of variation must we remember in planning the randomization?

Perhaps the most complete coverage of potential sources of variation is provided by the familiar five questions mentioned in Chapter I: *Who? What? Where? When? How?*

With these questions in mind we should try to visualize circumstances and events before and during the experiment, remembering that each sampling unit will meet the resultant (net effect) of a different combination of these variables. If the treatments to be compared are A and B, the randomization must determine whether the sampling unit that meets any particular combination of variables is an A-treated or a B-treated unit.

After contemplation of all this complexity it is consoling to remember that in a clinical trial extending over many months one simple initial randomization is often sufficient. However, many common types of medical experimentation appear less simple in design than clinical trials and some guidelines for randomization are helpful.

Q VI – 8. What are we going to randomize, and how?

Without any reference to a statistical test which we may later apply, let us imagine that we are inspecting the measurement data after an experiment that involved treatments A and B applied to different subjects. We try to see whether measurements within each treatment group agree closely with each other, and whether there is little overlap between the groups. That is, we use the intragroup variation as a kind of yardstick to measure the intergroup difference. Similarly, when we are looking at enumeration data, e.g., percentages of deaths and survivals, we look for similarity within the treatment groups and difference between them — a high percentage of deaths in the one group and a high percentage of survivals in the other.

We can trust our conclusions regarding the difference of the effects of the two treatments if we can be sure that, except for the treatments pushing the values apart, the randomization has been responsible for the presence of each value in its respective treatment group — that is, responsible for the intragroup variation that we use as our yardstick.

With this in mind we can try to formulate some general guidelines or rules for randomization.

Seven General Rules for Randomization.   These seven rules are followed by examples.

1. Be sure that your experiment design is simple enough for you to comprehend and carry through.

2. Randomize all the variation that you are going to use as a yardstick.

3. Do not randomize variation that you are not going to use as a yardstick. If you do, you will lower the sensitivity of the experiment.

4. Do not use randomization to make treatment groups *alike* in their characteristics. That is not its purpose. If you wish to make them alike, do so before the randomization, by a systematic restriction or subdivision of the population to be studied, or by making experimental conditions more uniform.

5. Avoid a confused mixture of random and systematic arrangements. It will lose more than it gains, because only bits of the data will be comparable.

6. If the experiment is to answer more than one question, consider whether more than one randomization will be necessary.

7. Remember that interclass variation + intraclass variation = total variation. Therefore, if a systematic design is to be used in order to remove interclass variation, so that treatments can be tested within classes, put as much of the total variation as conveniently possible into the interclass category.

Examples of Randomization.   In the following six examples no attempt is made to cover all the problems of design in the projects discussed, or to present alternative designs. The examples try to obey Rule 1, even though a more complex design might provide more information from the same size of experiment.

Ex. 1. A long-term animal experiment, e.g., comparison of foods or potential cancer-producing agents. The simplest design is to place the animals in their cages and randomize treatments throughout. Interanimal variation will include effects of cage position (light, temperature, humidity and ventilation), but the removal of cage-position effects would require a more complex design. If some or all of the cages contain more than one animal, it may be found that all the animals in certain cages have been assigned the same treatment; but we must not interfere with this randomization-effect by arranging, say, for 2 A's and 2 B's to be together in the same cage (Rule 5). Single-animal cages avoid such clustering and have other advantages also.

Ex. 2. Litter mates in an A-B long-term experiment. Each pair is a class or "block" and the sampling units are the individual animals within each pair. Our yardstick is the difference between readings on pairs, one difference from each pair. We know, for instance, that if A and B were merely letters assigned randomly and if every reading on a B-animal were subtracted from the reading on the corresponding A-animal, we would in the long run approach 50 per cent positive and 50 per cent negative differences; and for the purposes of our finite experiment we know how often various departures from the 50:50 ratio are met in samples of various sizes.

We are not going to use as our yardstick the interlitter differences that are going to affect equally both animals of a litter. Therefore we do not arrange the litters in random order in the laboratory (Rule 3); we arrange them in any convenient order. We reduce the possible differences between litter mates (except the differences that the treatments may cause) by keeping the litter mates close together. That is, we put much of the interanimal variation, which may be due to differences in location, into the interlitter variation, because we are not going to use this in the analysis (Rule 7).

Ex. 3. An acute experiment — comparison of A and B treatment on different animals. Treatment and observation on each animal will be completed in about an hour, but the whole experiment will extend over weeks or months. It is tempting to plan for an equal number of animals (say three) randomly assigned to each treatment on each day of the experiment, but unless we feel very sure from past experience that we can fill our quota each day the plan is risky. Some statistics books show how to analyze measurement data with unequal numbers of subjects in the treatment groups in different blocks (days), but apart from the complexity of the analysis it often involves assumptions that an experimenter would question if he could understand what they were.

The simplest procedure is to randomize in advance for the whole experiment (see *Ex. 5* under Examples of the Use of Random Numbers, p. 81). Even if this should assign the same treatment to all animals on one day we should resist the desire to tinker with the randomization (Rule 5). To avoid risk of bias through foreknowledge of the scheme of each day's work, someone who does not know the scheme can pick out the animals, or sealed envelopes can be used as in drug trials, one to be opened for each animal after it has been chosen.

Ex. 4. Intrasubject comparison of drugs A and B by cross-over design — a 3-month period on each drug. A certain measurement is taken at the beginning and end of each period, and the change in period (1) is compared with the change in period (2). It might be thought that the periods in each patient could be looked on as sampling units, analogous to litter mates or twins; but the difference, period (1) minus (2), might be positive (or negative) in all or nearly all the patients even if there were no drug difference. Therefore the experiment fits more clearly into the scheme of the null hypothesis if we consider the patients as sampling units, each presenting one measurement, a period (1) minus period (2) difference.

Then the "treatments" that we compare are the sequences, AB versus BA. Hence, we randomly assign these sequences (usually in equal numbers) to the patients. In the one sequence group, the difference (1) minus (2) means A minus B, in the other group it means B minus A. Therefore if, after the experiment, the two sequence groups differ in their (1)-minus-(2) differences more than we are prepared to attribute to the randomization, we attribute it to the difference in drug effects. (Further consideration of this design is best postponed until analysis of data is discussed — frequency data in Chapter XII, measurement data in Chapter XIV.)

Ex. 5. After an intersubject comparison of a drug with a placebo in rheumatoid arthritis, the patients' hand films were sent to a radiologist to determine whether there was less progression of the disease, between pre- and posttreatment films inspected side by side, in the drug-treated patients than in the placebo patients. The radiologist was not to know about the individual patients' therapies, but the question arose: Should the films be arranged in random order?

The random assignment of patients in the trial had randomized the relationship between the patients' order of entry and the treatments that they received. Therefore, to answer merely the question regarding treatment and x-ray progression of the disease, the radiologist could have examined the films in the order in which the patients had entered the trial, just as did the clinicians who assessed each patient at the end of his 6-month treatment.

However, there was an opportunity to inquire also into the relationship between the clinicians' findings and the radiologist's findings (Rule 6). Therefore, trends of various kinds had to be considered. In a trial in which suitable patients are scarce, a clinician, having utilized all the immediately available patients, is prompted to call in the patients who, although qualified in terms of the plan, may be somewhat different in type or severity from the patients admitted earlier. Again, the clinician's own standards of assessment may have altered during the trial, however closely he has tried to follow the prescribed system. The radiologist may also be the victim of nonrandom trends and fluctuations, e.g., an initial warming-up period, followed by a fairly steady state, perhaps later followed by monotony or fatigue, and at the end perhaps pressure to get the survey completed.

The trend or fluctuations in patient type would be combined with the clinical observer's trend in his reports. The radiologist's trends and fluctuations might, to a greater or less extent, coincide with or run counter to those in the clinicians' reports. Such complex phenomena are difficult to eliminate by analysis of the data. Therefore the film envelopes, each containing one patient's pair of films, were arranged in random order and then numbered 1, 2, 3, and so on, to show the order in which they were to be examined. This placed the radiologist's variation in random relationship to the variation in the clinical records.

Ex. 6. Observational variation estimated by duplicate readings. Probably the chief reason why many estimates of observational variation (experimental error or reading error) are too low is that duplicate readings are made one immediately after the other. To obtain a reliable estimate, the readings (two on each specimen) should be spread independently at random throughout the whole period of the experiment, or series of experiments, in which they are to be used (Rule 2). This can be done easily on preserved material like histologic specimens or x-ray films, but perishable specimens present difficulties. In the analysis of serum the difficulty can often be overcome by freezing and storing a sample of each specimen; but to avoid the effects of thawing and refreezing it may be desirable to store two samples of each specimen.

Q VI – 9. Are we going to examine our treatment assignments in order to see if the randomization has "worked well"?

Sometimes in reports on clinical trials the reader's attention is called to the evenness with which the randomization has distributed characteristics such as sex and age between the treatment groups. This may help to increase confidence in a technique that is still unfamiliar to many readers, but it is a somewhat curious ground for faith in a method that merely claims to approach equality of distribution of variables *in the long run*. How long the run must be, nobody can tell, and en route the randomization frequently produces inequalities that look impressive. Indeed, if we found in any small or moderate-sized samples exactly equal distributions of several variables that were independent of each other, we ought to suspect human interference.

Adjustment of Allocation after Randomization. If, after randomization, we detect an inequality of some feature between treatment groups, we may be tempted to make the groups more alike in this respect. If we are so tempted, we should remember the following five points:

1. If after randomization we examined a large number of independent features of the individuals in the treatment groups, we ought to expect the frequencies of some of them to differ greatly between the groups. If we call "rare" any difference that occurs in only 5 per cent of randomizations, we should expect about 5 per cent of these differences to be in the "rare" class.

2. In any particular experiment the purpose of the randomization is not to distribute individual variables (attributes or measurements), but the sampling units, each of which carries the resultant or net effect of a large number of different variables.

3. If we try to balance certain detectable features like sex or age and duration or severity of disease, it is not unlikely that we are throwing farther off balance some hidden features that may be far more important than those that we know about.

4. If we consider some features so influential that we wish the treatment groups to be homogeneous in that respect, we ought to use it as a basis for subdivision of our sample initially, and then randomize treatments within the subsamples.

5. If we have allowed any known feature (e.g., sex) to be randomized as part of the complex of variables, at the end of the experiment we can divide the data and compare treatment effects in the separate subclasses, e.g., males and females.

Q VI – 10.   How are we going to insure that the randomization will be solely responsible for bias throughout the experiment?

To answer this fundamental question we seek in vain for detailed rules. After grasping some principles we must apply our imagination to the particular circumstances of our experiment, and we must exert constant vigilance.

The Blindfold Method.   The best way of avoiding interference with the effects of randomization is of course the blindfold method — everyone who could in any way influence the results is kept in the dark regarding the treatment applied to particular subjects or specimens. Even in a blindfold drug trial there is no way, except education in scientific method, of preventing rank dishonesty, such as the illegitimate opening of the "emergency envelopes," i.e., the set of sealed envelopes, one for each patient, containing a statement of the compound that he is receiving, available in case he displays untoward symptoms and it is necessary to know whether he was receiving drug A or drug B. (He must, of course, be removed from the trial before the envelope is opened.)

Occasional leakages of information are bound to occur, for example when a pharmacist, having labeled a bottle with the patient's name forgets to remove the drug label before sending the bottle to the ward. Constant vigilance must be maintained by all participants.

Nonblindfold Experiments.   Some clinical trials cannot be run blindfold because the secondary effects of the drug under test reveal the drug — for example, the moon-like swelling of the face resulting from the action of the corticosteroids. When the drug under test has to be injected there is naturally some hesitation to inject a placebo solution because of the possibility of infection, although with standard precautions the risk is very slight.

The Revealing Labels "A" and "B."   It is surprising how many investigators think that they are conducting a double-blind trial when they use bottles of drugs labeled "A" and "B." If the observer sees, or thinks he sees, a difference in response between the A-treated and B-treated patients he is likely to be biased or to try to avoid bias. The difference in handling and evaluating the two groups may be subtle but very real. If the patients compare their experiences they, also, can produce biased responses. Moreover, if it is necessary in an emergency to find out what drug a patient is receiving, the drugs received by all patients in the trial will be revealed. Sometimes an attempt is made to mystify observers and patients by assigning two letters or label-colors to each drug; but this is still a treacherous "pseudo–double-blind" technique.

"Objective" Methods.   If an experiment is not blindfold the rule is that objective methods of assessment must be used; but in fact it is very difficult to insure that a method is in all respects neutral to the treatment that a subject is known to be receiving. Functional tests, such as the measuring of grip strength in rheumatoid arthritis by asking the patient to squeeze a rubber bag connected to a mercury manometer, are readily influenced by the attitude of the examiner. In questioning a patient,

even if we use a set form of words, our tone or attitude can be easily affected by our knowledge; and there is much to be said in favor of asking the patient to write the answers to printed questions without giving him any explanation or help.

A blood pressure reading that we might accept and record for an A-treated subject we may doubt in a B-treated subject, and we may repeat the reading. Do we really know that our results would be the same if we took a second reading on all subjects?

A number of men, half of whom had received a treatment that was a possible preventive of nasopharyngeal inflammation, were lined up for inspection of the nose and throat by a medical officer who was skeptical of the treatment. After the inspection was over, an attendant remarked: "Did you notice, sir, that you spent much more time examining the treated cases than the controls?"

In a certain clinical trial the nurses were required to report small skin hemorrhages that might occur. The drug was to be administered intramuscularly into the buttocks. In the planning of the trial one of the clinicians was strongly in favor of a placebo injection in the controls because this would automatically insure that all patients had an equal opportunity of skin inspection by the nurses.

Destruction of Random Order. In laboratory work randomization can be ruined by a technician who is either improperly instructed or is unreliable. For example, in a certain experiment cage positions had been randomized and then it was found that the technician had, for his own convenience, grouped the cages according to treatment. In this instance the fault lay with the investigator, who always wanted the validity of his results to be "proved statistically," but thought that randomization was a statistician's useless fad.

Q VI – 11. If we are trying to find whether there is a difference in the effects of two or more treatments of any kind, what are the two types of error that we may make in drawing our conclusions?

On the one hand, we may conclude that the treatments differ in their effects when in fact they do not. On the other hand, we may conclude that there is, for our purposes at least, no difference in their effects when in fact there is a difference. This truism is the basis for a rather useful distinction between Type I errors and Type II errors.

Type I Errors. Let us suppose that we make it a rule to classify as "rare" the extreme differences — those that occur in not more than 5 per cent of randomizations such as card shufflings. After a treatment comparison, if the observed difference in the outcome is in the 5 per cent rarity class, we conclude that something more than the randomization was probably responsible, and in an experiment in which the randomization has been solely responsible for all the bias, the "something more" means the treatment difference. We can now visualize all the experiments in our lifetime in which, although we do not know it, there is no difference in treatment effects. If we adhere to the 5 per cent rule we will commit a Type I error in not more than 5 per cent of these experiments.

More exactly, we ought to visualize the no-real-difference experiments conducted throughout the lifetime of an indefinitely large number of investigators, because any one of us may have bad luck in our randomizations — too many extreme differences. However, that need not worry us, because many of our experiments will be on treatments that do differ in their effects, and if we use the 5 per cent standard our total risk of erroneously inferring a difference will be much less than 5 per cent. If we use a 1 per cent standard of rarity, our risk will be less than 1 per cent.

In technical terms, the Type I error of a specified magnitude (e.g., 5 per cent or 1 per cent) is our risk of rejecting the null hypothesis when it is true; but it may be more useful to think of it as our risk of following a false clue.

Type II Errors. We must be rather careful in using this term. If an observed difference is not in our "rarity" class (5 per cent or 1 per cent or whatever we have chosen), we have no right to conclude that there is no real difference in treatment effects — we can never prove the null hypothesis true (Q VI – 1). We can merely say that the real difference, if it exists, has not produced a difference in our experiment that is big enough to satisfy our standard. Our verdict is "not proved," and in that verdict there is no error. However, after most experiments we act in some way or other as a result of our findings. If we act as if there is no real difference between treatment effects, when in fact there is a difference, we make a mistake, whether it has serious consequences or not.

We would like to know our risk of committing such mistakes, but the mere finding that a difference is not rare, on our 5 per cent or other standard, does not tell us our risk of making this other kind of mistake. To obtain a figure for this kind of error we need to ask a question such as: "If the real difference is such and such, and we take samples of size N, what is our risk of failing to detect a difference?" For instance, our knowledge of random sampling tells us what we will find if we have two large populations of subjects, A-treated and B-treated, like disks in two separate barrels, and if we then take from each population a strictly random sample of 20 subjects and repeat this process many times.

Let us suppose that the A-population contains 25 per cent X's (75 per cent not-X's) and that the B-population contains 50 per cent X's (50 per cent not-X's), that in each pair of samples of 20 we find the A-B difference in the numbers of X's and apply our 5 per cent standard of rarity. After repeating the process many times, we will find that we have judged the A-B difference "real" in only about 27 per cent of the sample-pairs. This is the percentage of our "successful" experiments, i.e., those in which we have detected something that exists in the populations. In the other 73 per cent of sample-pairs we have failed to find a difference that is large enough to meet our standard. We call 73 per cent our Type II error. It can be called our risk of accepting the null hypothesis when it is false, or our risk of failing to follow a true clue.

Lest we stray too far from the real world at this point, we should remind ourselves that when we are comparing A and B treatments, of any kind, on human or biologic material, we are not actually taking random samples from an A-treated and a B-treated population. As we proceed in a clinical trial, for example, the later patients may represent a somewhat different population from the one represented by the earlier patients with respect to their percentage of X's, even if they were all treated by A (or by B). All that we can hope to do is detect a kind of average difference, if one exists. However, the Type II error helps us in deciding what size of sample to take in order to have a good prospect of detecting a difference that we do not want to miss.

For instance, with samples of 100 and population percentages of X's 25 per cent and 50 per cent respectively (a difference of 25 percentage points) the Type II error is approximately 5 per cent. With populations containing 50 per cent and 75 per cent X's it is the same. As we pass farther from 50 per cent X's, but keep the sample size the same (or even somewhat smaller) and also the same population difference, the risk of error becomes less. Thus, with populations containing 5 per cent and 25 per cent X's and samples of 100 the Type II error is only 2 per cent. (The basis of these statements is revealed in Chapters XI and XII.)

The Power of an Experiment. In connection with the Type II error there is another rather useful term — "power." If our Type II error is 73 per cent, the percentage of "successful" experiments, 27 per cent, is called the "power" of that particular experimental procedure in the specified situation (composition of populations and sample size). If the Type II error is 5 per cent, the power is 95 per cent. The power is thus a numerical expression of what we have previously referred to as the "sensitivity" of the experiment.

It may be helpful here to mention a much-used symbolism, in which percentages are expressed as decimal fractions and Greek letters are employed. Thus, a 5 per cent Type I error becomes $\alpha = 0.05$. A 10 per cent Type II error becomes $\beta = 0.10$. With $\beta = 0.10$, the power is $1 - \beta = 0.90$.

Q VI – 12. If we intend to apply a test of "statistical significance" to our data, how will we know that it is a legitimate test?

A "legitimate" test is one that follows from the particular kind of randomization employed in the experiment. Having performed the actual randomization, we ought to know what series of randomization experiments would enable us to obtain the information that we need, about rarity of differences, and so on, without performing any arithmetical test at all. Then we ought to see how far the proposed test is equivalent to the series of randomization experiments, what assumptions underlie the test, and what is the evidence that these assumptions are safe with our data. These points are illustrated in later chapters; but here two general remarks may be made:

1. An investigator displays remarkable credulity, often unlike his other research behavior, if he performs (or requests, or demands) a statistical test without knowing its experimental equivalent, such as card shuffling.

2. Many research workers would be astonished if they knew the hidden assumptions in some of the tests and other mathematical performances that they take on trust. Sometimes they would see that the assumptions were inappropriate. More often, if they searched for evidence to justify the assumptions, they would find very little, either in their own data or in other data of similar type. They might then start to wonder what results they would obtain if half a dozen equally plausible assumptions were made, one after another, and used as a basis for the analysis of their data.

Q VI – 13. If a legitimate test is applied to our data and gives a verdict "statistically significant difference," what will it tell us?

Technical jargon, a useful shorthand, can do a great harm if its meaning, and especially its limitation of meaning, is not clearly understood. This seems to be the reason why the phrase "statistically significant" has done so much damage. The best way to elucidate jargon is to translate it. If a person says that a difference is "statistically significant," he means, or ought to mean, simply this: "Differences as large as this, in samples of this size, are so rarely produced by random processes alone, that I believe that this particular observed difference signifies (indicates, or points to) something in addition to a random process." This translation has purposely substituted "random processes" for "chance," because we are so often misled by colloquial meanings of "chance" — a mysterious force, or factors that we do not know about, or factors that we are unable (or too lazy) to correct for.

The 5 Per Cent Standard. It is for the investigator to decide what he will call "rare" in classifying random events. That matter is discussed under Q VI – 15. Here let us assume that he adopts the commonly used 5 per cent standard of rarity — the "5 per cent level of significance." To obtain an idea of what this means, let us consider the example given under Q II – 4. In 100 subjects (50 A's and 50 B's) there were, let us say, 35 "successes." If all 35 were in one group and none in the other, we would feel sure that randomization was extremely unlikely to be solely responsible. If 16 were in one group and 19 in the other, we would know that randomization would often cause such a trivial difference.

Somewhere between these two possibilities we must find a cut-off point such that all the more extreme differences must total to not more than 5 per cent of the total card shufflings. We could do this by actual card shufflings repeated, say, a thousand times; but we know so much about the effect of randomization in such simple cases that we can use the mathematical short cuts described in Chapter XII. Then we find that the required cut-off point lies between 13 and 12 successes in one sample (A or B) with the remainder (22 or 23 successes) in the other sample.

Hence, if the investigator's samples contained 12 or fewer of the 35 successes in one sample (and 23 or more in the other), he could say that the observed difference, if actually due to the radomization alone, would be in the "5 per cent rarity class of extreme differences." Translating this into jargon, he would say: "the difference is significant at the 5 per cent level."

The Probability P. To avoid the term "significant" the investigator could say "P is less than 0.05"; but this introduces another troublesome term, "probability." We are again misled by colloquial usage, especially the association of "probability" with the idea of prediction. Here, 0.05 is merely the decimal equivalent of 5 per cent, and we can define *probability* in this context as the relative frequency with which certain specified events (e.g., sample differences of a certain size or greater) occur in a series of randomizations, i.e., the frequency of these events expressed as a proportion of the total events produced by the randomization when it is repeated again and again. We are applying information that we possess regarding the effects of randomization, when it alone is acting, to the data from an experiment in which randomization was used, but to which something else (a treatment difference) has been added. We are not, as is a gambler, concerned with the use of the information for prediction.

We would perceive this more clearly if, whenever we saw "P less than 0.05" attached to an observed difference, we substituted a phrase like "Frequency in pure randomization experiments less than 0.05" or even "Randomization frequency less than 5 per cent."

Misconceptions Regarding "Significance" and P. When we conclude that a difference is "statistically significant" we should bear clearly in mind the following five points:

1. "Statistical significance" should never be used loosely, to mean proof of the reliability of the experiment or adequacy of sample size.

2. We must make our standard of "rarity" clear, either with each verdict or at the beginning of a report. Often "significant" and "not significant" are used without further specification to imply the 5 per cent level, while "highly significant" or "very significant" implies the 1 per cent level (P less than 0.01). This habit creates the impression that these purely conventional levels are almost laws of nature.

3. Statistical significance, even with a P value that contains many zeros after the decimal point, does not necessarily mean practical significance. There is often a reduction in human stature between morning and evening, but it is so slight in adults relative to their total length that for clinical purposes no allowance need be made for it. Some drugs, tested for pain-reducing properties, have produced statistically significant effects, but the effects have been too small to be of clinical value. We should always ask a question such as: "If there is a real difference in the effect of A and B, how large or how small may it be?" In the analysis of data, a significance test should not be the end of the road.

On the other hand, size alone does not indicate importance. When someone looks at a set of figures (usually his own figures) and says: "The difference is not statistically significant, but it is clinically significant," it is difficult to know what he means. He may be relating what he sees to other information that seems to point in the same direction, in which case he is making a statistical judgment. Or he may be impressed solely by the size of the difference. Or he may be retreating to unverified clinical impression.

4. Statistical significance is not a mathematical proof that a real (population) difference exists. If we were living in a world in which differences between drug effects did not exist, our drug trials, if we conducted any, would still produce differences with $P = 0.05$ or less, and they would do so in 5 per cent of our trials. Because drugs in the real world often differ in their effects, when we meet a significant difference in a particular trial, we are justified in having some confidence that further study of the same kind of patient under the same conditions would reveal differences in the same direction. But the P value tells us nothing about how often this will happen or fail to happen. It would not do so, even if our original samples had been random samples of their respective treatment-populations, and if we sampled again from the same populations.

5. P values tell us nothing about the nature of the association between the variables that we are studying, or about the size of the differences in effect between the factors under test.

Q VI – 14.   If a legitimate test is applied to our data and gives a verdict "nonsignificant difference," what will it tell us?

A translation of "nonsignificant difference" can be thus: "Differences as large as this, in samples of this size, are so often produced by random processes alone that these data do not convince me that anything more than a random process was responsible." "So often" means, of course, more often than the 5 per cent random frequency or other value that we have chosen as our standard. The verdict is simply: "Not proved." It is not a declaration that the factors under test have actually the same effect — that the two samples have come from the same population with respect to the dependent variables that we are studying. Nor is it a proof that the difference is "insignificant," i.e., of no consequence. It implies that, so far as we can tell from the data, a real difference, which we might find by taking larger samples, might be in the opposite direction from the difference found in our experiment.

Again, our experiment does not tell us much unless we ask a question such as: "If a real difference exists, how large may it be in either direction?"

Q VI – 15.   If we are going to apply a test of statistical significance, what level of significance will we choose?

Translated, this means: "What is our definition of 'rarity' in randomization experiments? What is our cut-off point in a distribution of random frequencies which will determine our rejection of the null hypothesis?"

We must, of course, make our decision regarding the cut-off point before we see, or even suspect, the results of our experiment. Otherwise, we may be biased, or our decision may be influenced by our fear of being biased. We may decide to accept the conventional cut-off point, P = 0.05 or, if we desire greater assurance, P = 0.01; but we ought always to know what our standard implies — what may be the consequences of our choice. Here we are helped by the concept of the Type I error, which is just another way of stating our standard of rarity. It specifies our risk of accepting as real the apparent evidence of a difference that does not in fact exist — our risk of rejecting the null hypothesis when that hypothesis is true. For example, it tells us how often we would accept one drug as more effective than another drug when we were comparing two drugs that did not in fact differ in their effects. In a series of laboratory investigations it tells us what proportion of the false clues we would follow.

We have to weigh this risk in relation to the particular circumstances of our study. There are no universal rules, but the following three points are worth noting:

1. It seems sensible to demand more convincing evidence (e.g., P less than 0.01 instead of 0.05) if the verdict of "significance" would run counter to previous experience or knowledge.
2. It seems sensible to accept less strong evidence (even P between 0.10 and 0.05) when the verdict would agree with other experience or knowledge.
3. The higher our standard of rarity — the lower the P value accepted as a cut-off point — the more likely we are to miss a real difference.

Even these simple guidelines are not easy to apply. Indeed, although the scheme of error risks (Types I and II) is a useful concept, it does not provide us with a definite numerical standard in most biologic or medical research, as it does in the sampling of industrial or agricultural products. In those areas the producer can find in dollars the cost of the two types of mistake that he may make in estimating, from a sample, the percentage of defective items (e.g., lamp bulbs that burn out too soon) in the whole batch — (1) underestimation, which will lead the consumer to seek a more reliable product; (2) overestimation, which will necessitate discarding the whole batch or selling it at a lower price.

Counting the cost in medicine, even in drug testing, is much more difficult. Even if an investigator says that he has set his risk of a Type I error (his significance level) at a certain value, the best way to discover his real standard is to see what he does after he has obtained his results. Having found a certain difference in outcome between two treatment groups, does he act as if it were due to the treatment difference, or as if it were fortuitous, or as if he really did not know?

Q VI – 16. If the verdict of a test is "significant" at our predetermined level, what will we do in consequence thereof?
This question, considered before we start the experiment, should prompt us to think again of the immediate purpose of our research — the direct

question that it is designed to answer — and to ask ourselves whether a verdict of "significant" under the circumstances of our experiment would give us an adequate answer. No specific guidance can be given, but it is helpful to reflect on six topics: (1) rare events, (2) credibility of interpretations, (3) multiplicity of causes, (4) associated agents, (5) group effects, and (6) experimental proof. Although some of the examples are taken from surveys or even from casual observations, and not from experiments in the strict sense, the message that they convey is equally important in experiments.

Rare events. Very unusual events can occur by chance, as is illustrated by the following three quotations:

Boswell in his *Life of Samuel Johnson* tells us that an acquaintance of Johnson "observed, as something remarkable that had happened to him, that he had chanced to see both No. 1 and No. 1000 of the hackney-coaches, the first and the last." "Why, Sir," said Johnson, "there is an equal chance for one's seeing those two numbers as any other two."

"The chance that a pack of cards shall be dealt in *any* assigned order is the same — less than one in a billion; we suspect a joke or a fraud only if the particular order in which the cards fall suggests design" (Greenwood, 1944).

"The 'one chance in a million' will undoubtedly occur, with no less and no more than its appropriate frequency, however surprised we may be that it should occur to *us*" (Fisher, *The Design of Experiments*, sect. 7).

These statements do not imply that, having met a rare event, we should never seek for causes other than chance; but they show that, however long we may seek, we may not find such causes, because they may not exist. It is well to recall this when we read letters in medical journals recording an unusually high incidence, in the same district at the same time, of a reputedly noninfectious disease such as appendicitis, or reporting the simultaneous occurrence of cancer in two or more unrelated persons in the same household.

Credibility of Interpretations. However much evidence there may appear to be in favor of a certain causal interpretation, we may find ourselves unable to accept the interpretation. As Greenwood (1944) pointed out, if we stuck postage stamps to the beds of some patients (without knowledge of patients or staff) and found that all those patients recovered, whereas all those without stamps died, we would nevertheless not attribute the recovery to the postage stamps, because the relationship would not be credible, or conceivable, or rationally acceptable.

The criterion of credibility can, however, sometimes mislead. For example, when Jenner used cowpox vaccine to protect people from smallpox, his evidence was rejected by some of his contemporaries because it was inconceivable that one disease should protect against a different disease (Greenwood, 1944). The rationality of the method was discovered much later when the viruses of the two diseases were shown to be related.

Multiplicity of Causes. In an abstract form we can describe a cause-

and-effect relationship by an expression such as: "If A, then X; if not A, then not X." Actual phenomena, however, are seldom as simple as this. When a person becomes infected by an organism we think of his illness as due to that organism; but it is due also to his lack of resistance, and this is due partly to environmental factors, including nutrition and numerous events affecting his health in the past.

In pure research we may try to discover all causal factors, but in applied research we commonly choose as the cause of a phenomenon one or two major factors, often those with which we can most easily interfere, in order to prevent or cure disease. There is danger in this, however, because there may be other equally important factors. For example, the spectacular success of bacteriology led us to concentrate on the "seeds" of disease, bacteria, and pay too little attention to the "soil," the patient's constitution, physical and psychologic.

Associated Agents. There is a well known story of a man who got drunk first on scotch and soda, then on brandy and soda, then on rye and soda, and then blamed the soda, ignoring the *associated agent* or *concomitant factor,* alcohol. This fallacy is common in medicine for two reasons:

1. Our ignorance. For example, certain of the benefits of cod liver oil were long attributed to the oil itself, whereas we now know that they are due to vitamins in the oil.

2. The complexity of phenomena. Most clinical treatments comprise many elements, which a clinician cannot study one by one, as would a laboratory worker. A physician can sometimes omit certain elements from his treatment and watch the effect of the rest, but the surgeon can hardly perform a series of "dummy" or partial operations from which various parts of the full operation are omitted.

For our immediate purposes, a wrong explanation of a successful treatment may not matter, but in the long run it may be very misleading. The important thing for an experimenter in any field to remember is that "Treatment A" means the composite of items so labeled.

The associated agent that most commonly misleads the clinician is *the patient's mind.* The psychologic element accounts in many instances for the following phenomena:

1. The success of a certain treatment with some patients although it fails with others. Many patients try to please, or at least to avoid discouraging, their physicians. Others resist his efforts, sometimes because it pays them, either psychologically or financially, not to get better.

2. The failure of a treatment in a certain patient after its initial success.

3. The success of a treatment in the hands of one physician, although it fails in the hands of another.

4. The success of some new and highly advertised remedies.

The risk of our being misled by the psychologic component of therapy is of course the chief reason for the use of placebos in testing drugs. When they are impossible we have to depend on two less reliable methods: (a) "objective" observations, often questionable because we seldom know the extent to which the mind can affect the body; and (b) long-term follow-up, which is useful because a psychologic effect is likely to wear off sooner than a physical effect.

Group Effects. Although an intergroup difference in outcome may be clearly attributable to the difference in treatment applied to the two groups, we must always remember that we are talking about groups. For example, a patient who had improved on the more effective drug A might have improved even more on the less effective drug B; and this is equally true if we have used each drug in succession on all patients in a cross-over design.

Experimental Proof. "In order to assert that a natural phenomenon is experimentally demonstrable we need, not an isolated record, but a reliable method of procedure. In relation to the test of significance, we may say that a phenomenon is experimentally demonstrable when we know how to conduct an experiment which will rarely fail to give us a statistically significant result."

If for the phrase "statistically significant" we substitute a word like "consistent" or "similar" this statement is remarkably like the assertions of some experimenters who distrust "statistical" methods and who repeat their experiments until they are convinced that they know how to produce a particular effect. It may, therefore, be a surprise to them, and also to some devotees of significance testing, to know that the quotation is from *The Design of Experiments* by the statistician who did most to develop and disseminate significance tests, R. A. Fisher (later Sir Ronald Fisher). To those who were directly acquainted with Fisher's attitude to these tests and his close contact with experimenters' problems, the quotation contains no surprise. It would, I think, be fair to express his concept of the function of significance tests as follows. They help us because they enable us to separate two classes of results: (a) those which, from the evidence of the particular investigation, could well be fortuitous; (b) those which would be hard to explain by random processes alone.

Q VI – 17. If the verdict of a test is "not significant" at our predetermined level, what will we do in consequence thereof?

Although we recognize that a verdict of nonsignificance simply means "not proved according to our standard of evidence (our chosen significance level)" we may act as if "not significantly different from" is synonymous with "the same as."

In a clinical trial two drugs may not have differed "significantly" in the features that we have studied. Perhaps we cannot wait for further evidence before using one of the drugs, or perhaps we have concluded that the difference, even if it exists, is probably not great enough to be important. In such cases our choice of drug will sometimes be determined by other considerations. For instance, if only one of the drugs produced undesirable effects, we would prefer the other one. Cost, difficulty of administration, our greater familiarity with the standard drug than with the new one, other people's experience with the new drug — these and other factors may influence our choice. If there were no objection to either drug, we would be likely to choose the one which, in the trial, seemed to be more effective.

An example of another kind of behavior occurred in an investigation of the treatment of traumatic shock during World War II. Dogs were experimentally injured by a certain technique and then 15 of them were kept at an environmental temperature of 95 degrees Fahrenheit, whereas 10 were "cooled to an equivalent degree." Of the warmed animals 11 (73 per cent) died; of the cooled animals only 4 (40 per cent) died. Pure random assignment of the 15 deaths among 15 animals labeled "A" and 10 animals labeled "B" would produce in about 20 per cent of the randomization experiments differences equal to and greater than those found in the actual experiment. In other words, the difference was far from significant at the 5 per cent level, because P was about 0.2. That is, if we accept the observed difference as indicative of something more than a random process, we are adopting a standard that would lead us to follow something like 20 per cent of false clues.

The investigators actually took that risk, although apparently unaware of it because the report did not mention a significance test. With a larger number of dogs they obtained clear evidence of the benefit of cooling. Therefore, disregard of the risk in this case was justified. Disregard of such risks, i.e., the acceptance of a lower standard of significance than usual, is always legitimate provided that the reason is well defined. The actual reason here is unknown, but it might be one or more of the following:

1. The possession of some other knowledge of the physiologic effects of cooling that would agree with, or explain, the observed difference.

2. The ease with which a larger experiment could be done.

3. The fact that if cooling did reduce mortality, it might be very important in treating human shock.

4. The large size of the difference, $73 - 40 = 33$ per cent. This apparently impressed the investigators, because when they first announced it they did not even mention the sample sizes. Such frequency differences are often impressive to laboratory workers who are used to small percentage errors in measurement data.

Q VI – 18. What will make us decide to terminate the experiment?

Fixed Sample Sizes. In the experiments discussed so far, the sample sizes are fixed in advance. When we have reached these numbers of subjects and apply an appropriate test to our results we know our Type I error. During the experiment, however, even if there is no real difference in the effect of the treatments under test, we nearly always observe fluctuations in the data. Sometimes one treatment seems to be favored and sometimes the other, just as if we had cards, some marked "S" and some marked "F," in a well shuffled set and turned them up one by one.

Let us suppose that as the experiment proceeds we get the impression that a treatment difference is emerging, that we then apply a significance test and find that P is less than 0.05. That result has no meaning with reference to our data. We have analyzed the samples, accumulated up to that point, as if they were strictly random samples, whereas we have in fact chosen them because of their contents. If we do this we will obtain far too many "statistically significant" differences in our experiments.

Indeed, we can obtain as many "significant" differences as we wish if we are willing to go on trying. This can be shown by using cards or random numbers as "subjects" of the "experiments," or by an arithmetical lay-out that represents the behavior of a random process. In these experiments there is no difference between the "treatments"; they are merely labels such as A and B. We make it a rule to stop the "experiment" whenever we have reached a verdict of "significant" at any predetermined level (e.g., 0.05), but to continue to use more "subjects" (cards or numbers) whenever we have not reached that level.

By this procedure we could reach a verdict of "significant" in all our experiments. Some of the experiments would be exceedingly long; but the spurious verdicts can start whenever a laboratory worker uses the "try, try, try again" method. Having found that the first batch of animals does not give a statistically significant difference, he adds a few more animals. If the verdict is still "not significant" he adds still more animals, and tests again.

Perhaps the damage done by this misuse of significance tests is not tremendous, because the investigator often gets tired after three or four tries. His true risk of Type I error may be about 10 per cent, instead of less than 5 per cent, as he thinks it is. The point is that his actual risk of error depends upon his impulse or whim in each individual experiment. This is one of the many ways in which the use of statistical tests in laboratory and clinical research makes the vaunted claims of precision for statistical techniques rather ludicrous; and the blame, I think, lies largely with those of us who have produced books of elementary statistics.

There is, of course, another danger in stopping an experiment because of the results that are emerging. If we have an impression that no difference between treatment groups is appearing and then we apply a test, we run the risk of having too many "nonsignificant" differences, when in fact a real difference in treatment effect is present.

These warnings do not imply that we must deprive ourselves of the right to stop an experiment whenever we wish, in view of what appears to be coming out of it, especially in relation to other knowledge that we possess, or because we see disadvantages in continuing it — for example, an excessive number of undesirable effects in a drug trial. It simply means that if we intend to play the "significance testing game" we must obey the rules. The sample size must be determined by something unrelated to the data that it is producing, unless we use the "sequential design" discussed below.

Samples Determined by Amount of Material and Time. In order to perform a fixed-sample-size experiment, suitable to give us an estimate of error risk at the end, we do not need to specify in advance the actual sample size. We can decide to put into the experiment all suitable subjects available during a certain period of time. The danger in this plan is, however, that the intake of subjects may be speeded up or slowed down as a result of the figures that emerge during the experiment. For example, a physician who sees no exciting difference between the effects of two drugs in a clinical trial may relax his efforts to secure suitable patients.

The Sequential Design. This method is much more akin to the experimenter's centuries-old step-by-step procedure than is the fixed-sample-size method, but it has been only recently developed as a systematic design, and it is still undergoing changes. When it was devised during World War II, it was for a time an official secret, because in the testing of materials and processes it enabled verdicts to be obtained from smaller samples, and therefore more quickly, than did fixed-sample-size methods. In many drug evaluations, a decision based on the fewest possible patients is desirable for ethical as well as economic reasons.

The distinction between the sequential design and the traditional step-by-step method of experimenters is that the sequential method enables us to set in advance our Type I and Type II errors, whereas the old method does not allow us to estimate our error risks either before or after the experiment. The sequential design does not graft the fixed-sample-size significance tests illegitimately on to the step-by-step method, but provides decision rules of its own. These rules are developed by complicated mathematical techniques, but that need not disturb us, provided that we know three things:

1. What the method tells us in terms of the random sampling of disks from a barrel.
2. The difference between our experimental circumstances and the disks in the barrel.
3. The limitations of the sequential method in medical research.

In Chapter XVI (sect. 3) is an example of the rules for a sequential experiment, and their implications in terms of random sampling are discussed. Here we look at the general procedure, as exemplified by a drug trial.

Sequential Drug Trials. We have randomly assigned patients to treatments A and B. When the result from the first patient comes in we hold it until we can pair it with the first result from a patient on the other drug. We then compare these two with respect to the measurement of drug effect that we have decided upon, the change in a certain variable since the pretreatment examination. If both patients show the same amount and direction of change they tell us nothing about the difference in drug effect if one exists, and we discard that pair. If we assess the patients broadly as "better," "worse" or "no detectable change," we may have many such "tied pairs." (The pairing does not imply initial matching, but this can be done if there is a good reason for it, and if it is feasible, e.g., if in an animal experiment litter mates are available.)

Each "untied" pair shows evidence that it is apparently in favor of A or of B. If the first pair shows an A-preference we can count it as a score of $+1$. If the second untied pair, obtained in the same way, also shows an A-preference, the score becomes $+2$; but if it shows a B-preference the net score is zero. We proceed in this way, and for each number of untied pairs the rules tell us whether (1) we have accumulated a large enough (plus or minus) score to say that A is significantly better (or worse) than B, or (2) the score is so small that we can pronounce a verdict of "no significant difference," or (3) we must continue the experiment.

Some Drawbacks of the Sequential Design. Before deciding to use a sequential design we must find out how much we are likely to save, in sample size, by doing so (see Chapter XVI); but even a great potential saving may not compensate for the disadvantages of the method. The principal drawbacks can be expressed in terms of a clinical trial, but translation into terms of any other kind of experiment will be obvious.

1. The original type of sequential design is "open-ended," i.e., although it usually requires smaller samples than the fixed-sample-size design, the experiment may continue indefinitely without reaching a verdict of either "significant" or "not significant." Modifications, called "restricted" or "closed" designs, have therefore been devised. Their minimal sample-size requirements are not as low as those of the open-ended design, but in using them we always know at the beginning the maximum sample size that may be necessary. Such knowledge is often very desirable in drug evaluation.

2. The sequential design is of no use unless the period of treatment of the individual subject is very short compared with the total length of the experiment. In a clinical trial if the treatment lasts only 2 or 3 days we can withhold patients until we have obtained definite results from the first dozen or more; but if the therapy has to last 6 months all available patients may have been admitted before the first few have completed their period of treatment.

3. A sequential experiment is intended to answer the specific question for which it is set up. If in addition we desire answers to some questions about other variables, and if those variables are closely related to the variable on which the sequential experiment was based, we will obtain too high "significance" estimates. We have decided to stop the experiment because of the result shown by the primary variable. Therefore, if we now treat the samples as in a fixed-sample-size experiment for comparison of other closely related variables, we commit the error already discussed in the section on Fixed Sample Sizes.

4. Whether sample size is predetermined or determined sequentially, a small sample contains less information than a large sample. Regarding the sequential design, a clinical investigator has written: "It seems to me unlikely to supplant completely the large-scale therapeutic trial. . . . When a new treatment is introduced for an important disease, assuming the treatment is not such a radical advance as to make formal testing unnecessary, there are several advantages in making a big study. First, . . . a big study permits of analysis to show the scope of the treatment within the disease. Secondly, a big study is often an advantage in permitting one to take stock of secondary aspects, such as complications of the new therapy, which may be of great importance" (Truelove in *Medical Surveys and Clinical Trials*, edited by Witts).

Q VI – 19. Are we going to make more than one comparison in the same data? If so, are significance tests legitimate?

We can look at two kinds of multiple comparisons: (1) Comparisons suggested by the data, (2) Preplanned comparisons.

Comparisons Suggested by the Data. Let us suppose that we had a set of cards representing treated patients, some cards marked "S" (Success) and others "F" (Failure), that we shuffled them and then marked half of them "male" and the other half "female" without regard to their S and F marks, then shuffled again and marked half of them "young" and half of them "old," then shuffled again and marked half of them "treated early" and half of them "treated late," then reshuffled them and marked half of them "sedentary work" and the other half "heavy work," then reshuffled them and marked half of them "brown eyes" and the other half "blue eyes," and so on, through many contrasts.

If we recorded the results after each shuffling we would sometimes find that many of the F's had been thrown into one class and few into the other class. If we applied a "significance" test in those instances we would find in some, or perhaps in all of them, a verdict of "significant" at the 5 per cent level, or even at a higher level. Indeed, we ought to expect 5 per cent of such shufflings to give such a verdict, because that is what "significant at the 5 per cent level" really means.

And so, if we make comparisons in any set of real data we can always expect to find some that are significant, even if there is no real association between the dependent and independent variables. If we pick out for testing only those differences that appear striking, we may find every time a "significant" difference. The real value of searching for big contrasts lies in the discovery of hypotheses to be tested by a new investigation. When we have the results of that investigation we must, of course, present them separately from the data that gave us the hint. If we pooled the new data with the first data, and tested the combined data, our test would be spurious. The samples would not be random but selected because of part of their contents, the part contributed by the first data.

Preplanned Comparisons. In a trial of streptomycin plus bed-rest against bed-rest alone, pulmonary tuberculosis patients were not divided into groups according to temperature (as an index of activity) at the beginning of the trial (Medical Research Council, 1948); but from the outset the investigators planned to divide the data into several initial-temperature groups in order to compare patients' progress in the different groups and also to see whether the streptomycin versus bed-rest contrast differed according to the initial activity of the disease. In such comparisons, if the relationships of the dependent variables (e.g., change in the patients' condition) and the independent variables (e.g., initial temperature) were purely fortuitous, no more than the usual 5 per cent of the comparisons would in the long run yield P values of 0.05 or less.

In clinical trials several measures of effect are commonly used — for example, in rheumatoid arthritis, strength of hand grip, number of painful joints, time required to walk 50 feet, and other measures. It is very unsafe to assume that these provide independent evidence of the effect of a drug on the phenomena that cause the symptoms or disabilities. Indeed, if there were perfect correlation among the measures of change, e.g., if an increase in grip strength of 40 mm. of mercury always accompanied a reduction in the number of painful joints by 10 and a reduction of 2 seconds in the walking time, a "significant" difference in any one of these measures would always be accompanied by a "significant" difference in the others. And yet all of these differences between the treatment groups might be due to the one, rather uncommon, random allocation of patients to therapies.

Although perfect correlation between the measures of change does not exist, some degree of relationship is commonly present, and allowance can, in part at least, be made for it. For example, we can ask: "If there were no drug-placebo difference in the change of grip strength, does it appear that there would be a drug-placebo difference in the change in numbers of painful joints?" Such questions are seldom of great concern in a drug trial; but in other experiments they may lead to important discoveries.

Q VI – 20. If we are comparing more than two treatments, how may significance tests mislead us?

It often seems desirable to compare, in one experiment, three or more treatments, each on a separate group of subjects. If we compare A with B, A with C, and B with C, with 20 animals in each treatment-group, it would seem that we can obtain three answers from 60 animals, whereas if we made the comparisons in three separate experiments we would require 120 animals. However, the matter is not so simple.

Comparison of Extremes.   First let us consider an experiment in which there is no natural grouping of the treatments, such as there would be if A and B were drugs, with C a placebo, or if A and B were chemicals of similar composition, with C differing in some specific way from both of them. Let us suppose that the results (e.g., percentage frequencies or average values) show the largest difference between A and B, with C intermediate in value. If we select the A-B difference, apply a two-sample test and pronounce the difference "significant" because P is less than 0.05, our verdict will be spurious. We are not comparing random samples but samples selected because of their contents. Our action is something like picking the winner *after* seeing a horse race. No one would accept our bet, but we may win acceptance for our significance-test verdict if we submit our report to the right journal.

The first thing to do in such a multiple-treatment comparison is to look at the intergroup variation as a whole and ask: "How often does a randomization like the one used in this experiment produce as large intergroup differences as this?" There are tests that help us to answer this question, and they are mentioned in Chapter XII (frequency data) and Chapter XIV (measurement data).

If we decide that the intergroup variation is not "significant" according to our standard, this may be all that we wish to know; or we may wish to pursue an interesting apparent difference in the data and devise another experiment to test its genuineness. If, however, we find that the intergroup variation meets our standard of "significance," we naturally ask: "Which treatments differ from which other treatments in their effects?" This kind of question is not easy to answer. Professional statisticians have proposed several different answers — different methods of analysis — and have, of course, argued with each other about them. Therefore, the rest of us should be chary of using any of the proposed methods. Each method may be correct in the circumstances, and with the assumptions, postulated by its proponent, but in biologic and medical research we often know little of the circumstances beyond what we see in front of us, and we often do not know what assumptions are valid.

If we have decided that the intergroup variation is "significant" and if we have to act on the result of the one experiment (e.g., to choose one therapy out of three or more), our "best bet," although we cannot attach a "probability" to it, is to assume that the most extreme difference represents a real difference. Here we are acting on the principle that a sample is more likely to be near to the center of its population than to be far off the center. We can trust this principle best if our samples are large, because a big difference between small samples can be less real than a smaller difference between larger samples.

All Possible Comparisons.   The suggestion that, for purposes of action, attention be confined to the extreme differences hardly satisfies someone who has put three or more treatments into his experiment, expecting to obtain a definite statement about each treatment. Having learned some simple two-sample tests, he may proceed to test each treatment against every other treatment in turn. Perhaps we can see the danger in this method if we imagine that someone takes a strictly random sample of the statures of the men in a certain city, and then compares it with random samples of men's statures from half a dozen other cities, one sample per city.

Let us suppose that the populations of all seven cities are actually identical with respect to men's statures, but that the investigator obtained from his first city a rather rare type of random sample, i.e., one whose average stature differs greatly from the true average of that city. He may then find "significant" differences between this sample's average and the averages in the samples from each of the other cities. He will, at least find P values that are smaller than what he would find if he had obeyed the rules that make the significance test valid, i.e., if he had taken a fresh random sample from the first city every time that he compared it with another city. Clearly, the same kind of thing can happen in a multiple treatment-comparison.

Multiple Intergroup Differences. In a comparison of three or more treatments (A, B, C . . .) a verdict of "significant intergroup variation" does not tell us a great deal. It justifies our belief that, if we could find (or build up) the corresponding treatment populations, we would discover that two or more of them actually differed with respect to the variable that we are studying; but this could be true in a number of different ways. The A, B and C populations might all differ from each other, or A and B might be identical but differ from C, or B and C might be identical but differ from A. In any of these situations the variety of combinations of possible population values might be infinite, so far as we can tell from our actual samples. Usually, therefore, if we wish to define more clearly the individual treatment differences after a multiple comparison of the type discussed here, we must perform more experiments.

We can proceed a little farther in the kind of experiment in which treatments A and B are alike in a certain respect and differ in that respect from treatment C, e.g., two drugs versus a placebo. In the analysis we start with a comparison of A and B. If they do not differ significantly we can pool their data and compare with the data from C — provided that we realize clearly what we are doing. In effect, we are saying: "We are not convinced that there is a difference between the effects of A and B. If A and B were actually equal in their effects, would this experiment indicate that C differed from them?"

It is important to realize that once we have used the information from our experiment in the analysis just described, if we use it over again to make some more comparisons (e.g., A versus C, or B versus C) we run into the same danger as in the imaginary stature-survey of the seven cities.

Let us suppose now that a test has shown that A and B differ significantly (A greater than B) and that the value (e.g., average) for C is lower than that for B. It seems appropriate to compare B with C and accept a verdict of "significant." If, however, the verdict is "not significant," we should realize that this verdict and the "A-B significant" verdict may have been due to the same cause. The effects of A and B may not actually differ, and both may differ from C, but the randomization may have, as it were, pushed the B-sample so far below the A-sample that it came near to the C-sample.

All these possible interpretations after multiple treatment-comparisons, of the kinds discussed here, are rather frustrating. The method does not carry one as far as might be expected. Factorial designs (Q IV – 8) carry us much farther.

Q VI – 21. How will we estimate what our results really tell us, numerically, about the population represented by our sample?

This question recalls the quandary discussed under Q III – 9. On the one hand, unless our sample of animals, patients or other sampling units is a strictly random sample of its population, we cannot derive from it a population-value estimate that has known reliability, i.e., an estimate with a known risk of error. On the other hand, in most medical research we cannot obtain strictly random samples of the populations to which we desire to apply our results; or, if we do possess samples that are close enough to random samples for our purpose, we do not know that they are. And yet we badly need to know how far we may be misled if we accept our sample estimates at their face value.

The Problem of Nonrandom Samples. In the Medical Research Council's (1948) 6-month clinical trial, comparing the treatment of pulmonary tuberculosis by bed-rest alone with the treatment by bed-rest plus streptomycin, there was a difference in outcome (statistically significant at the 5 per cent level) in the mortality (case fatality rates): 14 of the 52 purely bed-rest patients died, but of the 55 patients who received streptomycin only 4 died. No one would deny the clinical importance of this difference, but the next question should be: "What do the 4 deaths in 55 streptomycin-treated patients (7.3 per cent) tell us about the case fatality rate that would be found in a large population represented by these streptomycin-treated patients?" More precisely, we should say: "What case fatality rate might be approached if more and more of this kind of patient were treated in the same way?"

The basic features of the population are given by the description of the sample: patients of both sexes between the ages of 15 and 30 years inclusive, with bilateral pulmonary tuberculosis, bacteriologically proved and unsuitable for treatment by collapse of the lung (e.g., by introducing air into the pleural cavity). The definition was further restricted by the fact that the trial was conducted at seven specified hospitals in the United Kingdom during the year 1947. We would make the definition much more specific by adding many of the details recorded in the report, such as temperature on admission; but we would still have no absolute assurance that the 55 observed streptomycin-treated patients would be equivalent, for the estimation of possible error, to a strictly random sample of a population so defined. Indeed there was no such population, because during the period of the trial it was stipulated that all eligible patients at the seven centers be enrolled in it.

The 1948 and 1949 samples from the same centers and defined in the same way might indeed differ from the 1947 sample by more than random differences, i.e., they might represent different populations; but if such a possibility prohibited any sort of estimate from the 1947 sample it should by the same reasoning have prohibited the clinical trial itself, and it would prohibit most other clinical trials and many other kinds of experiments. The streptomycin investigators clearly refused to be blocked in this way, because they knew that the disease and other circumstances in chronic pulmonary tuberculosis do not change so greatly from one year to the next as to stultify their 1947 experiment.

Random Processes in Sample Formation. The more specifically we describe our sample, by race, sex, age, condition at start of therapy, strain of organism in certain diseases, and by other major factors that influence a patient's progress, the nearer we come to a situation in which the differences in outcome between successive samples, so defined and treated alike, are due to random processes, i.e., the action of a number of factors that are independent of each other. Some of the patients in the 55 who received streptomycin would be, from the start, likely to do well and others unlikely to do well, for reasons not yet discoverable by any method of investigation; but the presence of each patient in the sample of 55 would be determined by a combination of circumstances stretching far back in his own and his ancestors' history, a different combination for each patient. This reminds us of the mixing of disks in a barrel during a random sampling experiment.

We next visualize the patients in the hospital during the trial, subject to many forces, independent of the state of their tuberculosis and independent of each other. One patient cannot "stomach" the hospital food. Another reacts in the same way to a certain nurse. A third patient finds both delectable. We add to this picture a virus that produces an attack of influenza in one patient but leaves another unscathed, regardless of their attitudes to food or nurses. Then we add a physician who is very perceptive and skillful in attending to even minor elements in patient care, and another physician who is less so. We could continue to add factors indefinitely, each of which could contribute a little to help or hinder a patient's response to the streptomycin. Some patients would receive mostly helpful factors, others mostly hindering factors; many would receive mixtures of both kinds. Again we are picturing a more or less random process.

The streptomycin investigators could therefore have said: "Unless we trust, provisionally, the uniformity of Nature we can get nowhere in drug evaluation. Let us assume that there were no major differences between our group of 55 patients and other groups at other times and in other places. Even so, there would be differences due to random processes, because random processes are part of the uniformity of Nature. Let us find out how much or how little our 7.3 per cent case fatality rate in 55 patients would tell us if random processes were the only cause of intersample differences."

Systematic Differences. In this imaginary quotation the phrase "no major differences" is too indefinite to be synonymous with "purely random differences." The phrase "no systematic differences" is preferable. "Systematic" is used here in the same sense as when we speak of the systematic difference between two instruments designed to measure the same thing. We estimate its size by paired readings on the same material, one reading by each instrument; but the reading difference is not necessarily the same in all the pairs, because fluctuations of the instruments and observer can occur. We increase the precision of our estimate by taking the average difference from more and more pairs.

A systematic difference that would nullify the streptomycin data of 1947 would be the presence in subsequent years of patients whose tubercle bacilli were resistant to streptomycin, a phenomenon that has occurred during the use of many antibiotics. To translate the "systematic difference" into the terms of a disk-sampling experiment, when we first start sampling we can imagine that 10 per cent of the disks in our barrel are marked "D" (death) and 90 per cent "S" (survival). After a while somebody, unknown to us, slips into the barrel a batch of disks of which 40 per cent are marked "D." Our subsequent samples, although still strictly random, will be affected to a greater or less extent by the systematic change in the population.

Estimates of Population Values.   The disk-sampling experiment would provide the streptomycin investigators with the most useful form of question regarding the reliability of their sample: "If our sample of 55 streptomycin-treated patients, containing 4 deaths (7.3 per cent) were a strictly random sample of its population, what would it tell us about the percentage mortality in the population."

We could find the answer to this question experimentally. For example, we could put in a barrel several thousand disks, of which 20 per cent were marked "D," and take a thousand random samples of 55 disks. If we found that samples of 55 containing 4 D's or fewer were "rare" by our definition of the term, e.g., if they comprised fewer than 5 per cent (or 2.5 or 1 per cent) of the total samples, we would conclude that the mortality in a population randomly represented by the streptomycin-treated sample was unlikely to be as high as 20 per cent. Then we could do another sampling experiment on a population containing 15 per cent D's. If we found that 4 deaths in 55 was not in the "rare" class of sample from that population, we would accept 15 per cent mortality as a possible value.

Then we could take a number of other populations, working up from 15 per cent and down from 20 per cent, until we discovered a boundary or limit between the population percentages that we would reject as unlikely and those that we would accept as possible. Chapter XI shows that we do not need to perform the experiments with actual disks, because we can do them on paper by using the binomial expansion, and that even that labor is seldom necessary, because tables such as our Table I give direct answers about limits of population values. For example, if we use 2.5 per cent as our standard of rarity in random sampling, the answer to the streptomycin investigators' question is: The percentage mortality in a population randomly represented by a sample of 55 with 4 deaths (7.3 per cent) might lie anywhere between 2 per cent and 17 per cent. (The estimation of population values from samples of measurement data is discussed in Chapter XIII.)

Such estimates, made after any observation, are minimum estimates of our present ignorance because they allow only for random sampling variation. If, when we use our present estimate later on, there is also a systematic difference from the present conditions, the new population value may be far outside the limits that we have now estimated. But even our present minimal estimate of error is often very valuable. It may show that even at its best under present conditions a certain therapy would not be very effective; or that even at its worst it would be better than the therapy that we have hitherto employed. Often the chief value of the estimate is that it reveals how little our sample has told us.

Q VI – 22. Is a "null hypothesis" an appropriate concept for our experiment?

After a long chapter with the null hypothesis as its principal text, this seems to be a rather belated question. It has been delayed because it is necessary to see the implications of the null hypothesis before considering its applicability in particular cases. We can look at two types of cases: treatment comparisons and the study of observer and instrument differences.

Treatment Comparisons. It must be admitted that we seldom start an experiment with a completely open mind as to whether a particular hypothesis is or is not true. We often start a drug trial because the drug (or perhaps a relative of it) has apparently shown "promising" results in a few patients or animals. Our original hypothesis, therefore, might be that the difference in percentage of S's in an A-treated population would exceed the percentage of S's in a B-treated population by at least 20 percentage points. We could, however, test this by setting up a null hypothesis that the true difference was just below 20, say 19 percentage points. We could demonstrate, by a method based on the random sampling of disks from a barrel, how often various sample differences would occur if the 19 per cent hypothesis were true. We could classify as "rare" the largest differences (e.g., the upper 5 per cent), and then we would find out whether the A-B difference in our drug experiment was so large that it would be in the "rare" class. If it were so large we would reject the null hypothesis.

There are many such situations in which we can use our past experience, intuitions or convictions in the framing of a suitable null hypothesis; but we naturally ask: "Is there not some way in which we can express quantitatively our belief, based on previous experience, that a certain hypothesis is true (or false) and then combine it with a probability value that we derive from our experiment?"

Statisticians also have asked such questions, but the results so far have been chiefly rival theories. They are attempts to set inductive inference — the process by which we develop new knowledge — on a rational foundation, and to make it more efficient. Mathematical models are developed, containing such quantities as "prior probabilities" and "likelihoods." They necessarily involve assumptions and simplifications — exclusion of many of the complexities of the real world. To this in itself there can be no objection, because all mathematical models, such as $2 + 2 = 4$, are abstractions. The great distinction between the simple-addition model and the models proposed for inductive inference seems to be that we have learned by experience where the simple-addition model is applicable, what it does for us in the real world. Until proponents of theories of inductive inference ("statistical inference") can propose also some way of properly testing the theories in the real world, an investigator need not feel guilty if he disregards them, unless he is called upon to help in testing them.

Observer and Instrument Differences. Some workers who are, very rightly, concerned about problems of instrument differences and observer differences make careful studies of these. For example, two observers may make repeated blood pressure readings on a number of subjects, each observer using the same two sphygmomanometers. Unfortunately, however, they sometimes analyze their data by "significance" tests, i.e., they set up null hypotheses (no interobserver difference, no difference between instruments) and test them. One might say that they are thereby asking questions to which we all know the answers. Being acquainted with the material world, we have no doubt that any two instruments of the same kind, even of the highest quality and possessing Bureau of Standards certificates, would be found to differ in their readings of the same thing if we tested them very minutely. Being acquainted with human beings, we need not stipulate very minute testing in order to reveal the differences.

What we ought to be concerned about in such studies of differences is not statistical significance but practical significance, i.e., the importance of the differences in the work that the observers and the instruments are to perform. How much variation and bias can these differences introduce, and particularly how will they compare in magnitude with other variation, e.g., between subjects? Obviously, the closer we can come to exploring these questions under actual working conditions the better. In clinical research this may be difficult; but it is very unsafe to trust the transference to a working situation of the results obtained from a study conducted under artificial conditions. Such a study may be useful as a first step, but no more.

CHAPTER VII

INTERPRETATION AFTER A SURVEY

The term "survey" here as elsewhere in this book does not imply large samples. Most of the everyday clinical researches are surveys in whole or in part. The term includes also what may be called "pseudo-experiments," in which appropriate randomization has not been used or in which the randomization has not been solely responsible for the bias throughout the experiment. The difficulties and uncertainties of survey methods have been discussed at many points in previous chapters. Even in Chapter VI (Interpretation after an Experiment) most of the ideas (e.g., the null hypothesis) and certain of the methods (e.g., reduction of bias by blindfold observation when possible) are equally appropriate to experiments and surveys.

This chapter discusses some survey problems not previously mentioned. It is concerned chiefly with surveys that attempt to throw light on causal relationships, and not so much with the record-keeping type of survey that is useful for the production of a revised description of a disease or for administrative planning. The discussion will no doubt seem discouraging or skeptical, and it may be discounted by some readers as an experimenter's jaundiced view of survey methods. This view is, however, shared by a number of medical statisticians who are well versed in survey techniques. One of them expressed his feelings in the following way: "I have been teaching these techniques for years, and trusting them. Now I have discovered that the survey method is a very blunt instrument."

Q VII – 1. What is the most obvious risk in a cause-and-effect interpretation after a survey?

The "Post Hoc" Fallacy. If by conducting a survey we have found an association between two variables and then we accept this association, by itself, as proof of a causal relationship, we commit the fallacy of *post hoc ergo propter hoc* — "after this, *therefore* because of this" — sometimes more appropriately expressed as *cum hoc* (with this) *ergo propter hoc.*

111

This fallacy is perhaps the commonest fallacy in medicine, as well as in our everyday discussions of all kinds of phenomena, from economic depressions to the best way of making coffee. The first step toward avoiding the danger is of course the use of "controls," i.e., contrast-samples — to see whether, when "this" does not happen, "that" does not happen. But contrast-samples are not sure preventives, because "this" may in Nature and in human affairs be closely associated with something else that is the real cause of "that."

Statisticians in public health have long been aware that much of the evidence that apparently supported immunization against infectious diseases may be spurious because it has been of the "post hoc" type. In an epidemic, immunized persons have escaped more frequently than those who had not been immunized, but this may have been because more of the nonimmunized lived in slums where infection spreads easily, or because those who take care to be immunized take other precautions also, such as the avoidance of crowded places during an epidemic. It is only very recently that medical workers outside of public health, and members of the general public, have begun to realize that the only way to avoid this dilemma is a properly planned and conducted experiment.

Q VII – 2. What is the essential difference, with regard to causal interpretation, between a survey and an experiment in the strict sense?

As previously emphasized, interpretation after an experiment takes the "either-or" form — either the randomization alone or the randomization plus the factor under test. After a survey there are three possible causes of an observed difference: (1) random processes, (2) the factor under test, and (3) biases not solely due to random processes. In other words, after an experiment we can go beyond the proof of an association between two variables to a proof of cause, in the sense that we can attach to our causal inference an estimate of error — the frequency with which the observed effects are produced by randomization alone. In a survey we cannot go beyond proof of an association, because our error term is unknown — we cannot state the "probability" of *hidden* biases.

Hidden Biases. To obtain a sense of our ignorance of the numbers and magnitude of the hidden biases, let us suppose that we are planning a survey, retrospective, cross-sectional or prospective, in the search for a causal factor in a certain disease (X). With sufficient subjects, we might make our contrasting groups (A and B) alike with respect to all factors known or suspected to influence the occurrence of X, except the factor under test (A); but we should remember that factors previously hidden are continually being discovered — biochemical, genetic, environmental and psychologic factors — associated with the pathologic and other phenomena that we study. At any time a factor now hidden may be discovered — for example, F, a factor so closely related to X that, if we knew about it now, we would no more think of mixing the F's and not-F's in our study-samples than we think of mixing, say, children and adults in most studies of disease today. Indeed, there are likely to be many

F's. Causation in medicine is like an iceberg, mostly hidden from view, but we often behave as if what we can see is all that matters, and we disregard the submerged mass that may wreck our causal inferences.

Q VII – 3.   Are we going to apply a statistical significance test after our survey? If so, what will it tell us?

Significance tests after surveys can be very dangerous. If a group of heavy smokers and a group of nonsmokers are followed for 5 years and there is a higher mortality among the heavy smokers than among the nonsmokers, with a P value of 0.0001 attached to the difference, this does not in the least indicate that the difference in smoking habits was the cause. And yet in many surveys large and small, in medicine, sociology, psychology and elsewhere, P values have been so misinterpreted.

Because of such dangers some investigators now condemn the use of significance tests in surveys; but there is this much to be said for the tests. If there are many possible associations in the material that we are studying and we wish to follow the apparently promising clues by further studies, perhaps of different types, a significance test can be a great time-saver. An alternative method might be to follow only those differences that were greater than so much (say, 20 percentage points); but significance tests offer the advantage that they take sample size into account. However, background knowledge and insight are commonly more useful guides than any automatic rule based on a test.

Verdicts of "highly significant" should be viewed with special caution. When I see a survey-research P value containing three or more zeros, if the difference under study has not been fairly obvious before the study I am inclined to suspect the influence of selection factors in the sampling, or some hidden bias in the observational methods.

Q VII – 4.   What will be the logic of our inference after a survey?

The logic of many surveys can be described as reasoning from circumstantial evidence. Therefore it is well to remember that in courts of law sometimes all the circumstances have pointed to the guilt of the accused, until some little fact has been unearthed and has set him free. Sometimes this important fact has not been found until after he has been imprisoned or executed.

General Guidelines. Although in a survey we cannot, as in an experiment, make causal inferences with specified risk of error based on knowledge of random processes, it would be very useful if we had rules of procedure for the conducting of surveys, and for reasoning from the data, that would insure that a certain specified percentage of our total surveys would give correct verdicts. There are no such rules. All that we can say regarding procedure is that we presumably stand the best chance of success if we (1) follow as closely as possible the methods of good experimentation, and (2) test the same hypothesis in as many different ways as possible.

This does not mean repeating the same procedure on similar groups of subjects under similar conditions. It means thinking out various consequences of the same hypothesis and exploring each one, as does a clever detective. As a simple example, in large-scale studies a prospective survey and a retrospective survey may help to support each other because, although both contain biases, some of the biases differ in the two methods. Mere repetition of the same procedure on similar groups is like the method of building up clinical knowledge that was stigmatized by a physician who said: "We make the same mistake a thousand times and call it clinical experience."

The Nature of Association. In the interpretation of survey results it might hardly seem necessary to mention that, if there is truly an association between A and X, A may be the cause of X, or X may be the cause of A, or both may have a common cause. And yet this concept was apparently unfamiliar to a physician who brought to a statistician some figures which showed very clearly that, in fatal cases of a certain disease, the higher the doses of penicillin the greater was the prolongation of life. Inquiry revealed, however, that it was the physician's standard procedure with all cases of that disease to increase the dose of penicillin progressively until recovery or death.

In some instances the only connecting link between A and X is *the passage of time.* A number of infectious diseases (measles, scarlet fever and others) are much milder than they were at the beginning of this century, and this is counted by some people as one of the triumphs of modern medicine. They apparently do not know that the decline started long before artificial immunization and antibiotics were available.

Graded Trust in Surveys. Even rather superficial contemplation reveals some of the factors that determine the readiness and strength of our acceptance of survey evidence regarding causal relationships. These factors include:

1. The speed with which X follows A.
2. The high degree of association — if A, always (or very commonly) X; if not A, never (or very seldom) X.
3. The simplicity, directness and reliability of the evidence.
4. The plausibility of a causal connection and the absence of any other equally plausible explanation — a rather shaky foundation for belief.

Surveys that search for causes of disease differ from each other greatly with respect to these four factors. The famous investigation by which the London physician John Snow traced an outbreak of cholera in 1854 to the Broad Street pump provided immediate, abundant, simple and (as it now appears to us who know about the water-borne *Vibrio cholerae*) very plausible evidence (Mackintosh, 1955; Hill, 1953, 1955).*

---

* It is interesting to note that the story of the Broad Street pump, as it is usually told, terminates by improving on truth with fiction. Even an exceptionally well informed and critical microbiologist, addressing the public, wrote that Snow "controlled the outbreak by the mere artifice of removing the handle from the pump." As Snow himself pointed out, the cholera mortality had, from unknown causes, decreased greatly before the handle was removed (Hill, 1955). This is worth remembering when we propose, or read about, an "experimental confirmation" of an inference drawn by epidemiologic (survey) methods.

The detection of the source of some particular physical disorder in a certain job in an industry does not usually entail much debate about possible biases. And if, having spotted and removed the apparent cause, the investigators find that the disorder disappears, they do not worry about the "post hoc" fallacy.

By contrast, the recent surveys relating smoking to lung cancer, and various studies of the causation of cardiovascular disease, have raised doubts regarding interpretation, largely because the first three factors listed above did not have compelling force. For very valuable discussions of research methods in both these fields, reference should be made to *Medical Surveys and Clinical Trials* (Witts).* Instead of discussing them here we can look at a project that at the outset appeared much simpler.

In a proposed study of exposure to x-rays as a possible cause of leukemia, radiologists employed in the Armed Services during World War II were to be followed for perhaps two decades after the end of the war. Other doctors in the Services at the same time were to form the contrast-sample. In a population of war veterans, difficulties of follow-up are much less than in other groups; but other difficulties quickly presented themselves: (1) In two decades many things can happen, including exposure to other leukemia-causing factors, whatever they may be. (2) The low incidence of leukemia would require large numbers of subjects. (3) Although presumably radiologists would in general be more exposed to radiation than other doctors, the amount of exposure could be only guessed at, and some of them might have had very little. (4) Although the causal connection between radiation and leukemia was plausible, it was also quite conceivable that some doctors, less physically robust than others, had chosen radiology as a profession in order to avoid excessive strain. What the connection between physique and cancer might be, we do not know; but in our vast ignorance we cannot afford to ignore the possibility.

Emotions and Proofs. In a book entitled *Epidemics and Crowd Diseases,* published in 1935, the late Professor Major Greenwood wrote as follows regarding artificial immunization: "Honourable and able men have differed passionately in their opinions of these methods; vaccination against smallpox has been blessed and blamed with theological vehemence; more modern applications of this principle have been defended and attacked with equal fury. The reader and I are of course greatly influenced by this emotional atmosphere. No intelligent person supposes that logic determines practical issues . . ." (Greenwood, quoted from Brit. Med. J. Editorial, 1962).

Even after a therapeutic or prophylactic trial, involving randomization, double-blind procedure and vigilance throughout the experiment, disputes may arise regarding the practical application of the results. The dispute may be concerned with the amount of the potential benefit obtainable

---

* If, after studying the section referred to, a reader is not averse to contact with a publication which some authorities would probably assign to a medical Index Expurgatorius, he can turn to a letter addressed to the editor of *The Lancet* by Dr. Joseph Berkson (1962).

from the treatment, or it may go much deeper. The disputants may all agree that, in the particular experiment, a causal relationship has been established, and the dispute can then often be described as a controversy about the representativeness, in composition and circumstances, of the sample on which the experiment was performed — whether it is in all relevant respects sufficiently like the populations in which the results are to be used.

Sometimes such differences of opinion stem from differences in previous experience; but whenever we detect in ourselves or others a strong emotional element in such controversies we should suspect nonrational sources of belief.

If nonrational factors can influence what people believe after an experiment, it is all the more likely that they will do so after surveys related to health or other human affairs. The attitudes of various investigators toward evidence from surveys of various kinds would form the subject of interesting but very difficult psychologic and sociologic studies. The association between cigarette smoking and lung cancer can be plausibly explained as a causal relationship; but this is not a very strong statement to make in an effort to induce people to avoid smoking cigarettes, and perhaps that partly explains the attitude of certain scientists who were not themselves involved in research on smoking and cancer.

Those scientists were all well aware of the fact that association by itself does not prove a causal relationship. They would doubtless have pointed it out if they had been reviewing reports of researches on birds or butterflies; but when certain statisticians pointed it out in relation to researches on smoking and cancer they reacted as if the statisticians doubted the roundness of the earth, and as if such doubts were dangerous. On the editorial page of a leading scientific journal one writer even implied that financial support from tobacco manufacturers had perhaps influenced a statistician who expressed dissatisfaction with the nature of the evidence that was currently accepted as a proof that cigarettes actually caused the cancers.

This kind of behavior makes us wonder what is "proof" and what is the difference between "belief" and "acceptance of proof." Even with a scanty knowledge of the history of human thought we can see different definitions of these terms at different times and in different places. The definitions seem to depend largely on what is held to be very important by the particular society — for example, the health of the soul in medieval Europe, physical health, or at least the avoidance of physical disease, in some Western societies today. To those who are concerned about the welfare of their fellows in terms of their society's most esteemed ideal, anything which will, or may, promote that ideal is "good," and it seems to be but a short step from "the good" to "the true." Certainly, people are not likely to give up a pleasure unless they believe, without a flicker of doubt, that its danger is real and great. In the eyes of some people, therefore, anyone who raises doubts in such matters is subversive. Some of the discussions that follow the next question may invite that accusation.

Q VII – 5.   How may differences in admission rates (selection rates) produce spurious results in a survey?

In a survey the *admission rate (selection rate)* of subjects with a certain characteristic (A) is the proportion of the total A's in the population that come into the survey. If there are 1000 A's in the population and 100 of them get into the survey, the admission rate is 10 per cent. A "spurious result" in this context is a finding that is not true in the parent population. It may be a spurious association between characteristics or a spurious absence of association.

Bias Due to Admission Rates.   It has long been recognized, perhaps since hospitals were first started, that diseases differ greatly in their hospital admission rates. That is, hospital populations are biased samples of the general (diseased) population in terms of the relative proportions of different diseases. However, it was not until a paper by Dr. Joseph Berkson of the Mayo Clinic appeared in 1946 that we started to realize that this bias could vitiate studies of association between diseases, and between any other variables, when the studies were made on hospital patients. Even now, many years later, many people do not appreciate this danger, not only in medical surveys but in a survey of any kind unless strictly random samples are obtained from the parent population.

Berkson illustrated the mechanism of spurious association by a search for a relationship between diabetes and cholecystitis (gallbladder inflammation). There was such a strong impression of this relationship that some surgeons were removing the gallbladder in the treatment of diabetes. To test the association, hospital records were used. The comparison of diabetics with all nondiabetics was, of course, unsatisfactory, whatever results it might have shown, because some of the nondiabetic diseases might themselves be positively associated with cholecystitis, or some of them might for unknown reasons be negatively associated with it, i.e., they might contain an unusually low frequency of cholecystitis. Berkson therefore took as his contrast-sample the records of patients that showed a condition that could not reasonably be thought to be associated with cholecystitis — eye defects (refractive errors) of the sort for which patients come to a clinic for glasses.

The fourfold contingency table (diabetes versus refractive errors; cholecystitis versus no cholecystitis) showed a higher proportion of subjects with cholecystitis in the diabetic group than in the refractive-error group, and the difference was statistically "significant" (P less than 0.05). Then Berkson demonstrated that such an association could be entirely fallacious owing to a very simple mechanism, a kind of "interplay of admission rates." This particular example is somewhat complicated; therefore we will start with a very simple imaginary one.

A Simple Interplay of Admission Rates.   In a population let there be 40 A's and 40 B's. In each of these two groups let there be 10 X's and 30 not-X's; i.e., there is the same degree of association of X with A and with B. The A's and B's need not be equal in number, but for simplicity we make them so. For simplicity also we imagine that there are only three diseases and that there are no AB's. In the population we have, therefore:

$$AX: 10; \text{A–not-X}: 30$$
$$BX: 10; \text{B–not-X}: 30$$

Bias due to interplay of admission rates occurs when three conditions are fulfilled:

1. The admission rates of A and B are different.
2. The admission rates of X and not-X are different.
3. If a person is an AX (or a BX) he has a greater chance of admission than if he were simply an A (or simply a B, or simply an X).

Let us first imagine that the admission rate for B, by itself, is zero. This disorder (say, a cold in the head) does not itself bring a patient to the hospital where the survey will be made. B's come in only if they are brought by another disease, X in this case; therefore 100 per cent of the B's in the survey will have X. If the admission rate for A is anything greater than zero, some A's will come in that are X's and some that are not-X's. Therefore fewer than 100 per cent of the A's will be X's, and we will find a closer association of X with B than with A; but it will be spurious in the sense of not being true in the parent population. (The matter of "statistical significance" does not concern us here. We would always find a significant difference by taking a large enough sample under the same conditions.)

Let us now give B an admission rate of its own, but lower than that of A. For example, let the admission rates be as follows: A, 60 per cent; B, 20 per cent; X, 50 per cent. The not-X condition has no admission rate of its own.

Looking back at the population, we see that into the hospital will go the following patients:

AX: 60 per cent of 10 (because they are A's) = 6, leaving 4 behind.
   50 per cent of the remaining 4 (because they are X's) = 2
   Total AX's = 8
A–not-X: 60 per cent of 30 (because they are A's) = 18
   NOTE. – The same figure (8 AX's) is obtained if we let X take in 50 per cent of 10 (leaving 5 behind) and then let A take in 60 per cent of the remaining 5.
BX: 20 per cent of 10 (because they are B's) = 2, leaving 8 behind.
   50 per cent of 8 (because they are X's) = 4
   Total BX's = 6
B–not-X: 20 per cent of 30 (because they are B's) = 6

Therefore in our survey we will find:

	X	Not-X	Total
A	8	18	26
B	6	6	12

The percentage frequencies in this table are as follows:

8/26, i.e., 30.8 per cent of the A's are X's
6/12, i.e., 50.0 per cent of the B's are X's
Difference = 19.2 per cent

As in the previous example, X afflicts a higher proportion of B's than of A's. If the totals were large the difference would be very impressive and highly "significant," but totally misleading as regards the parent population, in which X occurs just as often among A's as among B's.

The mechanism is clear. The A's and the B's, if they are also X's, have an additional chance of getting into the hospital; but A, having a higher admission rate than B, takes in a higher proportion of its victims than does B. That leaves more B's to be taken in by X. It appears as if the higher admission rate of A had *pushed* X's into the B group; and I have found this simile the easiest way of remembering the effect.

The trouble caused by this mechanism arises of course from the fact that we do not know the number of A's, B's and X's in the population; if we did, we would not need to make the hospital survey. For the same reason, we cannot give factual examples of the damage that the mechanism has done. Perhaps that will be possible when people who are making population studies discover hospital admission rates and then demonstrate their effects on surveys made within the hospitals.

In the meantime, we can take fictitious illustrations. For instance, if in the above example the A's were persons with coronary heart disease, B's were persons with bronchitis, X's suffered from bunions and not-X's did not, we could demonstrate a greater frequency of bunions among bronchitic patients than among coronary disease patients.

When we are trying to visualize the admission-rate phenomenon, we must remember that persons do not usually present themselves for medical attention with diagnostic labels but with signs and symptoms. When they are thoroughly examined many disabilities or abnormalities are noted, and often more than one diagnosis is reached. We must remember also that numerous factors, not only the symptoms, determine that a person goes for medical attention to a certain doctor or hospital at a certain time.

Arithmetical Exercises. The effects of the interplay of admission rates can be demonstrated by mathematical symbols, but many of us in medicine find it easier to become acquainted with such a phenomenon by working out some simple arithmetical examples. For convenience, we repeat the figures given above. Population frequencies: AX, 10; A–not-X, 30; BX, 10; B–not-X, 30. Selection rates: A, 60 per cent; B, 20 per cent; X, 50 per cent; not-X (per se), zero. This will be referred to as our "original example."

Ex. 1.   Double the B-population — BX, 20; B–not-X, 60. Retain all the other figures. Show that the percentage frequencies in the survey are the same as before: 30.8 per cent of A's are X's; 50.0 per cent of B's are X's.

Ex. 2.   Give not-X an admission rate of its own, as if it were another disease — 25 per cent, i.e., less than that of X. Retain the other original figures. Show that in the survey 27.6 per cent of A's are X's, 33.3 per cent of B's are X's — a smaller difference than in the original example, but in the same direction.

Ex. 3.   In the population let there be 15 AX's and 25 A–not-X's. Retain the other original figures, including the zero rate for not-X by itself. The actual association of X is now greater with A than with B. Show that in the survey 44.4 per cent of A's are X's, but 50.0 per cent of B's are X's as before. The bias has not only masked the real (population) association, but has produced the opposite association in the survey.

Imaginary Concrete Examples.   Although we cannot show how the interplay of admission rates has actually produced fallacious inferences, we can show how they could do so if we make suppositions that are true to our experience. For example, people with severe attacks of a certain disease are more likely to go to a doctor than are people with mild attacks, and in some diseases men and women differ in their readiness to seek medical aid. Assuming the same degree of association of X with A and B in the population, the admission rate of A greater than that of B, and the rate for X greater than the rate for not-X, we can replace the letters A, B, X and not-X by specific entities or characteristics and show how the mechanism described above would lead to fallacious inferences.

Ex. 1.   A's are females; B's are males with the same disease. X's are severe cases; not-X's are mild cases. Inference: The disease is more frequently severe in males.

Ex. 2.   A's are younger persons; B's are older persons with the same disease. X is a complication that arises during the course of the primary disease. Inference: The complication is commoner in older patients.

Ex. 3.   In a certain region, where there are people of different racial origins, different socioeconomic groups, with different dietary habits, there are several hospitals. In one of them, owing to financial, social or geographic reasons, the admission rate for people who consume vegetable fat (A's) is higher than the admission rate for people who eat much animal fat (B's); X is coronary disease and not-X is another disease (or group of diseases or accident cases) used as a contrast-sample in a study of coronary disease in relation to dietary fat. For simplicity, the admission rate for the not-X's can be assumed to be the "basic" admission rate for any sick person in the particular group (A or B); the admission rate for X, as in the original example, is higher. Inference: Coronary disease is more frequently associated with an animal-fat diet than with a vegetable-fat diet.

Ex. 4.   A retrospective or cross-sectional survey is conducted in order to discover if there is a relationship between a certain habit (heavy drinking, eating or smoking) and a certain disease (A) in contrast with some other disease (B). The X's are abstainers, more careful about their health and more likely to go to a doctor when they feel that something is wrong with them than are those who indulge in the habit. The indulgers must therefore be lettered "not-X." Inference: There is a higher proportion of abstainers in the contrast-group, i.e., a higher proportion of indulgers in the disease under scrutiny (A).

Ex. 5. Two diseases, A and B, are compared with respect to the presence (or average level) of a certain serum protein, X. The substance itself would not be considered likely to influence a person's tendency to seek medical aid; but all that is required for the production of an admission-rate bias is that X be associated with something that influences the admission rate. For example, X and not-X might predominate in different age groups. Or X might be associated with some feature or stage in the two diseases under study that would increase the admission rate of X's. Or the presence (or high level) of X might be due to some metabolic or excretory defect which would increase the likelihood that a person suffering from A or B would go to a doctor or would require longer treatment.

Speculations of this kind have shown that admission-rate biases could affect studies of anatomic collections, prehistoric remains, body build and blood groups (Mainland, 1955 b).

Autopsy Admission Rates. For more than 30 years it has been recognized that autopsy records are dangerous sources of data regarding the association between diseases, for other reasons than admission-rate bias. Berkson (1955) tells the story of a discovery, reported in 1929, of an apparent antagonism between cancer and tuberculosis. In a very careful investigation the autopsy records of 816 cancerous subjects were matched on a one-to-one basis by sex, color, age and date of death with records of noncancerous subjects, and it was found that active tuberculosis was recorded for only 6.6 per cent of the cancerous group but for 16.3 per cent of the noncancerous subjects.

After careful consideration of possible flaws in the evidence, it was decided that there must be a biologic antagonism between tuberculosis and cancer. "An experiment with animals was set up and an extensive program of treating cancer patients with tuberculin was instituted." Then a serious flaw was thought of — the possibility that cancer killed its victims quicker than did many of the other diseases, and therefore gave a person less time to develop florid tuberculosis such as was found in members of the noncancerous group. The concept of a cancer-tuberculosis antagonism was quickly dropped; but we ought not to forget the story, because the biostatistician responsible for the research method and the conclusions was one of the most penetrating thinkers in his field.

The actual flaw in the tuberculosis-cancer study may not have been the suggested difference in length of exposure to risk. As Berkson discovered in the middle 1930's, it may have been some kind of admission-rate bias. In terms of our simple example, if A were cancer, B were the other diseases used as controls and X were tuberculosis, the cancer could, as it were, push the tuberculosis into the control group. Doubtless the phenomena would not be as simple as this, and it is desirable to realize some of the complexities of the factors that influence percentage frequencies found in autopsy records.

Hospital autopsy data are influenced not only by the selection factors that bring patients to a particular hospital but by the factors that bring patients, already in the hospital, to the autopsy table, or keep them away from it. Death itself is the first factor. Referring to our basic example of admission-rate bias, let disease A kill a higher proportion of its victims than does disease B. Let X be some condition, equally common in the A's and B's, such as a kidney condition that tends to tip the scales against some patients. Then, even if all dead patients come to autopsy, X will be found more frequently among the B's than among the A's.

The other potential bias-causing factors include the resistance to autopsy that is displayed by relatives and undertakers, the persistence of some physicians when requesting permission for an autopsy in particular diseases or particular cases, e.g., those that have puzzled them in the patient before death. It is therefore interesting, but rather futile, to speculate on the possible causes of a particular result obtained from a study of autopsy records. The following actual result is offered for such speculation. Although coronary heart disease, diagnosed clinically, was commoner among men than among women, in a certain autopsy study it was found with equal frequency in the two sexes.

Sometimes a study of autopsy records is defended by the statement: "We know that autopsy studies are liable to numerous biases; but all that we claim to show is an association, or a lack of association, in an autopsy population." But surely, for medical purposes, we study the dead in order to learn about the living, or to obtain some useful hints regarding further studies on living human beings or animals. After an autopsy study of an association between diseases, or between diseases and other variables, it seems that, whichever way the autopsy results point, we may find the opposite information in life. We have learned a great deal about disease by the autopsy method; but we ought not to impose upon it a task for which it is unsuitable.

Admission Rates in Prospective Studies. Let us suppose that we wish to find out whether the occurrence of a certain disease is associated with some characteristic (e.g., a dietary habit, a physiologic or anatomic feature). We obtain a group of persons with the characteristic and another group without it, or possessing it in lesser degree, but like the first group in other relevant characteristics, e.g., sex and age range. We follow both groups for a certain period and find the incidence of the disease that we are studying.

If the two groups differed in their admission rates to the survey this would not by itself introduce an admission-rate bias in our conclusions about association of the disease with the variable under study. To produce such a bias, the X versus not-X difference in rates would be necessary, i.e., the persons who were going to develop the disease would have to possess a different admission rate from those who were not going to develop it. A prospective study appears so like a true experiment that we may trust it too readily. Even our present scanty knowledge of disease-determining factors and of attitude-determining factors ought to make us cautious.

We recognize that the occurrence of a disease is determined not only by agents from the outside but by the constitution of the person who meets the agents. We recognize that "constitution" means not the body alone but the psychophysical make-up of a person. And we recognize that the psychophysical make-up determines a person's attitude, including his degree of willingness to enter, and continue in, a prospective survey.

Various observations suggest how the interplay of factors might occur. For example, in one city a chest x-ray diagnostic screening service was offered free of charge to anyone who would come to a tuberculosis clinic. The employees of a large department store responded abundantly, whereas a university faculty paid little attention to the appeal, although the clinic was on the campus. Other examples of group differences in attitude have been noted in several medical follow-up surveys in Britain and the United States — a greater lapse-rate in the higher socioeconomic classes (Fletcher and Oldham, *Medical Surveys and Clinical Trials* edited by Witts). We now add to these attitudinal differences the fact that different socioeconomic, ethnic, geographic and occupational groups differ in the incidence of certain diseases and also in characteristics such as dietary habits, physiologic and anatomic features.

All that would be necessary to produce an admission-rate difference between the X's and the not-X's would be an association between (1) some constitutional feature that promotes or hinders the occurrence of the disease and (2) some attitudinal feature that would determine the response to an appeal to enter our survey and continue in it.

Sometimes there may be an even more direct connection between liability to disease and a person's willingness to submit to medical inquiry or examination. In a certain chest x-ray survey in which reasons for refusal were sought, fear of discovery of disease was found to be the chief deterrent. In some persons this might be groundless fear, but in others it might be due to recollection of some symptoms or the knowledge of the occurrence of a particular disease in the subject's family.

By using various possibilities of interplay of factors we can invent a variety of possible outcomes of our prospective survey on the association between a certain disease and a certain dietary habit. Let us imagine that those who indulge in the dietary habit are more cooperative and therefore have a higher admission rate than the abstainers. The indulgers are then the A's of our original example, and the abstainers are the B's. Let there be, equally common in A's and B's, some people who will develop the disease within the period of our survey. Some of them, owing to suspicions of their own health or knowledge of the disease in their families, do not enter the survey. Therefore, those who will not develop the disease have a higher admission rate; they are the X's in our original example. As a result of the survey the unfortunate indulgers will find that those who warned them long ago about the danger of the habit were apparently in the right, because a higher proportion of them have developed the disease.

In a survey that depends on volunteer subjects, attitudes alone do not determine enrollment. Circumstances of various kinds make it easier for some subjects to cooperate than others, and these circumstances may be associated with the features that we propose to study.

We might think that we could avoid all these problems by a compulsory survey, enrolling and following all employees in a certain industry or the members of some other clearly defined community. But when we start to wonder why the various individuals and groups of persons (e.g., job groups in an industry) came to be where they are, we see that the risk of admission-rate bias is still with us.

Perhaps if we were more accustomed to thinking genetically we would have less difficulty in accepting the possibility of associations that seem illogical. It is not inconceivable that on the same chromosome there should reside a gene that is associated with the development of a certain disease and also another gene that influences in some way the factors that bring a person into a survey or keep him out of it. That is, there may in some instances be a genetic basis for the admission-rate bias.

Admission-rate Bias in Measurement Data. It was mentioned earlier that the bias can affect not only frequency data (presence-absence of X) but measurement data (difference in average level of X in A's and B's). By extension therefore it can affect our efforts to discover a relationship between two sets of measurements. For example, let A_1, A_2, and so on, be ages and X_1, X_2, and so on, be levels of bone density determined by x-rays (Mainland, 1957). The bias can occur if (1) admission rates differ with age (students are commonly easier to enroll than faculty members), and (2) men with certain characteristics that affect bone density (dietary habits, health care, body build) are easier to obtain than men with other characteristics.

Q VII – 6. What are we going to do about the risk of bias due to interplay of admission rates in our survey?

If we are "practical" people, or "action-oriented," we may dismiss the danger as something invented, or at least greatly exaggerated, by a statistician. Let us assume, however, that we take it seriously. We have to admit that there is no certain prevention or cure; but there are certain precautions that we can take, along the following lines.

First, we ought to consider the purpose of the survey. If we are seeking for a sequence rather than a consequence, we may be little concerned about the risk of bias. A physician may observe that patients who have had a certain chronic disease for more than 5 years when they first come to him commonly do worse under treatment than those who had the disease for only 2 years. This may be due to some hidden interplay of selection factors, or even to a much simpler bias — the cases of longer duration may have been from the start the more resistant cases, that have gone from one doctor to another before reaching him. Whatever the cause, the observed association may help him in planning therapy.

It is when we are searching for a causal connection that we must consider carefully the risk of admission-rate bias and, of course, other biases also. We may help ourselves by questions like the following:

1. What factors could conceivably make the admission rates of A's and B's differ from each other, and in what direction?

2. What factors could conceivably make the admission rates of X's and not-X's differ from each other, and in what direction?

3. What would be the effects on our survey data of the various interplays between admission rates visualized in (1) and (2)? (There may be complex variants of the simple scheme that we have discussed here.)

4. Are some of the factors mentioned in (1) and (2) very unlikely to be present in our survey?

5. Can we obtain from any source some idea of the magnitude of admission rates concerned? If so, can we say that if a certain result is obtained from our survey it is very unlikely to be attributable wholly to admission-rate biases?

6. Can we devise two or more surveys under different conditions to test the same hypothesis?

Q VII – 7. Under what conditions can we omit a contrast-group in a survey?

In a pilot study, preparatory to an experiment or to a survey that will contain contrast-groups, we often use only one group of subjects, in order to become acquainted with the methods, the difficulties and the orders of magnitude of the variables that we plan to observe, e.g., a suitable dose range for an unfamiliar drug, and so on. If we are establishing physiologic or biochemical norms by examining a selected group of subjects, we do not introduce a contrast-group, but we are, or ought to be, building upon many comparisons already made between healthy and diseased subjects.

In clinical work one might say: "If I am merely trying to find out what percentage of successes I obtain with a certain treatment, surely I do not need controls." On the surface this looks reasonable; but let us see what a thoughtful surgeon wrote about the "statistics" of successful treatments (Ogilvie):

"Such experiences, indeed my whole experience, have left me with profound mistrust of statistics. I have not published mine since I was young and credulous; indeed, I do not know them now unless I ask my registrar to look them up for a particular purpose . . . Personal statistics . . . are either too good to be true or too true to be good.

"Those who see statistics in the making are well aware how errors may creep in or be pushed in . . . The ailing may be transferred to another ward, another block, another hospital, there to die; they may develop complications and be entrusted to the care of a physician and disappear from the surgeon's series; the unsuccessful cases may be indexed under another diagnosis, or appear in the list of operations done by the assistant . . .

"The surgeon who never does a severe operation has the fewest deaths, but he saves the fewest lives. The man who limits his operations on hypertension to a small group of young people who respond well to all tests has a wonderfully low death rate and high cure rate, but he passes by all those who need help most. The surgeon who closes up a high proportion of his cancer laparotomies as 'inoperable' and reserves his resection for the early growths can show a fine record on paper; how will he himself show up before the recording angel? . . .

"One gastric surgeon surprised the world some years ago by recording 500 gastrectomies for ulcer with 0.6% mortality. Fine! He then reached a total of 1,000 cases with a mortality of 0.6%. Grand! A little later he popped up with 2,000 with a mortality of 0.6%. Marvelous! He now has 3,000 with a mortality of 0.6%. Incredible! . . . It is clear that to this man, a skilled surgeon, the figure of 0.6% is a symbol, a creed, a banner beneath which he goes into battle. It is his story, and he is going to stick to it. As for myself I shall leave him stuck. The only figures which I find statistically significant are those recorded anonymously and analyzed impartially by someone with no personal interest in the verdict."

Q VII – 8. Are we going to use a previous series of cases in evaluating a new treatment?

An increasing awareness of the defects of the "previous series" or "past-and-present" method has been the reason why clinicians have turned to true experiments, which involve *contemporaneous* or *concurrent* controls, i.e., contrasting treatment groups, of which all members are investigated within the same period. Even if a previous series is not vitiated by all the features mentioned in the passage quoted above, there are many possible differences, unrecorded and unremembered, between one series of patients and a subsequent series — in type of patient and methods of selection, auxiliary treatments and general handling, e.g., preparation of patients for surgical operations. Methods in medicine are changing so rapidly that even the very recent past may be invalid as a standard of comparison. In many diseases, diagnosis is now made at an earlier stage than formerly, and therefore appropriate treatment can start earlier. Antibiotic drugs now prevent many deaths resulting from infection after surgery; therefore a new surgical technique for cancer may be associated with a longer average survival time than a former technique.

It is regrettable that the impressive term "historic controls" has started to appear in medical literature. At best, these cases still form a "previous series." Sometimes the term means nothing more than poorly documented statements of someone's experience.

We may condemn the "previous series" method, but can we escape using it? Every year, hundreds of new drugs are produced — often old drugs slightly modified, but with claims to virtue derived from animal experiments or from trial on a few human patients. Adequate experiments are impossible for more than a small fraction of these products. Even apart from the large amount of time and effort required for a proper trial, and apart from the scarcity of trained personnel, only a limited number of patients are available at any one time.

We can therefore sympathize with the administrators of an agency that is engaged in testing anti-cancer drugs. The agency is not only faced with numerous compounds but is subject to strong public pressure for massive and speedy action. It was rather natural for such an agency to decide upon coarse screening, with few patients on each compound, and with only "historic" controls; but the decision can have consequences that are not reassuring to the proponents of controlled trials. Clinical investigators have expressed great satisfaction because a statistician in the agency had shown them that in anti-cancer drug testing "no controls need be run" and that "samples of 14 patients are sufficient."

Actually, the statistician's perfectly correct statement was of the following nature: If a strictly random sample of 14 patients was taken from an indefinitely large population of cancer patients treated by a certain compound, and if none of the 14 showed objective and unequivocal signs of improvement, then there would be a 95 per cent probability that such signs would not be found in more than 20 per cent of the whole population.

The meaning of the probability statement regarding the population percentage is discussed in Chapter XI. Here we note some more basic questions which the enthusiastic clinical investigators did not mention: "Is a change in a patient's condition to be accepted as 'unequivocal' only if it has never (or hardly ever) been seen before? If so, what will be the evidence that it is really very rare?" "What exactly will be the standards in each particular type of cancer against which the changes in the 14 patients will be gauged? How 'objective' will they be?" "If measurements (blood counts, sizes of surface tumors or of x-ray shadows) are to be the criteria, how will it be found out what allowance to make for observational variability?" "How will it be proved that measurements are not affected by the optimism, pessimism or excessive caution of an observer who knows what compound a patient is receiving?"

Q VII – 9. Are we going to use patients as a contrast-group in a survey?

In studying problems of disease we would often like to have healthy subjects as a contrast-group; but healthy subjects are often difficult to obtain, and to retain if the study involves follow-up. Moreover, willing volunteers may be aberrant subjects (Q III – 3). We are therefore frequently driven to use other patients for contrast.

Often a single contrast-group is created by taking all other available patients who are like those with the disease under study in sex, age

range, and some other relevant features. But this gives us a very heterogeneous group, with different biases affecting different subgroups (diseases), and we have no right to imagine that if we take sufficient patients,
with a sufficient variety of conditions, the biases will cancel out for our
benefit. It is much more desirable to take two or more of these subgroups — indeed, as many as possible — and place them alongside our
primary group.

It is interesting that the laboratory atmosphere of fussiness about
controls often fails to accompany a laboratory investigator when he goes
out to find samples among human subjects. A biochemist, wishing to
compare the concentration of a certain serum protein in a particular
disease with its concentration in healthy subjects, obtained samples of
blood from a blood donor clinic. He contrasted the average concentra-
tions of the protein in the two groups and, having attended a course in
biometry, he proposed to apply a "significance" test. When he was asked
how much was known about the effects on this protein concentration of
such factors as sex, age, diet, drugs and exercise, he confessed that little
was known in this regard. He stated, however, that he proposed to use
the significance test just as if he were comparing some measurement in
one animal species with the same measurement in another species. One
may justifiably wonder how far biology had penetrated into the course in
biometry that he had suffered.

Q VII – 10. Are we going to use official vital statistics in connection with our study? If so, what precautions should we take?

Sometimes we are tempted to compare our own figures with national
or regional vital statistics, particularly death rates and disease incidence
rates, but the coarse classification of those data (by sex, age, color,
country or state) leaves them still too heterogeneous to be very useful for
comparison with our particular group of diseased subjects. However,
the official figures look like appropriate sources of information in many
studies. Therefore we should realize that anyone — clinician, laboratory
worker or "nonvital" statistician — who contemplates using such figures
for any purpose whatever ought to acquaint himself with:

1. The factors that can influence a physician when he is creating a
"statistic."

2. The kinds of things that happen between the physician's pen and
the seemingly authoritative official publication.

3. The details given in the introduction to any table of vital statistics
that the investigator may intend to use.

Even after taking these precautions I do not feel safe until I have
consulted a well informed official in a Bureau of Vital Statistics. However, a preliminary view of the pitfalls can be obtained by considering
(1) mortality rates and (2) life expectancy figures.

Mortality Rates. The general (overall or so-called "crude") mortality
rate or death rate is expressed as so many deaths per thousand persons

living in a certain region in a certain year. When the population is divided into different subclasses or "species" by sex and by age (commonly in 5-year intervals), the rates are called "specific" rates — sex-specific and sex-age-specific. Within the total population and also within subclasses, the deaths are also listed by cause, and at this stage it is often desirable to give rates per hundred thousand population because the numbers in the numerators are small.

In the numerators of the rates appear the medical practitioner's contributions, conveyed by death certificates; but his diagnoses are classified according to rules adopted by international agreement (although not, by any means, obeyed in all countries). The denominators of the rates are official estimates of the appropriate populations exposed to the risk of dying.

Death Certificates. In addition to such factors as carelessness, culpable ignorance and dubious information regarding the age of the deceased, there are special sources of error in death certificates. Here are three examples:

1. The frequent difficulty of precise diagnosis of cause of death. Autopsies have shown that, although death certificates based on clinical observation are commonly correct in broad classifications by system (e.g., cardiovascular-renal disease), they are much less accurate with regard to particular organs or lesions in an organ. (It should be noted in passing that autopsies cannot be taken as reliable sources of information when a disease is biochemical rather than anatomic.)

2. The pressure on physicians to state a specific cause of death. If he says, "I am not sure" or "Nothing definite except old age," an autopsy is required by law; and this is disliked by relatives and undertakers.

3. Unwillingness to cause offence, distress or inconvenience. For example, fear of causing offence can cause under-reporting of syphilis as a cause of death. Errors due to such influences could be reduced by the adoption, as in New York City, of a certificate in which the statement of cause is detached and kept confidential by the health authorities. Even this would not remove a difficulty faced by practitioners in England. If they certify, as the cause of death of a child at birth, "intracranial injury" or "asphyxia" (two of the commonest causes) a coroner's inquest will often be ordered. A physician can hardly be blamed for substituting the safer term "prematurity" or "atelectasis" (imperfect lung expansion) in order to avoid parents' distress and his own frequent attendance at court (B. D. Corner).

Classification. As our knowledge of disease and the experience of vital statisticians grow, classification must change, and so must the rules for treatment of the numerous certificates that contain two or more causes of death ("joint causes"). *The International List of Causes of Death,* used in the United States since 1901, has been revised every ten years, and every revision makes it difficult to compare present figures with those of the past.

The sixth revision (1948), the *Manual of the International Statistical Classification of Diseases, Injuries and Causes of Death,* issued by the World Health Organization, introduced great changes. In New York City a comparison was made (Erhardt and Weiner) between the new system and the one previously used there (fifth edition of the *International List,* and a United States *Joint Cause Manual*). The deaths occurring from January to August, 1949, were classified by both methods. Differences in numbers of deaths attributed to various diseases were expressed as percentages, the denominators being the numbers determined by the previous method. Causes that showed great "decline" were nephritis (70 per cent), diabetes (55 per cent) and syphilis (32 per cent). Great "increases" were shown by rheumatic fever (44 per cent), diarrhea and enteritis (39 per cent) and influenza (31 per cent).

Population at Risk. We must remember that the population is an estimate; and, although the details of method do not concern us, we should note two general points:

1. The more specific a death rate, the more useful it is, but the less reliable is its denominator. Intercensal estimates for regions, age groups and occupations are less dependable than estimates for a whole country.

2. Death rates (and other rates) classified by region depend on the rules, sometimes local rules, observed in tabulation. A very different picture is presented according to whether deaths from tuberculosis or insanity are recorded by location of institution where death occurs, or by place of residence. "Manhattan has more hospital facilities than its sister boroughs. The result is that less than 80 per cent of the deaths in Manhattan are of persons who reside there, and only 65 per cent of the births are to mothers who live on Manhattan Island" (Mustard). This statement was published in 1948, but a few years of hospital building can change such percentages.

The same kinds of bias, from reporting, classifying, and the estimation of populations, affect other figures, such as disease incidence rates. Moreover, although in the United States, Great Britain and a number of other countries it appears that nearly all deaths are reported to the authorities, this cannot be said of all the diseases that practitioners are required by law to report, i.e., the "notifiable" diseases, mostly of an infectious type.

Life Expectancy. This is one of the most misunderstood products of the vital statistician. It is estimated by the "life table" method described in books on public health statistics, a rather complicated procedure. In principle, however, the "life expectancy" or "expectation of life" at each age is simple. In a table for 1948, opposite age zero the life expectancy for white persons in the United States was stated to be 65.5 years in males and 71.0 years in females. These are essentially the *average ages at death* of the white males and females who died in 1948 (after certain adjustments for the age-composition of the population). Opposite age 20 in the same table were the figures 49.0 years for males and 53.8 years for females. These represent, for people over age 20 who died in 1948, the average number of years that they had lived beyond that age.

The figures therefore do not really tell us anything about the living people who were born (or were aged 20) in 1948. They would be real forecasts only if the death rates remained the same until all these people had died, and death rates are never constant.

Life expectancy figures are used for the comparison of mortality at different periods. For example, in the middle of the nineteenth century the figure at age zero was about 40 years (Dublin), a difference of about 25 years from the 1948 figure. This figure, however, does not show (1) that a child nowadays can expect to live 25 years longer than his forefathers, or (2) that anyone today lives any longer than the oldest persons in a former period, or even (3) that a larger proportion of people reach old age than in former times. Several thousand people living to the age of 45 instead of dying before the age of one year can easily raise the average age at death. Life expectancies of people who have reached the age of 70 show little change over long periods.

Because of the possible confusion in meaning, and for other reasons also, sex- and age-specific death rates are commonly preferable to "life expectancy" in the comparison of mortality. This does not imply, however, that the life table method of studying deaths (or other events) in a succession of equal periods is suspect or of little value. Life expectancy is only the last column in the life table. Previous columns show such information as the numbers of subjects at the beginning of each period to whom the event under study had not yet happened, and then the proportion of those initially available subjects to whom the event happened in each period.

When corrected by, or constructed from, records of insurance policyholders, "forecasts" from life tables provide a starting point for the establishment of insurance premiums. Without any such implied prophecy, the life table method is useful in research on duration of life (or of freedom from symptoms) after medical treatment. It can be used also in animal research, for example to display, month after month, the incidence of tumors in mice treated with a potential cancer-inducing substance.

The Value of Official Statistics.   An experimenter is apt to turn with skepticism from the statistics produced by health authorities. But when he tries to imagine our condition if we had no such statistics he will probably agree with the late Professor Greenwood (1943) that here "the perfect is the enemy of the good."

Imperfect though vital statistics were in 1857, it was only through them that Florence Nightingale could show that the mortality of soldiers, selected for physical fitness and living in English barracks during peacetime, was far greater than the mortality of civilians of all ages, fit and unfit, living alongside the same barracks. It was such figures that drove the authorities to institute reforms (Woodham-Smith).

A laboratory worker may be appalled at the gigantic errors of bias revealed from time to time in vital statistics. Cases of malaria reported annually in the United States fell from 48,610 in 1946, through 17,317 and 9797, to 4239 in 1949 (World Health Organization Report, 1950). The striking decline was found attributable very largely to a change in diagnostic methods. Certain health authorities had started to require demonstration of the malaria parasite in the blood before accepting a diagnosis of the disease. Other currently accepted figures doubtless contain similar errors, but without the figures we would have no idea of the magnitude of the problem or whether, as in this instance, a change in method was worth the effort.

For research workers, official vital statistics have their chief value as evidence of apparent differences and trends, suggesting areas in which special investigation is desirable.

Q VII – 11. If, instead of taking a particular hypothesis to clinical records, we search among them for possible relationships, are there any fruitful methods of procedure?

Routine clinical records have many defects (see Chapter IX), but they can be used as starting-points to generate hypotheses for further special studies. There are no rigid rules of procedure, but a few hints may be helpful.

1. If from the outset we use all the available records and test on them a large number of hypotheses — those based on previous impressions and those suggested by the records themselves — we are almost bound to find a number of "statistically significant" differences; and then the only way of trying to weed out those that are due to random processes is to obtain new data. We can do a first-stage weeding, however, if we start with a *strictly random sample* (a quarter, a third or perhaps a half) of the total records. On this sample we can make as many comparisons as we wish. Then we can take the most suggestive of the results — differences that are statistically "significant," or unusually large, or very important if genuine — and introduce them as hypotheses to be tested on the remaining records (the second phase of the study). We must not, of course, pool the two sets of records in analyzing or reporting our results.

2. In the first phase of such a survey it is permissible to work from effects to possible causal factors, instead of in the usual reverse direction.

3. When we are seeking for a relationship between two variables it is useful to remember the advice given by an experienced physiologist to a younger man who had failed to obtain an effect from a certain dose of a compound injected into animals, and was puzzling over the dose to try next. The older man remarked: "Make the difference big enough. Try multiplying by 10." If in our preliminary studies we are seeking for the possible influence of a variable A, which is present in different degrees in different subjects, we should try to compare extremes — subjects with much A against subjects with little or no A. We can use the same method if we are working from effects to possible causes.

4. Although we may feel that it is a pity to "waste" any of our records, the matching process mentioned under Q IV – 4 may be much more productive than mass contrasts of heterogeneous data.

5. At every step in our study, and in every other kind of study, we should think about the kinds of biases that might be present, and we

should try to detect them. Someone has aptly called biases in an investigation "contaminants" — "positive" contaminants which create false evidence of a relationship, and "negative" contaminants which mask true relationships. The rule is therefore: Continually seek for contaminants.

Q VII – 12. In view of the uncertainties of research by survey methods, ought we to avoid these methods as much as possible?

If we did so — if we tried to confine ourselves to experimentation in the strict sense — we would have to give up most of our research on human beings. And then, having obtained results from experiments (animal experiments and such experiments as are feasible and permissible on human beings), we would have little assurance that these results would apply in the outside world. All experiments, even clinical drug trials, are simplifications, abstractions from phenomena in the everyday world.

It is true that the admission-rate bias, the incidence-prevalence fallacy (Q V – 8) and the numerous other biases or contaminants are very discouraging; but this is partly due to our attitude. We are anxious for results that can be applied immediately, or at least very soon, so that we can "cure" diseases or tell people how to live longer by avoiding this and that. Likewise in the laboratory we desire clear, positive, publishable results. Biases are therefore "bad" things because they hinder us. We could make more progress in knowledge and understanding if we ceased to look upon the bias-causing factors as pathologic factors. They are natural phenomena and we could learn much by studying them.

To take as an example a problem that appears to be one of pure clinical pathology, let us suppose that we have found in hospital patients a higher level of serum protein X in patients with disease A than in patients with disease B, and that other workers, using similar material, have confirmed our finding. The difference may indeed be directly related to the differences between the two diseases. On the other hand, it may be due to the selection factors that determine the constitution of hospital samples of A's and B's. To explore these factors we would have to get samples outside the hospital, but the exploration could lead to rich discoveries regarding the behavior of diseases in the population and regarding the behavior of people themselves. Medical training does not fit us for such studies, and we would have to seek the cooperation of behavioral scientists — sociologists, psychologists and perhaps cultural anthropologists. It would be beneficial to many of us in medicine to come into contact with meticulous experimentally-minded workers in those disciplines, especially the workers who appreciate the embryonic nature of their science.

Such a search for selection factors would be frustrating, perhaps for a long time a mere gathering of hints and partial insights, which would lead to more questions. It is not a study for a young medical graduate who has to achieve quick success in clinical or academic life; but it seems to be the only way in which we can hope to sharpen the blunt tool of survey research in medicine.

CHAPTER VIII

SAMPLE SIZES

If we review previous discussions (especially under Q VI – 11) we will find that they have almost covered the substance of this chapter; but the question of sample size is so important that it deserves a chapter of its own.

Q VIII – 1. How large should our sample be?

Nowadays this question is often asked by investigators, and that is a sign that statistical thinking is leading to prudence; but before we can answer it we must ask ourselves four other questions. For convenience they are discussed in terms of an intergroup A-versus-B experiment with prefixed and equal sample sizes, and with results expressed as percentage frequencies of X (e.g., improvement) and not-X. The principles apply, however, equally to paired comparisons, to surveys, to unequal samples and to measurement data.

The four questions are:

1. What assurance do we require that, if there is no real A-B difference in effect, we will not be fooled by our randomization? That is, what level of statistical significance (Type I error) do we choose?

2. If treatment B is really superior to A, how great must this superiority be in order to be of interest to us? That is, what is the smallest difference that we would consider important to detect? By "real" superiority we mean that if we could experiment on an indefinitely large population we would find that B produced a higher percentage of X's than did A.

3. If the amount of difference, stated in answer to Question 2, really exists (or would be found if we had a population to work on), what assurance do we require that our experiment will produce a statistically "significant" difference in outcome? In other words, if the specified real difference exists, what assurance do we desire of a "successful" experiment, rather than a waste of time, effort, money and perhaps of patients' or animals' suffering? Technically, what Type II error do we choose? — What power do we demand in our experiment?

4. What data do we have regarding the percentage of X's to be expected in either an A-treated or a B-treated population?

When we think about these questions, three things become rather obvious from our general knowledge, and they can of course be demonstrated experimentally:

1. If we demand a greater assurance of not being fooled by chance differences (e.g., the 1 per cent level of significance), we will require larger samples than if we are satisfied with weaker evidence (e.g., the 5 per cent level).

2. If we seek evidence of small differences in effect, we will need larger samples than if we are content to detect only large differences. Incidentally, it should be noted that "detect" here does not imply that the samples will show the actual (population) difference, but merely that they will show a difference in the same direction as the population difference and large enough to meet our standard of "rarity" in randomization.

3. If we are willing to take a 50:50 chance of detecting a difference when it exists, we are running considerable risk of waste effort. If we have only that likelihood of detecting the difference that we are primarily interested in, we have still less assurance of detecting a smaller difference.

An 80 per cent power sounds fairly high, but if we express it as a 1-in-5 (20 per cent) chance of failure it does not sound so encouraging. Most experimenters demand a much higher power, such as 95 per cent (a Type II error of 5 per cent).

We may have little idea of what to expect as the percentage of X's in either an A-treated or a B-treated population. If so, it is safest to assume that one of them would contain 50 per cent X's because, as is shown by Table V (discussed below), this assumption will give an over-estimate rather than an underestimate of the required sample size.

Q VIII – 2. Having decided on the difference to be detected, and on our Type I and Type II errors, how are we to find our required sample sizes for a binomial two-treatment experiment or survey?

Table V contains information for equal A and B samples containing up to 100 individuals (see Appendix). For example, let us stipulate that if the proportion of X's in the A-population were 25 per cent and the proportion in the B-population were 67 per cent, we wish to be assured that 95 per cent of our experiments would be successful. By "successful" we mean that they would produce a contingency table (A, B; X, not-X) containing more X's in B than in A, and that the difference would be significant at the 5 per cent level. Taking our population values to Table V, we find under $N = 50$ that the percentage of successful experiments (the power of the experiment) would be 98.8. Therefore we would require almost 50 subjects in each sample.

Examination of other parts of Table V reveals, as we would expect, that for a given sample size and any particular percentage of X's in the

A-population, the higher the percentage of X's in B, the greater is the power of the experiment.

The mathematics used in constructing the table will be better understood in the light of Chapters XI and XII, and will be described in Chapter XII; but the experimental equivalent was indicated in Q VI – 11.

Q VIII – 3. If our data are to be measurement data how will we estimate required sample sizes?

This is no easy problem. If, for example, we intend to compare the averages of two samples of measurements (A and B), we need to have first of all a fairly good estimate of the intersubject variation in either an A- or B-population, and in much medical research we do not have such information at the outset. Even if we had this information there would have to be carried through a rather extensive calculation for our particular problem, corresponding to what was performed for any pair of population values in Table V. A simple way of getting around the problem is suggested in Chapter XIV.

Q VIII – 4. If we wish to use a sequential design how are we to estimate the required sample size?

The essence of sequential design (Q VI – 18) is that there is no prefixed sample size. However, before setting up the design we must answer the four questions listed under Q VIII – 1. Then, having chosen from a book such as that of Armitage (*Sequential Medical Trials*) the numerical values that will give us the stop-and-go signs in our experiment, we can obtain from the same source an estimate of the maximum sample size that we may need.

Q VIII – 5. If we have to use unequal samples is there risk of bias?

In the simple analyses that are most commonly used in medical research, such as contingency table analysis and the comparison of two samples of measurements, inequality of sample size does not itself create bias; but the reason for the inequality may do so — for example, the refusal of a certain type of person to cooperate in a study. In many of the more complicated designs, such as the factorial design (Q IV – 8), balance must be maintained by equality of the samples or subclasses.

It can be shown experimentally or arithmetically that, in general, equal-sized samples are more profitable than unequal samples. That is, if we divide a particular number of individuals into equal samples and apply to our results "significance" tests in the usual manner, our experiment will provide a more sensitive test of a treatment difference than if we divide them into unequal samples. Sometimes in a survey one group is much smaller than another, or there may be some other reason, such as scarcity of a test compound, for dividing the total group unequally. Then we ought to use a larger total than would be given by Table V. The exact number can be calculated for any particular case, but usually it is not considered necessary to be so precise.

Q VIII – 6.   Do small samples introduce greater risk of biases than large samples?

An obstetrician was talking about a report on the use of a certain hormone to prevent abortion in 19 women who in previous pregnancies had always aborted. The treatment was apparently successful in all the women, but the obstetrician said: "It may have been a fluke. They ought to have tried more cases." About 15 years later, a clinical pharmacologist, discussing the sequential design, said: "Do not the small samples introduce a greater risk of runs than the larger samples required by the prefixed sample size design?"

The pharmacologist had in mind properly conducted experiments, whereas the obstetrician was referring to a trial that was hardly an experiment at all. And yet the obstetrician's comment would have been just as pertinent if the hormone had been tested in a properly conducted trial containing a contrast-group which had not received the hormone, and had proved beyond any reasonable doubt that the hormone reduced the incidence of abortion in the women who received it.

The point at issue is generalization to the population represented by the sample chosen for the experiment. The obstetrician, it is true, equated "fluke" with "chance," and he could have been given two pieces of information:

1. From "pure chance" samples (strictly random samples), however small they may be, we can argue to their parent populations with a risk of error which we can set for ourselves in advance.

2. The "flukes" and "runs" of cases that seem impressive to clinicians, and even to animal experimenters, are often paralleled by the sequences met by anyone who plays with random numbers.

But these remarks would have missed the point. The obstetrician was not thinking of "chance" in the strict technical sense. What he apparently had in mind — and the pharmacologist certainly had — was the question of nonrandom runs, i.e., clusters due to sampling from a group restricted in type, or place, or time.

Intuitively we feel that if we take a large sample — if we spread our net more widely — we are more likely to obtain a "representative" sample, something nearer to a random sample of the population. This is not necessarily so. Let us suppose that the first 50 cases in a study represented what may be called the "general run" of cases of a certain disease or injury, and that then something happened, such as the spread of a disease in one institution or an accident involving a considerable number of men in one factory. These cases might contribute a large part of the next 50 cases, but they might differ in severity or various other respects from the first 50 cases. This kind of event might not occur again for a long time. Therefore the first 50 might be more like a random sample of cases than would be the sample of 100.

Another example was mentioned earlier. As time goes on in a clinical trial it may be more and more difficult to meet our quota of suitable patients. Therefore we may call in patients who come to see us rather infrequently, because their condition does not fluctuate much or for some other reason. They may meet the required specifications for the trial, but may differ in various undetected ways from patients who attend more frequently and who are more typical of those to whom we would apply the results of the trial. A similar kind of thing can happen in animal experiments and in almost any kind of survey in which subjects are not overabundant.

One very great advantage of a large sample is the opportunity it affords to study differences between subgroups; but even for this purpose one large sample may not be as informative as a number of smaller samples studied at different places and times.

Q VIII – 7. Will our available subjects and other facilities enable us to obtain a sample that is large enough for our purpose?

Inspection of Table V often causes us to make our purpose much more modest. Instead of hoping to detect a difference of 10 percentage points we may decide to be content with 30. But however modest our aim, it seems almost inevitable in clinical research that we will find fewer subjects than we expected when we started our study. Our difficulty is not unique; I am informed that it is not an uncommon experience in sociologic and psychologic studies.

It has been suggested that the anticipated number of patients in a clinical trial should always be divided by 2 to give a more likely estimate. My impressions from work in chronic disease drug trials is that 4 would be a still more realistic divisor.

For any kind of clinical study, perhaps the best estimate of numbers of suitable patients (case loads) could be obtained if the principal investigator went through his case records for the previous several years in the company of a very meticulous colleague, along with the statistician, if one is to be involved in the study. These three searchers should have in front of them the detailed plan of the study, and regarding each of the previous cases that appeared to meet the specifications they should ask a series of questions such as the following: "If the study had been running when this patient was here, would he have met the specifications exactly?" "Had he any disqualifying features?" "Are the records complete enough to permit us to answer those two questions?" "Would the patient's own physician have agreed to his inclusion in the study? How do we know? Can we find out?" "Would any factors such as the internal politics of this institution, or attitudes of staff members to experimental treatments of patients, have impeded our enrollment of this patient?" "What has been the fluctuation of qualified patients during the past few years?" "If we could obtain for the study as many patients as we need, would we have to reject some because the work or space required would be too great?"

Such an inquiry would probably accomplish more than a safer estimate of the future sample size. For instance, it might cause bewilderment regarding the exact definition of the population that would be represented by the sample – a very salutary effect.

CHAPTER IX

COLLECTING, RECORDING AND EXAMINING THE DATA

Everything that has been said in previous chapters has a bearing on the collection of the data, which is the body of investigation; but some of the topics deserve further emphasis and illustration, and some further details of method have to be mentioned. The questions in this chapter can be grouped around the more general questions: *Who?* (Q IX – 1, 2); *What?* (Q IX – 3); *When?* (Q IX – 4-8); *How?* (Q IX – 9-27). *Where?*, referring to location, is implicit in many of the questions.

Q IX – 1.   Have we overlooked any of the influences that observers and other personnel may have on our investigation?

We must remind ourselves continually that each participant in a study is a different person. The teachers, the subsequent experience, the temperament and thought-habits of every physician influence his observations, diagnoses and other inferences. A statistician may be an astute critic, but once he has made what he thinks is a discovery he is likely to become as emotionally involved as anyone else.

"Even in such routine matters as recording long lists of numbers or other simple data, it has been demonstrated that the mistakes which are made are usually more numerous in the direction personally favored by the recorder. No human being is even approximately free from these subjective influences; the honest and enlightened investigator devises the experiment so that his own prejudices cannot influence the result. Only the naïve or dishonest claim that their own objectivity is a sufficient safeguard" (Wilson, 1952).

If the investigator has a good reputation we are inclined to accept his conclusions, but we must remember that an authority is no better than his evidence, and his evidence should include his method of neutralizing his own bias.

The numerical effects of interobserver differences are touched upon in later questions; but we must keep in mind broader effects also. For example, there are two legitimate methods of deciding upon the dosage of a drug in a clinical trial. It may be stipulated that all patients shall be maintained on four 200-mg. tablets of drug X (or its equivalent placebo) daily. Or it may be considered desirable to imitate more closely the conditions of ordinary clinical practice by allowing the clinical observer to regulate the dose according to his opinion of each patient's need or tolerance. We must, however, note two consequences of this latter regimen:

1. Generalization of the results of the trial is less secure than after a fixed-dose trial. Another physician, even if he treated the same patients, might well have a different opinion regarding their needs and tolerance.

2. If we try to connect dosage with response we are arguing in a circle.

Q IX – 2. If more than one observer will be involved, how may their differences affect the results?

In some laboratory procedures any well trained observer will obtain the same readings as any other, or the differences may be so trivial as not to affect the final figure obtained from an experiment; but this does not hold as universally as might be expected, even in the laboratory; and in clinical trials it is seldom true. Therefore, it is commonly stipulated that any one patient must be examined by the same observer throughout the trial.

Then the question arises: "What is to be done when the observer cannot come to the clinic at the proper time, or is sick or on vacation or away at a medical society meeting?" It is impossible to obtain a reliable correction term, which one could apply, say, to the number of painful joints, or to the blood pressure reading, obtained by a substitute observer and thus convert them into the regular observer's figures. The inter-patient variation will be increased by the introduction of the substitute, i.e., the sensitivity of the experiment will be reduced; but in a properly conducted double-blind trial the randomization will still be responsible for the bias. There is, however, one way to minimize the increase of variation, and that is to arrange for two observers to work together, one being the chief observer on some patients, the other on other patients. The unavoidable absence of one partner has then less effect on the readings.

In some kinds of observation, such as the reading of x-ray films, two or more assessors sometimes work independently, to produce more reliable results. When there is not complete agreement the disputed films or other specimens are often re-examined and discussed until agreement is reached. This may, however, simply result in deference to the most experienced or most dominant observer. In this connection Fletcher, in *Medical Surveys and Clinical Trials* (Witts), has called attention to two points that are often overlooked: (1) If other specimens, on which observers have already agreed, were re-examined the verdicts might be changed. (2) Forced agreement may obliterate useful evidence — the very fact that the verdict on certain specimens was doubtful.

Q IX – 3.   If we are conducting an animal experiment how may the condition of the animals affect our observations?

Up to now, the emphasis in all our sets of questions has been largely on human beings. Here we turn to animal subjects. Much laboratory work in medicine is based on chemistry and physics, and that is perhaps why many investigators have treated their animals almost as if they were inanimate objects. There is now a growing suspicion that the results of many animal experiments, although accepted in good faith by the observers and by the readers of their reports, have been vitiated by factors that were not gross enough to cause obvious disturbance or death — for example, minor infections and intestinal and skin parasites. The problem is, however, much broader than this, as some quotations from various sources will show.

In a foreword to the Universities Federation for Animal Welfare (UFAW) *Handbook on the Care and Management of Laboratory Animals,* Himsworth wrote as follows:

"No man wittingly brings about the failure of his own work. The great difficulty in all scientific research is to exclude complicating factors. Pain, suffering and illness are such factors. Only insofar as these are either excluded or kept under control can the research worker hope to achieve the object of his investigation."

The results of experiments are affected not only by the temperature and amount of light to which animals are subjected, but by such factors as the number of animals in a cage and the type of cage (Chance).

In rats that were given frequent gentle handling by the experimenter there was superior food utilization and greater weight gain than in rats that were infrequently handled, although the rats that received the extra handling exhibited much more activity and curiosity than the unhandled group (Ruegamer and others).

The UFAW *Handbook* points out that "there appears to be room for a great deal of research into the psychological conditions that make happy and contented stock." In the meantime, to increase their acquaintance with animal psychology, laboratory workers could profitably dip into the writings of experimental psychologists, such as *Behavior and Neurosis* by Masserman.

Q IX – 4.   How may unidirectional changes affect our observations?

"Every characteristic by which a group of persons is commonly classified, except their sex and race, can change with time" (Sartwell and Merrell).

In numerous other questions we have seen how easily we may fall into traps if we are not constantly on the watch for time relationships. The present question is concerned with sequences that are essentially irreversible, such as life from conception to death. In this connection two points must be remembered:

1. Individuals vary in the speed of aging, although we have so far no good measure of this.

2. It is not only the individual but the environment that changes with time. An American man of 60 in the year 1960 was not only older than a man of 20, but he grew up in a different era of hygiene, diagnosis and therapeutics, and he lived through a major war and an economic depression which the younger man escaped. Similarly, a man aged 60 in 1960 was different in his life experience from a man aged 60 in 1910. He might be even constitutionally different, because he might have died if he had been exposed to the same risks of infection as the man of an earlier generation. For these reasons, subjects in large surveys are often grouped by date of birth; i.e., comparisons are made within *cohorts*, which are groups of individuals born in the same year or within a few years of each other.

The span of time over which a change occurs may be of any length. The blood pressures of 483 persons, read on two occasions 40 to 80 hours apart, were generally found to be lower on the second visit than on the first — a phenomenon that could be ascribed to a "desensitization to the sphygmomanometer" (Comstock and Kendrick). Even in a very brief experiment we should never assume that a trend is absent or unimportant. A series of frog muscle contractions, produced by electrical stimulation of the motor nerve, can be influenced by progressive changes in the state of the muscle, and each contraction may be affected by its predecessors.

Changes over a period of years or centuries are called "secular" changes (Latin, *seculum*, an age). These changes may appear unidirectional but may be in fact reversible. At various periods in the past, some infectious diseases, such as scarlet fever and measles, have become rare and trivial in severity, and then some years or decades later they have again become prevalent and severe.

Q IX – 5. How may fluctuations affect our observations?

Fluctuations can be roughly classified as (1) periodic or rhythmic, or (2) irregular.

Periodic or Rhythmic Fluctuations.   These can be illustrated by three types:

1. Short-period fluctuations, e.g., the heartbeat and breathing.

2. Diurnal fluctuations, e.g., in body temperature and in the incidence of accidents on the roads and in factories. Human stature (and recumbent length) shrinks by day, and although this is usually unimportant in the routine measurement of adults, neglect of it can introduce serious bias in children's records. In one group the diurnal loss was equivalent to three months' gain by growth (Kelly, Souders, and others).

3. Seasonal fluctuations, e.g., in the Northern Hemisphere the incidence of poliomyelitis increases in the late summer and early fall.

These three types of fluctuations remind us that rhythm is a universal phenomenon, with examples ranging from the periodicity of sunspots and the spinning of electrons, to seasonal budding and leaf-fall, and human waking and sleeping. Investigation often reveals unsuspected rhythm; e.g., when perforations of gastric and duodenal ulcers (7829 cases) were classified according to the days when they occurred, fewest were found on Sundays and Mondays, and there was a fairly steady rise during the rest of the week (Jamieson).

In an experiment we do not, of course, need to detect rhythms in order to control by randomization the bias that they may produce. Indeed, the search for cycles can be risky, even for professionals such as economists. To take a crude illustration, we might try to find out whether there was a relationship between the phases of the moon and some particular type of event. Taking the span of several years, we could start with the day of the full moon, and if we did not find a clustering of the specified events on those days, we could go to the next day, and then to the next day, and so on. Giving ourselves twenty-eight chances, it would be rather surprising if we did not find some apparent clustering, even if the events were purely random.

Even in laboratory work we can deceive ourselves in this way. If we detect what appears to be a clustering of events, e.g., unusually high readings at a certain point in a series, we must safeguard ourselves by taking this suggestion as a specific hypothesis to other series of the same kind.

Irregular Fluctuations. All phenomena are more or less subject to small irregular fluctuations, but we must not assume them to be "random" in the strict sense. Two more marked types of fluctuation in the clinical field are sometimes ignored:

1. In most diseases, even those that run a generally downhill course, the sufferer's condition fluctuates in severity, and he is most likely to seek medical aid at times of greatest severity. Shortly after receiving treatment he may improve, but this would often have occurred whether he had received treatment or not. This phenomenon has been taken as evidence of benefit from treatment, especially in diseases like rheumatoid arthritis that are characterized by remissions, i.e., the disappearance of symptoms for months or even for years. This is one important reason for the use of placebos in drug testing.

2. When hospitals are crowded, only the most severe cases of a particular disease may be admitted, whereas when more space is available milder cases may be admitted also.

Q IX – 6. How will we correct for unidirectional and fluctuating changes?

Previous discussions have indicated the first two of the three general methods of correction for changes associated with time:

1. Systematic design of the investigation.
2. Randomization.
3. Analysis of time relationships in the data.

Systematic design includes subdivision (stratification) of the material into smaller time intervals than the total span — for example: subdivision by age ranges and classification of patients according to duration between onset of disease and start of therapy. It includes also the cross-over design, one group with treatment sequence AB, the other with the sequence BA (Q IV – 6).

Even in a simple survey, such as the comparison of blood flow by thermocouple on hand and foot, if we cannot make records at the two sites simultaneously we risk confounding sequence and site unless we use a cross-over design, with random assignment of sequences to subjects. It is not enough to make a few trials of each sequence and, finding "no differences of any consequence," to assume that this will be true for our complete investigation.

If three areas or factors are to be contrasted, the six sequences ABC, ACB, BAC, BCA, CAB and CBA can be used on an equal number of subjects, but even this amount of systematic arrangement can be complicated in analysis, and the loss of a single set of readings can unbalance the scheme. Unless we wish to make a special study of sequence differences, it is usually best to decide by random allocation the sequence in each subject, without attempting to balance the numbers allotted to the different sequences.

During the analysis of the data some methods mentioned in Chapter XV can be employed to reduce the effect of the time factor. For example, the interval (I_1) between the onset of disease and the start of treatment may be related to the interval (I_2) between the start of treatment and the disappearance of a certain manifestation of the disease. If we are comparing two groups, A and B (e.g., treatment groups or males and females), with respect to the interval I_2, we can answer the question: "If both groups had the same average I_1 what would be their difference in average I_2?"

Q IX – 7. Are we going to deceive ourselves by starting to time a phenomenon at the wrong point?

Here is a simple example which is not always remembered by optimists in cancer research. If we measure therapeutic effect by duration of life after start of treatment we can obtain an entirely spurious impression that therapy is more effective than formerly, simply because diagnosis is now made earlier in the disease and treatment is started earlier. Our starting-point should be in the time-scale of the tumor itself, but this is impossible to determine. Even the stage of progression of the tumor, by histologic methods or extent of anatomic spread, is usually an arbitrary and coarse measure.

The prevalence-incidence fallacy (Q V – 8) is another example of a wrong starting-point. To study one of "Nature's experiments" we should have started at the beginning (time T_0) when all subjects were present, not at the present time (T_1) when only a selected group remains for us to study.

A more complex example is the following. In 1925 a large survey revealed that among infants who were born within 1 year after a preceding birth the mortality rate was about one and a half times the mortality rate of infants born after an interval of 2 years or more. The author concluded that the short interval was responsible, perhaps through the influence of frequent births upon the mother's health; and this has been used as a strong argument for "child spacing." In 1944 another investigator found similar differences in mortality, but pointed out a serious fallacy in the explanation.

Although a child who is born after a 6-month gestation can survive, a premature child is more likely to die in infancy than is a full-term child. Let us call the time of birth of a previous child T_0 and divide the succeeding period of 12 months into four 3-month intervals by the points T_3, T_6, T_9 and T_{12}. Then it is only the children who are conceived between T_0 and T_3 who can be born as full-term infants before T_{12}. All those who are conceived between T_3 and T_6 and are born before T_{12} will necessarily be premature and will have the consequently increased mortality. Many of those conceived in that interval may, however, remain in utero after T_{12} and be born as full-term infants in the second year.

As usual, if we visualize an imaginary experiment the problem is clarified. In fact, the mere asking of the right question, as an experimenter would necessarily do, would have started the investigator on the right lines: "Is there a higher mortality among infants *conceived* at X months after a previous birth than among children *conceived* at X + Y months after a previous birth?"

Q IX – 8.   How will we correct for differences in length of exposure to risk?

In an experiment we can decide how long the subjects shall have an opportunity to meet certain events or develop certain phenomena. We can do likewise in a prospective study if we can maintain contact with our subjects. In using records or other historical information (e.g., clinical records, employees' records, or information about how long a person has lived in a certain district) we have to take what we meet, and usually we meet widely different periods of exposure to risk.

One way of trying to overcome the difficulty is illustrated by expressions like "number of cases of tuberculosis per thousand person-years of exposure to contact with an open case," and "number of accidents per hundred thousand man-hours" in a certain machine operation. The denominator of such an expression is the sum of the individual exposure times of all the subjects under study.

This method should not be used without thought. It implicitly assumes a linear relationship between time and exposure to risk — that a unit of time entails the same risk in all subjects and regardless of whether the unit is at the beginning, middle or end of the subject's exposure. Exaggeration helps to show that this assumption may be unsound. One hundred man-hours of flying, if two pilots each flew for 50 hours, would hardly be equivalent to 100 man-hours to which 100 pilots each contributed one hour.

If the numbers of subjects are large it is possible, by the methods that are mentioned in Chapter XV, to show the actual relationship between duration of exposure and the occurrence of events. This is work for specialists, but in all our observations we must try to avoid being misled by differences in exposure time.

We may laugh at the remark, "Newsboys have a lower average age at death than bank presidents," but many of us fall into the trap against which the remark is a facetious warning. Reports on the follow-up of patients (Q V – 7) are often rendered meaningless by neglect of the warning. Even if the report states an average length of follow-up it brings us no nearer to any real population to which the figures could apply; nor is it of use in comparing two reports of the same kind. For example, the same average follow-up, 24 months, could be found in a series followed for periods varying from 6 months to 10 years and in a series followed for 20 to 26 months. Even if the maximum and minimum are given as well as the average, or even if the follow-up period of every subject is listed, we can learn little or nothing unless we are given the state of affairs at certain specified points in the survey.

Q IX – 9.   Are we going to use routine clinical records in our investigation?

The personal bias in some clinicians' records was discussed under Q VII – 7. Here we are concerned with the quality of the information that they contain.

Fictitious Data. Hospital records are known to contain ambiguous and often incomplete data, and grossly misleading laboratory reports (see *Ex. 4* under Q IX – 14); but chiefs of service are perhaps less aware than their juniors of the risk of purely fictitious entries. A hospital record room sends a case history back to the ward because a blood pressure reading has been omitted. The required reading was not made, and the patient has gone home; but the report reappears in the record room with a blood pressure inserted. A patient's record contains a blood sugar estimate, although it is later found that no sample of blood was obtained from him and that the figure does not belong to any other patient. Almost as fictitious are some percentage differential leukocyte counts, which are assumed by the physician to have been derived from 300 cells, whereas in fact only 50 or 20 cells have been counted. Even conscientious interns have sometimes been driven to this subterfuge in order to accomplish the excessive blood counting imposed on them.

Hospital charts still commonly contain a space for respiratory rates, although physicians seldom use the figures. At some hospitals where the figures were always duly recorded, inquiry revealed that the respiratory movements were seldom or never counted. Even the simplest statements in a record may be untrustworthy; for example, a patient's age may remain the same, year after year, copied from one set of records to the next.

These various fictions may indeed not affect a patient's welfare greatly, for a doctor who knows his patient well needs few notes. Most disconcerting, however, is the fact that, although many clinicians readily admit that individual routine records are often undependable, they are equally ready to draw conclusions from a table of percentages or other figures derived from a mass of such records. However large the mass may be, systemic errors (all in the same direction) do not "average out"; and those defects that do not cause bias — some of the omissions and the large variable errors (of the ± type) — cause serious lack of precision.

Most of the people responsible for hospital and clinic records are not trained investigators, and moreover the pressure of routine work is commonly heavy. From experience gained in the making of clinical records myself, in watching others make them, and in trying to use them, I have come to believe that the only records trustworthy for anything more than superficial impressions, or as hints for further research, are:

1. The records made meticulously by a physician regarding his own patients because he wishes to learn from them.

2. Records kept regarding a particular group of patients by a suitable and adequately instructed person, specially assigned to the task.

Patterson (1954) rightly regretted the appearance of a tendency to place "too much emphasis on the prospect of research work being made possible by elaborate systems of record keeping which would enable clinicians to get all sorts of statistical material on request." As he says, "The fundamental duty of the records officer is to produce the record when it is wanted, the whole record, and at once."

Anyone who still has hopes of using hospital records as a basis of comparison for a new therapy could profitably read about the investigation made by Densen and his collaborators on the records in two hospitals of high standing. Also pertinent are some experiences in an attempt to evaluate retrospectively the value of cortisone in rheumatoid arthritis by information gathered from the records at twenty-nine clinics (Mainland, 1955 a).

Q IX – 10. Are we going to use questionnaires in our investigation? If so, what problems will arise?

The first problem will be that most of us do not know how to construct a good questionnaire, whether we are clinicians, laboratory workers or, with some exceptions, statisticians. The exceptions are those persons who have learned from behavioral scientists who have specialized in this area, and also from practical experience, how to put questions to people which will elicit answers that will not fool the questioner.

Most clinicians spend their professional lives asking patients questions; but their questions are not usually those that are best answered by "Yes," "No" or "Don't know." More valuable than these monosyllables is often an indirect answer or a bit of volunteered information, or even an exclamation or gesture, which can lead the inquirer to ask another question, and another and still another, until an idea is formed as to what is wrong and what the patient needs — a kind of hypothesis which may be tested by treatment of the patient. When we are studying a disease, or more correctly a group of diseased persons who have a certain common characteristic (a common label), our method must be different. For example, we must find out how many of the group answer "Yes," "No" or "Don't know" to a certain predetermined question. Then we must find out how many of those who answered in each way to this question, answer "Yes," "No" or "Don't know" to a second predetermined question; and so on.

This might appear to be an easy problem. It is far from easy to obtain reliable answers even regarding factual matters. The impediments can be classified, although with overlap, under four headings:

1. Questions and the questioner.
2. Defective recall.
3. Emotional factors.
4. Ulterior motives.

Questions and the Questioner.   Whether the questions are asked by an interviewer or presented in a list to be filled in by the respondent, the answers can be affected by the form and wording of the questions, their sequence, the length of the series, and the attitude of the interviewer or of the person who presents the list, even if he gives no help in the interpretation of the questions. Specialists in this field have learned how difficult it is to frame a simple question that will be interpreted by the respondents in the same way as by the questioner. They have discovered more subtle things also, such as the phenomenon of "response sets." For example, if the first few questions elicit a "No" answer, the answers to subsequent questions may tend to be "No" also, even if, to be consistent, the respondent should answer "Yes." He has developed a negative "set" or attitude.

Despite their knowledge, the more experienced specialists admit that they have still much to learn. Among other things that seem to need more study is the effect of the length of questionnaires. As one who consigns to the wastebox all questionnaires except those that he feels compelled to answer, I am amazed at the magnitude of some questionnaires which some young psychologists and sociologists impose on patients, with the approval of the collaborating physicians; but perhaps some patients welcome the attention. Indeed, in one study of the problems of the aged, obvious therapeutic benefit was conferred on a group of old men by extensive and repeated interviews conducted by attractive young women, whether the resulting thick book of answers from each respondent had any research value or not.

Mail questionnaires are less likely to have this therapeutic effect; and here brevity is essential, to promote response if for no other reason. Bradford Hill (1951 a) half-humorously but very wisely suggested a maximum of five questions; but he showed how, without exceeding that number per person, suitable design of the survey makes it possible to obtain answers to more than five questions.

Defective Recall.   Patients' power to recall accurately events and dates is much less than many physicians seem to believe. Sometimes it is possible to make independent checks of respondents' statements, for example by statements from other members of the respondent's family and by hospital records and industrial lists that show absenteeism. In most cases, however, all that we can say is that X (an event, habit, or attitude) was *reported* by *p* per cent of the A's and by *r* per cent of the B's. Therefore, while collecting the information we should try to find out if there would be any likelihood of greater under-reporting (or over-reporting) in one group than in the other.

Emotional Factors.   When fearful of a particular diagnosis or bewildered when it is made, no person should be expected to answer objectively. Even in healthy persons the questionnaires themselves may produce symptoms (Glaser, 1954; *British Medical Journal* Editorial, 1954).

Sometimes unpleasant knowledge can be thoroughly suppressed, as in a certain community health survey in which one man stated that he had never had a coronary attack, although it was discovered later that he had been treated for one in a hospital and had known at the time that there was no doubt about the diagnosis.

Ulterior Motives.   Hope of gain or desire to please are motives familiar in everyday clinical practice. A more subtle factor that may affect any respondent's statements is his concept of his relationship to others, i.e., his own view of the role that he plays.

The difficulties of creating a good questionnaire should make us refrain from the attempt unless we can secure expert guidance; but we cannot do any research without planning data sheets of some kind, and in clinical research these present some of the same problems as questionnaires.

Q IX – 11.   What are some of the precautions that we should take in planning data sheets?

Hill (1951 a) declared that in the planning of a questionnaire, for every question that a planner proposes to ask a respondent he should ask himself at least three questions. This advice is equally important in the planning of data sheets (record forms) either for an experiment or for a survey. Here are six questions that we should ask ourselves:

1. Will the instructions for observation and recording be clear and sufficiently detailed?

When a committee was planning an attempt to gather, by transcription from records at a number of clinics, evidence on experience with a certain drug, a member of the committee remarked that if many instructions were sent the transcribers would not read them. As it turned out, the few instructions that were issued were often ignored. The analyst had to make many calls for elucidation, and her fear of undetectable errors grew ever stronger.

Even in multiclinic drug trials, in which the observers' interest is generally much greater than in transcribing from past records, misinterpretation and neglect of instructions are common. That is one reason why a pilot study (Q II – 10) is so useful. It not only reveals to observers the extent and serious effect of inattention to details, but shows the planners the defects of their data sheets.

Even if one person is going to plan and conduct the whole research he ought to write out full instructions for himself. He may remember exactly what to do during the period of a short investigation, but it is surprising how quickly many of us forget details of a procedure that we think has become reflex.

2. What are all the possible answers to each question on the data sheet? Are they shown alongside the question, to be circled or underlined?

The choices offered should include every possibility and should be mutually exclusive — for example: Y(Yes), N(No), D(Doubtful), NI(Not investigated). "Check if present" is not a safe form, because the absence of a check mark may mean "not present" or "not investigated" or "present but not recorded." In a diary to be kept by a patient it is not safe to request "No. of pills taken," unless it is shown that "zero" must be recorded if none are taken.

Data sheets often contain spaces headed "Other" or "Additional Remarks," sometimes with the instruction to "Amplify on reverse side." If the information thus obtained is used in the actual analysis of the data (e.g., group comparisons) it conduces greatly to bias, because responses vary from zero to abundant detail. It may, however, give the analyst insight into the quality of the observer's work, sometimes by contradicting the answer given to one of the specific questions. It may, also, give hints of some phenomenon that should be studied systematically.

3. What are the various possible interpretations of each question by the persons who will make the observations and write the answers?

4. What are the various possible interpretations of each answer?

5. Is the order of the questions sensible?

In the examination of patients the most "sensible" order of procedure is, in general, the one used in ordinary clinical practice, which tends to minimize disturbance of the patient. It is not good technique to jump from one part of the body to another and then back to a region previously examined. Nor is it desirable, as a rule, to jump from questioning to physical examination and back again, although in ordinary practice a doctor often finds it helpful to do so.

There are also more subtle psychologic points to notice. For example, on the final visit in one double-blind drug trial in which I was involved the physician and the patient were both asked to report their impressions regarding the patient's improvement since the beginning of the trial. When the trial was over I was much annoyed to find that I had overlooked the order of the questions, first the patient's impression and then the physician's. As it turned out, the patients' responses were much more optimistic than those of the physicians. Either the physicians were unaffected by the patients' responses or had purposely discounted them.

When the sequence of observing and recording is decided upon, it should be adhered to in all subjects. Departure from this role increases intersubject variation.

6. Will the data sheets be sufficiently pretested?

Pretesting is the only way in which we can have confidence regarding the matters alluded to in the preceding five questions. Even long before a formal pilot study we should, in studies concerned with human beings, test our proposed instructions and questions on colleagues, nonmedical acquaintances and subjects like those who are going to be studied, including the less intelligent and less cooperative.

Q IX – 12. How will we try to prevent defects in observing and recording?

Perhaps the best way to remind ourselves, and all others associated with an investigation, of the importance of meticulous attention to details, is the frequent quotation of a statement made by Hill (1951 b) with reference to multicenter trials: "Every departure from the design of the experiment lowers its efficiency to some extent; too many departures may wholly nullify it. The individual may often think 'it won't matter if I do this (or don't do that) just once'; he forgets that many other individuals may have the same idea."

Those who plan a clinical study may point out alliteratively in the instruction sheets the great need for each statement to be *correct, complete* and *clear*. They may stipulate that before each patient leaves the clinic the data sheets shall be checked for omissions, obscurities and obvious mistakes by (a) the observer, (b) the nurse-secretary in the study, and (c) the clinic chief or his deputy, and shall be signed by each of these individuals. Whether this helps materially to improve the quality of the data I do not know. The clinic chief's signature, I suspect, is in some cases equivalent to the validation rubber-stamped on many unread documents today. The procedure was used in a clinical trial on rheumatoid arthritis recently conducted by the Cooperative Clinics Committee of the American Rheumatism Association (Mainland, 1961; Mainland and Sutcliffe, 1962). All cases from one clinic were discarded because of numerous departures from the protocol which at that clinic was considered unnecessarily elaborate. The other ten clinics took the project seriously, and it is of interest to note what can be achieved in the minimizing of omissions, whatever the immediate mechanism of this achievement may have been.

The condition of 68 joints, with respect to pain and swelling, was to be recorded in each patient by circling Y(Yes), N(No) or D(Doubtful) before treatment started and again after 6 months — a total of 15,368 items in the records. In all these there were only 10 omissions (0.07 per cent) and one observer out of the total 34 was responsible for 9 of them (on three patients). We must remember, of course, that absence of omissions is not synonymous with correctness of entries. This is especially true if an observer, having circled a number of Y's, asks his secretary to circle the N's at all the other joints.

Q IX – 13. How will we minimize misstatements in recording?

This question refers to a particular kind of defect — mistakes like circling "Yes" instead of "No" on a record form, misreading an instrument or recording the wrong figure, mistakes in copying and the like. The first step toward prevention is the appreciation of how common such mistakes are, and of how serious their effects can be.

In the trial of two widely different dosage levels of the same drug in patients with cancer of a certain gland, the data sheets requested statements about the presence or absence of metastases in bones. Without any intention to test accuracy of reporting, a question in another part of the record happened to refer also to these metastases, and when the statistician scrutinized the data she detected inconsistencies in the records of 11 of the 96 patients in the trial. Inquiry prompted the observers to re-examine the films and they discovered that in these 11 patients metastases had been recorded as present when they were absent, or vice versa, not because of doubtful x-ray shadows but through sheer error.

It does not appear very heinous if we make only one or two mistakes in each set of eight-page data sheets, but it is easy to build up a 10 per cent frequency of mistakes in one or more of the criteria that are being used to assess a drug effect. There may be an equal likelihood of erring in the postive or negative direction, or there may be bias in one or other direction. To obtain some idea of the effect of an unbiased 10 per cent error, let us assume that with drug A, if we had an unlimited number of patients and made no mistakes, we would find improvement in 50 per cent of them, deterioration (or no change) in the other 50 per cent, and with drug B these figures would be 85 per cent and 15 per cent respectively.

Let us now imagine a population of 1000 A's. There are 500 improved cases, but by mistake we classify 50 of them as "not improved," and we classify as "improved" 50 of the 500 that are actually not improved. In spite of our mistake we still have 500 patients in each category. However, with 1000 B's the results do not balance. Of 850 improved patients we classify 85 as "not improved," leaving 765 properly classified; and of the 150 who are not improved we classify 15 as "improved," leaving 135 properly classified. The results are:

Improved $765 + 15 = 780 = 78$ per cent
Not improved $135 + 85 = 220 = 22$ per cent

The A and B population percentages of improved patients with which we are now working are not 50 per cent and 85 per cent, but 50 per cent and 78 per cent. The difference may not appear very important, but when we look at the "power" of our experiment, by the method outlined in Chapter VIII, we find that the effect is not so trivial. Without discussion of details, we can make the following statements:

With population percentages of 50 and 85, more than 95 per cent of our experiments with samples of 50 would be successful, i.e., they would demonstrate B-better-than-A differences significant at the 5 per cent level.

With population percentages of 50 and 78 per cent, only about 75 per cent of our experiments with samples of 50 would be successful.

To retain the 95 per cent power we would have to increase our samples by more than half. With the same 10 per cent error frequency, but with other population percentages, we would need to double our samples to retain the 95 per cent power.*

Incidentally, this example illustrates two very general and important effects of random mistakes in classifying:

1. Whatever proportions of X's and not-X's we start with, the mistakes tend to convert them to a 50:50 proportion.
2. Consequently, although the mistakes are random, we form a biased estimate of population values unless the true value starts as 50 per cent. Thus, the 85 per cent was not changed to 85 ± some error term, but was reduced to 78 per cent.

In preparing questionnaires for psychologic studies, it is customary to insert questions that will provide checks on accuracy and consistency of responses. It appears ridiculous that such safeguards should have to be contemplated for reports on straightforward observations made by persons labeled "investigator." And yet all of us are liable to make mistakes that astound us if we discover them. Therefore we must institute rigid precautions. The simplest way to minimize mistakes in observing and recording, and also to guard against omissions, is an arrangement whereby someone who is meticulous reads to the observer each question in the data sheets, records the observer's response and then reads it back to him, so that he can check it.

Q IX – 14. Will our observational methods be sufficiently accurate for our purpose?

This is a complicated question, and the best introduction to it is perhaps a series of examples of observational error.

Examples of Observational Error. During recent years radiologists and clinicians have shown an increasing readiness to investigate and reveal the defects of observational methods in which they had placed great confidence. Much attention has been paid also to errors in clinical chemistry.

Ex. 1. X-ray detection of pulmonary tuberculosis. In a survey of chest films prepared for detection of tuberculosis, five experts examined the same films of 1256 men (Birkelo and others). Among the results were the following:

On the first round of observations one observer classified only 59 films positive for tuberculosis; another found 100 positives.

Agreement of all five observers on positives: 27 films.

Found positive by only one observer: 47 films.

When the films were reassessed later by the same five observers there

---

* I am indebted to my former colleague, Miss Lee Herrera for elucidation of this topic.

were many reversals of verdict. Expressed as percentage change per observer, some of the reversals were as follows:

First positives classified as negative by the same observer — Minimum: 7 per cent; Maximum: 41 per cent.

First negatives classified as positive by the same observer — Minimum: 6 per cent; Maximum: 19 per cent.

One observer, with 59 first positives, missed four of them the second time, but added 23 which he had previously called negative.

Ex. 2. X-ray assessment in a clinical drug trial. In the trial of streptomycin plus bed-rest against bed-rest alone in pulmonary tuberculosis (Medical Research Council, 1948), two radiologists and a clinician assessed the films independently, blindfold regarding the therapy of individual patients but apparently aware which was the earlier film. The categories were: Improvement (Considerable; Slight or Moderate), No Change, Deteriorioration (Slight, Moderate; Considerable). "No Change" might signify no appreciable change in the picture, or improvement in one part of the lung offset by deterioration in another part.

The assessors differed appreciably in grading by subgroups (considerable versus slight or moderate) and in the "no change" assessment, but agreed more closely in the distinction between "improvement" and "no improvement." For example, in the comparison between status on admission to the trial and status at end of the fourth month in the total 97 patients the assessments were:

Assessor	Improvement	No Change	Deterioration
X	53	8	36
Y	56	14	27
Z	53	9	35

Ex. 3. Questioning on history and symptoms. This example is taken from an instructive discussion of investigational error in a search for the presence of pneumoconiosis in coalworkers (Cochrane and others). Four physicians, A, B, C and D, interviewed among them 993 men, each physician seeing a different subgroup, about one quarter of the total. The age distributions of all subgroups were similar, and there was no reason to suspect strong selection factors. The percentages of men reporting histories of bronchitis, pleurisy and pneumonia differed little between the subgroups. For history of dyspepsia, however, the frequencies ranged from 9.9 per cent (Dr. A) to 26.9 per cent (Dr. D). Regarding current symptoms there were also great differences. For sputum the range was from 13.0 per cent (Dr. A) to 41.9 per cent (Dr. D); for cough, from 23.4 per cent (Dr. A) to 40.3 per cent (Dr. C).

For tightness of chest and pain there was fair agreement between the groups and there was little difference regarding the frequency of dyspnea (difficulty in breathing) probably because the men were asked questions that were aimed at assessing the degree of breathlessness in terms of four simple categories.

Ex. 4. Gross errors in clinical chemistry. Many physicians have long been aware that they could not trust the reports from certain laboratories or certain technicians; but the widespread occurrence of gross errors was not appreciated until a survey was made in 1946 of 59 hospital laboratories, chiefly in Pennsylvania. Solutions of known composition were distributed, and some of the results are shown here (Belk and Sunderman):

Substance	As Prepared (per 100 ml.)	Allowable Error(±)	As Analyzed Extreme Values	Number of Estimates Satisfactory	Estimates Unsatisfactory*
Calcium	6.6 mg.	0.5 mg.	3-17.7 mg.	14	29 (12)
Urea nitrogen	45 mg.	5 mg.	5-60 mg.	14	27 (13)
Sodium chloride	456 mg.	15 mg.	350-775 mg.	30	14 (2)
Hemoglobin	9.8 gm.	0.3 gm.	8-15.5 gm.	17	34 (11)
Glucose	60 mg.	10 mg.	40-571 mg.	33	19 (5)
Serum albumin	4.6 gm.	0.3 gm.	1.5-10 gm.	9	35 (7)

*Of the unsatisfactory estimates, the numbers that showed "gross error" are given in parentheses.

The "allowable errors" had been "arbitrarily selected by the referee as being limits that should be maintained for satisfactory practice." (For sodium chloride the authors' correction of the published figure is given here.)

There is no reason to suppose that surveys in other states or countries would have revealed a very different picture. Suggested causes include inadequate training and scarcity of technicians, partly due to low salaries. Improvement has occurred in some laboratories since the report was published, but gross defects still remain.

Ex. 5. Errors in blood counts. Some specialists in the field of blood diseases have misled us in two different ways:

1. By too vague standards. "One will soon recognize the uselessness of exaggerated exactitude . . . A mathematically exact determination of the 'actual' leucocyte count is an impractical dream; for clinical purposes, approximate enumeration is sufficient, guarding against gross mistakes by adequate care" (Schilling). This is a good general principle, but not of much value to anyone who is comparing two actual blood counts.

2. By impossible claims of precision. In the red cell count the random error of observation, expressed in the form of a quantity called the "standard error," which is mentioned in Chapter XIV, has been stated to be 1.4 per cent of the observed count, or less. Proper investigations have shown that it is 8 or 10 per cent (Berkson and others; Biggs and MacMillan). "The 'accuracy' of the skilled haematological technician is a product of the method of training. It is usual to set a standard of agreement between repeat counts which must be achieved before a worker's results are considered reliable. Since this standard is invariably one that cannot be reached by accurate counting, the technician learns to count very rapidly and to make unconscious adjustment in a series of counts to

ensure that all will agree with the first" (Biggs and MacMillan, pp. 273–274).

The standard error of 1.4 per cent arose from the belief that the number of red cells counted in five separate squares of a counting chamber should not differ by more than 18; that counts showing greater variability indicate incomplete mixing in the pipette and should be rejected. In reality, perfect random scattering would cause differences of up to 40 cells and occasionally more.

Nowadays the red cell count is often supplanted by hematocrit readings or hemoglobin determinations; but the long persistence of a method with fake precision tends to make one a little cynical regarding clinical laboratory science.

Ex. 6. Errors in body measurement. To clinicians who are conscious of the crudeness of their observational methods it may be some consolation to know that when anthropometrists (persons specially trained in measurement of the human body) examine their techniques they do not find any reason for complacency.

When 21 anthropometrists measured the wife of one of them, the differences between the highest and lowest measurements were: stature (21 observers), 1.8 cm.; hand length (13 observers), 2 cm.; transverse chest width (15 observers), 4 cm.; pelvic breadth, between iliac crests (18 observers), 5 cm. (Steggerda).

From a thorough study of variation in stature measurement Boyd concluded that a trained observer, employing a standard technique and measuring each person twice, should expect to find differences up to 1.5 cm. between the two readings, and even greater than that in about 5 per cent of the pairs.

Terms Relating to Observational Error. In discussions of observational error a number of technical terms are employed, and it is desirable to look at some of them, to see if they, or the concepts that underlie them, could help in problems such as have been illustrated in the foregoing six examples. The terms are: validity; systematic and variable errors; reproducibility; sensitivity and specificity; precision and accuracy.

Validity. The concept of validity is simple enough (Q II – 3), but to establish or measure the validity of a test or observational method is not easy when we are using the test or method to tell us about something that we cannot, or cannot easily, find out directly; and this is often the case in clinical research.

In *Ex. 1* (x-ray detection of tuberculosis) the great variation among observers' verdicts shows that the method must have low validity; but how would we determine its degree of validity? In many cases of tuberculosis detected by x-rays there are no other definite signs or symptoms, and the detection itself leads, or is intended to lead, to prevention of further development of the disease.

In *Ex. 2* (x-ray assessment of change in a clinical trial) some confirmation of the x-ray verdicts might be obtained by noting what had happened clinically (weight change, temperature, sputum) during the same period of 4 months; but the reason for x-ray examination is that it tells us more directly what is happening in the lung than do any of the clinical phenomena.

This example introduces also another aspect of validity: the validity of an observation as a prediction. By following the patients after the fourth month it would be possible to measure the prophetic value of the x-ray verdicts at the fourth month — unless, of course, a change in treatment was made in accordance with those verdicts.

Systematic and Variable Errors. A rather old distinction is the one between "systematic" errors ("fixed" errors, or errors of "bias") and "variable" errors ("accidental" or "random" errors). In its elementary form this terminology implies that each thing measured has a "true" size. Then the systematic error can be defined as *the error that affects uniformly all measurements of the same thing by the same observer, instrument and technique.* Variable errors, on the other hand, are *differences between repeated measurements of the same thing by the same observer, instrument and tchnique.*

These concepts are rather useful starting points, but observation is much more complex than they seem to imply. What, for instance, was the "true" stature of the anthropometrist's wife in *Ex. 6?* By making many measurements of her stature, each of the observers could have built up his own "population" of readings, and it is not unlikely that two or more of the observers would have arrived at different average statures. This suggests that here, and in very many other situations, it would be more realistic to talk of "systematic differences" between methods and/or observers, rather than "systematic error."

In some situations there is a standard method with which readings made by other methods can be compared. For example, if a quick and simple colorimetric method is used for a certain chemical determination it may be standarized against actual chemical analysis. But even here there is no single value for the systematic error. A large number of pairs of readings must be made, and in each pair the difference between the two methods must be found. Then the average of these differences is a kind of net systematic error, but the variation among the differences is equally important, or even more so.

The anthropometrists' stature readings illustrate some other important points. If one of the observers had made a large series of readings on the same woman, the variation among them would have represented his variable error in the measurements of that woman's stature. There are at least two factors that we can imagine contributing to it:

1. Variation in the subject's stance (posture), even when a standard position was prescribed.
2. Differences associated with passage of time, such as fatigue and boredom of the observer and subject.

There would also be a number of small independent factors influencing different readings to a different extent. We can call them "the random element in the variable error," but it is obviously inappropriate nowadays to use "random" as synonymous with the whole variable error.

The concept of systematic and variable error can be extended to qualitative data of the "present-absent" type. If one of the physicians in questioning coalworkers about cough (*Ex. 3*) missed a certain proportion of those who in fact had cough, that would be his systematic error of underestimation. Here, we suppose, a "true" value could be obtained, perhaps by inquiry among members of the family and fellow-workers. By contrast, in the x-ray detection of tuberculosis (*Ex. 1*) the "true" value (with and without tuberculosis) would be unknown. Again, the concept of systematic differences between observers is more appropriate than systematic "error." The idea of estimating an individual's systematic error by his divergence from the consensus of "experts" is sometimes appropriate, but hardly in this case, in which the experts disagreed with each other, and also with themselves.

Reproducibility. This term, or "repeatability," is often heard. It may mean simply low variable error, but when it refers to the use of the same method by different observers it implies also smallness of systematic differences between observers.

Sensitivity and Specificity. These terms are commonly used in connection with diagnostic tests, but they are applicable to any type of observation.

In terms of diagnosis, if a condition is present, the test ought to give a positive result. If it gives a negative result it is a "false negative." The frequency of false negatives is the number of negatives expressed as a percentage of cases in which the condition is present, and the higher the frequency the less *sensitive* is the test. In general terms, the more frequently a method distinguishes between things that really differ (e.g., blood pressures or stages of a disease) the more sensitive is the method.

When a diagnostic test gives a positive result in the absence of the condition that it is intended to reveal, the result is a "false positive." The frequency of false positives is the number of positives expressed as a percentage of cases in which the condition is absent; and the higher this frequency the less *specific* is the test. Again, the same concept can be applied to other types of observation.

The percentage frequencies of false negatives and of false positives can both be called systematic errors; but the variable error of the method can increase both of these, and contributing to this error is the variability of what is being tested, e.g., fluctuations in level of a serum protein, while the condition of the subject remains essentially unchanged. There are, however, two other factors at work:

1. The inability of a method to detect less than a certain amount or degree of the variable that it is to record. This increases the proportion of false negatives.

2. Overlap of the frequency distribution of the variable under test in different conditions, e.g., different diseases, or states of disease and health. This increases the proportion of false positives. Where there is such

overlap we have to decide what shall be the boundary between "positive" and "negative," e.g., a certain dilution of blood (titer) when the variable is a serum protein. Hence it often happens that there is some inverse relationship between the frequency of false positives and the frequency of false negatives, and this is somewhat analogous to the relationship between Type I and Type II errors (Chapter VI).

Precision and Accuracy.   If the variable error of a method is low, we can speak of the method as having *high precision.* If at the same time the systematic error is low (or there are only small systematic differences between observers) we can call the method *highly accurate;* and it was in this inclusive sense that "accurate" was used in the question that opened this discussion. "High" and "low" are, of course, relative terms. Their absolute values depend on circumstances, and on the purpose of our observations. Depending on circumstances, also, accuracy may or may not include validity.

Handling the Problem of Accuracy.   From the foregoing discussion it might be thought that an enormous amount of investigation on observational error would be necessary before we could start any research. Certainly, we ought to pay more attention to it than we often do, and in the "epidemiology" of chronic diseases the unreliability of methods of observation is one of the major impediments; but in the projects that most medical workers pursue the problem is not overwhelming. Although each project requires special consideration, the following five reflections may be helpful:

1. We must not be misled by those who say that the unreliability of x-ray and clinical observations is not serious because in the assessment of patients a comprehensive picture is obtained, in which individual observational defects lose their weight. Be that as it may, in research we have to study individual variables.

2. In view of the gross errors in routine laboratory work, we ought not to undertake serious research involving laboratory data unless we are assured that the laboratory work will be constantly of high quality.

3. In a properly conducted experiment the randomization controls the biases that may be introduced by methods and observers. It is when we come to estimate population values after the experiment, and to make comparisons with other people's work, that the bias (systematic error) of our method may mislead us.

4. With measurement data it is possible to make a comprehensive analysis of observational variation, showing the contributions from various sources: between observers, between instruments and between readings by the same observer using the same instrument. We can thus estimate the amount of reduction of variation that we would achieve by taking the average of a number of readings, by using only one instrument and by using only one observer. The method is called "components of variance analysis." To do this properly, however, is usually a big undertaking. So, also, is any attempt to find reliable correction terms for observer

differences and instrument differences. In most small-scale work it is
preferable to use the same observer and the same instrument throughout,
and to allow the fluctuations of the observer and of the instrument to be
pooled with the intersubject variation.

5. We should not reject a method of measurement (or other assessment)
merely because the variation between readings on the same subject
appears large. The question is: When we take samples (e.g., A-treated
and B-treated) of size N, will the variation between the subjects in these
samples (which includes *intra*subject variation) be small enough to
allow us to detect an A-B difference of the size we wish to detect? (see
Chapter VIII).

There is a growing literature on observational error and variation, of
which a valuable classified bibliography is given by Fletcher and Oldham
in *Medical Surveys and Clinical Trials* (Witts).

Q IX – 15. If we are going to estimate observational variation will our estimate include all its components?

It was pointed out earlier that all factors responsible for observational
variation must have an opportunity to affect our estimate of it. Here
is an example of failure to adhere to that rule (Mainland, 1954).

When a physiologist was planning a series of experiments that would
employ mixtures of a radioactive sodium salt and a radioactive potassium
salt, he ran preliminary tests on solutions of those two salts. On receipt
of a sample of each salt from the atomic energy laboratory, solutions of
the two salts were made and mixed in a certain ratio. Then duplicate
determinations on aliquots of the mixture were made by Geiger counter.
The procedure was repeated when other samples of the same two salts
were received from the same laboratory, but it was found that the results
were too discordant to be explained by the variable error estimated from
the duplicate determinations. The physiologist suspected differences
arising at the source of supply, but he had, of course, failed to see that
his duplication was only partial. It had not included the dissolving,
dilution and mixing of the salts, and thus it had omitted to measure a
large part of the error.

Q IX – 16. How will we know that an event reported in a clinical experiment has really happened?

We might add: "How will we know that an event not reported has
not happened?" and, "How are we to know about these events in any
kind of experiment?"

The general answer is, of course, that there must be confidence in the
dependability of participants, their full understanding of what is required,
and a maintenance, throughout the experiment, of a sense of the importance of the study and of the participants' roles in it. The particular point
of the question is, however, that in a clinical experiment patients are
participants and we often cannot be sure that a patient has taken the

prescribed drug or the prescribed amount. This is particularly true of outpatients, but not invariably false for inpatients. To ask a patient to return the unused pills or capsules is not a sure check; nor is the testing of the patient's blood (or urine) for the drug on each visit to the clinic, because knowledge of the approaching visit may prompt a neglectful or recalcitrant patient to take his medicine. Until the problem is solved the safest title of an A-versus-B trial would be "Prescription of A versus Prescription of B."

Q IX – 17.   Are we aiming at too great precision?

In striving for precision we may overreach ourselves and lose more than we gain. "A simpler and less specific test applied to a larger number of subjects may provide more information at less cost than an elaborate test on a smaller group" (Fletcher and Oldham in *Medical Surveys and Clinical Trials*, edited by Witts).

Although perhaps appalling to a laboratory worker, sometimes the best question to ask a patient in a clinical trial is: "Do you feel better this week than you did last week, or worse, or about the same?"

Attempts at precision can even lead to bias, as in scale reading.

Interpolation in Scale Reading.   In reading all kinds of scales, such as rulers divided into centimeters and millimeters, burets, and electrical indicators, it is customary to interpolate by eye between the marks on the scale. Many laboratory workers, throughout their careers, trust their interpolations, although it was shown long ago that such faith is an illusion.

Table 1. Final Digits in Interpolation by Eye

(*Yule, from Yule and Kendall*)

Observer	A	B	C	D
Total No. of Measurements	1258	3000	1000	1000
Final Digit	Frequency per Thousand Measurements			
0	158	122	251	358
1	97	98	37	49
2	125	98	80	90
3	73	90	72	63
4	76	100	55	37
5	71	112	222	211
6	90	98	71	62
7	56	99	75	70
8	126	101	72	44
9	129	81	65	16
Total	1001	999	1000	1000

Table 1 shows the results of an inquiry into the accuracy of inter-polation. Observer A measured drawings by a transparent scale divided in millimeters, judging by the eye the last decimal figure, between the millimeter marks. Thus, if a reading was 3.64 cm. the 4 would indicate that the line on the drawing seemed to lie four-tenths of the distance from 3.6 to 3.7. Observers B, C and D made human head measurements and estimated by the eye between centimeter marks on a scale. In all four sets of measurements, the final digits were eye estimates, and there should have been approximately equal numbers in each of the classes, 0, 1, 2, . . . , 9 — about   100 of each digit per thousand measurements.

The personal idiosyncracies of the observers were so marked that the final digits were quite misleading; and these observers were not excep-tional. If, therefore, there is no vernier attachment on a scale, the sensible rule is: *Read only to the nearest scale division.* When a value is so near to the middle of a scale interval that allocation to the mark above or below is difficult, it matters little where it is placed. In a series of readings one can allocate such values alternately to the higher and lower marks, or even allocate them at random.

The rule stated above is observed by some workers, but may disturb precisionists. If they persist in the interpolation habit, it would be reason-able to expect them to demonstrate that, in the end-result to which their individual measurements lead, their habit gives them greater accuracy than if they read to the nearest scale division. Perhaps the habit is often harmless, but it seems a little ludicrous to indulge in a somewhat time-consuming practice of pseudoprecision.

Q IX – 18.   How will we insure, for all sampling units, an equal exposure to observation?

Under Q VI – 10 it was mentioned how a clinician recommended a double-blind trial with placebo injections in order to insure, literally, equal exposure of all patients' gluteal regions. In animal experiments two operative procedures may differ greatly in length and thus give unequal opportunities for observation. Ways must be sought to avoid bias.

Equality of observation is one reason why the intervals between exami-nations should be the same for all subjects in a clinical trial, but some latitude must be allowed. For instance, if examinations are made at 4-week intervals and the clinic meets once a week, deviation of ±7 days may be necessary and allowable in a 6-month trial, but this should be the maximum. The effect of departure from schedule may be merely random increase of intersubject variation, but it may also contain an element of bias. For example, a patient on one of the drugs may feel little benefit and make no strong effort to return on the proper day.

Q IX – 19.   Will we be consistent regarding precision in the various parts of the investigation?

We would look askance at a person who measured part of an object to the nearest quarter-inch and the remainder to the nearest 0.1 inch, and then added the two lengths; but we sometimes do equally foolish things in the laboratory. In an investigation of salt exchanges between the intestine and blood in animals, the experimenter said that he felt that the error of his chemical analyses should be kept low, "about 2 per cent." Apparently he would have been ashamed to publish results containing a greater error than this, and he asked how often he should repeat each analysis in order to attain that precision.

Naturally, we wish to use chemical methods that are dependable, in the sense of not introducing every now and then a grossly discordant estimate; but the actual precision to be demanded depends on the other sources of variation in the experiment. In the investigation of salt exchange the variation in results would depend largely on the variation between animals, or between different experiments on the same animal. Even at an early stage of an investigation, and without resort to "components of variance analysis" mentioned under Q IX – 14, it often becomes obvious that the biologic variation will be much greater than the variation in chemical analysis. When that is so, increase in the chemical precision, either by improved methods or by more determinations on the same specimen of fluid, does little to reduce the variation in the experiment as a whole.

Q IX – 20.   Are we going to be deceived by the structure of our measurements?

Complex Measurements. The measurements that we analyze at the end of an investigation are often not the original direct measurements, but adjusted, derived or compound measurements (ratios, products, indices and the like), and unless we are careful they may lead us astray. A familiar compound expression for the surface area of the human body is the DuBois formula: Area $= 71.84 \times \text{Weight}^{0.425} \times \text{Height}^{0.725}$. Obviously, we could not discover anything new about the human body by measuring the heights and weights of a group of men, estimating their areas by this formula, and then plotting areas (Y) against heights (X), but we may fall into the trap when both X and Y are derived measurements, and we have used a common factor in constructing both of them.

Even more subtle was the mechanism that for a time deceived those who were analyzing the data from a clinical trial in which aspirin and cortisone were compared in the treatment of rheumatic fever. The drugs appeared to have a different effect on the measurements obtained from electrocardiographic tracings, and then it was discovered that the physicians had followed the customary procedure of adjusting the measurements according to pulse rate, and that, since the two drugs affected the pulse rate differently, a spurious difference in the electrocardiographic data had been produced.[*]

Percentage Changes. Perhaps the simplest example of adjustment of measurements is the habit, deeply engrained in medical investigators, of expressing a change (in measurement or frequency) as a percentage of

---

[*] For this example I am indebted to the late Marjorie T. Bellows, Chief Statistician, American Heart Association.

the initial value. Sometimes this is an attempt to measure an effect by an appropriate yardstick in order to obtain a more sensitive indicator. At other times there is merely a feeling that the same amount of change, measured in absolute units, ought to be given greater weight if the starting point is low than if the starting point is high.

Precautions with Complex Measurements. Two rules will help us to avoid pitfalls:

1. Before creating such measurements we should see our reasons clearly.
2. Even if such measurements are desirable we should explore the relationships of the original measurements thoroughly.

For example, if we propose to express changes in percentage form, we should first determine whether the magnitude of the change is in fact related to the magnitude of the initial value. If we find such a relationship and decide to use percentage change as our expression, we should, nevertheless, go back to the original measurements (or frequencies) whenever we propose to study the relationship between the change and some other variable. Even then, we should beware of a built-in relationship, due to observational error. If an initial value is too low it will tend to make the "change" too great, and if the initial value is too high it will tend to make the "change" too small.

There are many different ways in which we can concoct complex measurements that appear to have meaning to us. If a statistician tears them apart as unworkable or misleading, we should be grateful, even if we do not clearly understand his reasons. If, however, he himself starts to produce derivatives from the original measurements, we should insist on finding out what he is doing, but we should have the patience to listen to him, so that we will know whether his products are appropriate or not.

Composite Indices in Clinical Assessment. The editor of a medical journal once remarked that "physicians are arithmetically minded but not statistically minded." His comment could have extended far beyond the medical profession. Quantitative methods have been so successful in all fields of activity that many people have come to believe that if a number is attached to something the number must have a meaning — that we know more about the thing than if we merely describe it, or say that it is bigger or smaller than something else. We are encouraged in this worship of numerology by the ease with which numbers can be manipulated to produce other numbers, such as averages and indices.

When a physician tries to assess the overall condition of a patient by combining the evidence from a number of different criteria there is a special temptation to apply to each measure a score and then average the scores. During recent years American rheumatologists have paid a good deal of attention to such schemes in the assessment of activity of disease in patients with rheumatoid arthritis — part of an effort to make clinical assessments more objective and more communicable by quantifying them. This is a praiseworthy objective, but we ought not to imagine that a numerical expression *per se* can achieve it.

Criteria of rheumatoid activity have included the following: duration, in hours and minutes, of the general bodily stiffness present on waking in the morning; average number of aspirin tablets consumed per day; strength of hand grip in mm. of mercury; number of joints painful on pressure; erythrocyte sedimentation rate. All these are measurable entities; but sometimes qualitative criteria have been introduced into the same scheme, e.g., pain, classified as: none or slight; present only on movement; present at rest; wakens patient from sleep. A scoring system (sometimes merely 0, 1, 2, 3) is applied to each criterion, and each patient obtains an average score. The averages can, if desired, be classified in ascending order of activity, e.g., none, mild, moderate, severe.

There have been considerable disputes about the desirability of such schemes, about methods of evaluating them, and about the assignment of appropriate weights to the various individual components of the indices. Some details may be instructive, because the problem of overall assessment occurs everywhere in medicine.

Attempts at Evaluation of Indices. The following are a few of the ideas and methods used or proposed for evaluating indices of activity in rheumatoid arthritis:

1. It has been stated that, if the various components of an index agreed closely with each other as they rose and fell in individual patients, this correlation would be a strong argument in favor of the index. On the contrary, the closer the correlation, the less would be the need for observing more than one of the components. Moreover, disagreement among the components would not in itself prove that any of them were useless. They might be measuring different phenomena or mechanisms; but if so, what would an average score tell us?

2. Composite indices have been used in drug trials, and if a particular index has shown a clear-cut difference in drug effects that index has been approved by the investigators. Obviously, this would be valid only if an independent method had established a drug difference in the same trial; and in that case one might wonder why the index should be used at all.

Even if an index were properly validated in one drug comparison, it would not necessarily be reliable in the comparison of two other drugs, which might differ from those in the previous trial in their effects on the individual components of the index. Incidentally, the individual effects would be what a physician would wish to know in prescribing a drug.

Difficulties arise even when, in any one drug trial, we seek to compare different indices, or the same index with different systems of weighting the individual components. Let us suppose that we know, by an independent method, that drug A is superior to drug B. What right have we to suppose that an index that maximizes the A-B difference in outcome is nearer the truth than an index which records a more modest distinction?

3. Studies in observational variation have been used in support of

composite indices. It can be shown that, although each individual component has a large variability, the variability of the composite index is smaller. Perhaps the best way to counter this argument is to point out what would happen if we included some more items in the composite index — variables that had nothing to do with the activity of the patient's arthritis, such as pelvic width or a few numbers assigned to each patient from a table of random digits. These "measurements of activity" could be given scores like the other components of the index, and then the average of all the components could be found. The effect would be to pull in those indices which had previously been outliers, i.e., to reduce the observational variation.

Principles of Evaluation.   Only if we make a clear statement of what an index, or any other technique, is supposed to do for us, can we hope to find out how well it performs. Regarding composite indices of rheumatoid activity, there seems to be general agreement that in clinical trials the separate measures of effect must be studied. Even they are composite; for example, weakness of hand grip results from lack of muscle force, pain, swelling, stiffness, deformity and the patient's mental attitude.

Two proposed uses of the composite index are:

1. Assessment of individual patients in ordinary clinical practice — (a) status on first arrival, (b) change between one visit and the next, or through a succession of visits.
2. Communication — for example, in reporting the initial disease activity in a group of patients in a clinical trial or other study.

In the handling of an individual patient an overall assessment, either impressionistic or by composite index, can be used for prognosis and as a guide to therapy. It appears likely that a physician would pay more attention to his patient's individual peculiarities than to the index, and would disregard the index if it differed from his own impression. However, let us imagine a physician who decided to use the index as a predictor, or as a therapy indicator, or for both purposes. How could he test its value?

Treatment of patients would undoubtedly be influenced by their condition. The physician would presumably prescribe more powerful drugs (or higher doses) to those with high activity indices than to those with low indices. Then, no matter what happened to the patients (improvement, no change, or deterioration), he could not say how good or how bad the index was, either in prognosis or as a guide to therapy.

The only way to answer such questions regarding any measure of effect, individual or composite, is by a trial in which the therapy of individual patients is not influenced by the activity of their disease. In its simplest form, the trial would contain a high-index group and a low-index (or moderate-index) group. Within each group two therapies, or two doses of the same therapy, would be randomly assigned.

The second possible use of a composite disease-activity index, i.e., for communication, recalls the classification of a disease by stages of progression (Q IV – 4) in which physicians imagined, for about a decade, that they knew what each other was saying, whereas in fact they could not have used the scheme unless each of them had supplied his own mental correction terms to make patients fit into it.

When physicians use a composite index of rheumatoid activity they often report that it is the scheme devised by Dr. X, with certain specified modifications; but beyond these recorded changes there are often unreported differences in technique, e.g., in the method of measuring hand grip, and in the way of questioning patients about the duration of morning stiffness.

The first step in testing a scheme of communication is to decide, exactly and in detail, what scheme shall be tested – a decision to be made by a representative body of those that would use the scheme. At this stage, some of the items proposed for a composite disease-activity index would probably be dropped by common consent, e.g., if the information was difficult to elicit from patients.

The test itself would involve several hundred patients at all stages of the disease, and with widely different degrees of activity. Ideally, each patient should be examined by all members of a representative group of physicians working independently of each other; but this is obviously impossible, for at least three reasons: (1) In rheumatoid arthritis and many other diseases there are not enough patients at any one time and place. (2) The burden of repeated examinations would be too heavy on the patients. (3) When a patient has given a particular answer to a certain question he is likely to repeat that answer to another observer who questions him immediately afterward.

A partial solution of these problems could be found by organizing the tests within a number of different centers. Patients would be randomly divided in equal numbers into two or more groups, one group for each observer. If the index scheme were reliable, the observed results should not differ more than the randomization could easily account for. An initial matching of the patients before randomization, by someone who was not going to take part in the study, would increase the sensitivity of the test.

The important point to appreciate is that, before any scheme of classification, either an index or anything else, is recommended for general use, much thought and much hard work are required.

Indices for Prediction of Fitness. The foregoing remarks should not be taken as a condemnation of all composite indices. In efforts to determine the suitability of persons for various occupations, psychologic tests are given and a composite index or rating may be formed. Its validity can be tested to some extent by watching the performance of persons after they have been assigned to jobs. Similar schemes, involving physical and socio-emotional assessments, can be used in connection with the return to work of persons who have been disabled by accidents or disease.

Q IX – 21. How, in general terms, are we going to handle our data during analysis?

The most hopeful answer is: "We are going to keep as close to the data as we possibly can." When an investigator comes to a statistician for a preliminary discussion of his research plans and within fifteen minutes starts talking about IBM punch-cards and about raising money to pay a company to put the cards through a machine, the prospect of sound research is not bright.

Various kinds of mechanical analyses have their place in some researches, but the first machine that we should usually think about consists of our hands and a set of ordinary index cards, 3″ × 5″ or 5″ × 8″ depending on the number of entries. Although sheets containing data from many individuals are useful for an overall view, cards are much more useful for grouping the subjects in numerous different ways, and even a thousand cards are not too burdensome for many analyses.

The figures that we are analyzing represent the patients, animals, things or processes that we are studying, and the more familiar we become with them, the more likely we are to know about their interrelationships, oddities and defects; and the more likely we are to catch hints of explanations and clues for further research. We should, of course, make our arithmetical labor as light as may be, and often a minimal requirement is a desk calculator with a ten-digit keyboard, for multiplication and division. Clerical help may be necessary, but even a clerk reduces our direct experience of the data.

Many of us learn to reduce, by triple checking, our mistakes in recording, copying and calculation only after discovering in our records a serious blunder when it is too late to correct it. Similarly, we may learn the need for perfect legibility of figures by having to discard the results of hours or weeks of experimentation because a digit has been changed by writing over it, instead of striking it out and writing the correct figure. (Illegible words can perhaps be excused because the context is a guide, but illegible figures are unforgivable.)

Tricks that help in calculation are best learned by practice, with personal help from more experienced workers, but two general pieces of advice can be given:

1. If possible, check calculations by some other method than was used in performing them — e.g., add figures in a table vertically the first time and horizontally the second time; check division by multiplication.

2. See if your result is sensible, as judged by your knowledge of the data and by rough calculation.

Q IX – 22. What are we going to do about "significant figures" and decimal places?

Students who have learned in mathematics or laboratory classes something about "significant figures" and the number of permissible decimal places are often somewhat confused when they meet statistical analyses.

The confusion does not seem to be any less in the minds of some of them who become laboratory professors.

The number 57.6, if it implies "between 57.55 and 57.65," is said to have three "significant" figures, i.e., figures that mean something. So also have 5.76 (between 5.755 and 5.765) and 0.00576 (between 0.005755 and 0.005765). This term must not be confused with "significant" in the statistical sense. Rules have been developed regarding the number of figures that can be considered significant in various calculations — how the number changes in different steps of calculation, and how many figures are therefore permissible at the end. These rules are, however, of little or no importance to an experimenter, as will be seen from a consideration of how many decimal places should be carried.

Students in laboratory classes are often told that they should not express results with more decimal figures than are justified by the precision of the individual measurements. This is based on a good general principle — "Do not pretend to know more than you really know" — but when it leads an intelligent teacher of biochemistry to criticize the average value of a set of readings because it contains more decimal figures than each of the individual readings, there must be something wrong. A little experiment with random numbers may reduce the confusion.

Five numbers were taken, as they came, from a column in a table of random numbers, and then decimal points were inserted: 5.843, 3.086, 0.466, 5.746, 9.519. Average = 4.932. Each number was then rounded to the nearest second decimal figure: 5.84, 3.09, 0.47, 5.75, 9.52. Average = 4.934. This is only 0.002 above the average obtained from the original measurements. If, therefore, we had rounded 4.934 to 4.93, we would have been claiming less precise information than we could justifiably claim. We would have needlessly sacrificed precision. Even with such a small sample we are more likely to gain precision than to lose it by taking more decimal figures in the average than in the components. The same effect has been shown by experiments with actual measurements instead of pure numbers.

This is a relatively trivial matter; but not so trivial are the misunderstandings displayed by some teachers of physics and some medical laboratory workers who criticize statisticians for expressing quantities to four or five decimal places when they are derived from values that have only two places. Such critics apparently overlook two features of the calculations:

1. The precision of statistical results is not expressed by numbers of decimal places, or by "significant figures" as described above, but by statements of how far a sample estimate may lie from the value in the population represented by the sample.

2. Reduction of figures can lead one far astray. To illustrate this very simply, the square root of 486.4 is 22.05448. If we retain only one decimal figure, as in the original number, the square root becomes 22.1 and the square of 22.1 is 488.41, i.e., two full units larger than the original. In

a long computation this kind of error, although not so obvious as in this example, can become serious. To be safe, we should carry more figures than will be required at the end. As a rough guide in simple computations one can say: "Carry at least two more decimal figures than are required in the answer."

Q IX – 23. What guidelines should we follow in preparing tables and graphs?

Courses and textbooks in public health statistics give much detail regarding the construction of tables and graphs, but a clinician or laboratory worker seldom needs such varied and complex information and skill. The best way to learn good methods is by criticizing others' products and imitating the best of them. One should ask, for example: "Do the headings and subheadings of the table minimize the reader's need to refer to the text?" "Does the graph serve the main purpose of a graph, i.e., to clarify the relationship?" Many graphs that arrive at a laboratory of medical statistics do the reverse. They may contain ten or a dozen criss-crossing lines, in a variety of colors, with individual subjects distinguished by symbols such as large dots and small dots, circles, squares and triangles. Investigators often seem to be unaware of the tricks that the eye can play in creating a pattern or in masking a real trend.

Dangers of Graphs. "Diagrams prove nothing, but bring outstanding features readily to the eye; they are therefore no substitute for such critical tests as may be applied to the data, but are valuable in suggesting such tests" (Fisher, *Statistical Methods for Research Workers*, sect. 7).

"Graphs should always be regarded as subsidiary aids to the intelligence and not as the evidence of associations or trends" (Hill, 1945).

It would be well if these two quotations were posted, and read, in every laboratory and on the title page of every scientific journal, because graphs, by their vividness, can mislead even more easily than figures.

To reduce expense, editors of journals often prefer graphs to tables, and an author's opposition to editorial pressure should be based on sound argument. Few graphs enable a reader to deduce an investigator's actual figures, yet these are what a serious reader or another investigator wants to see.

Unless we scrutinize graphs very carefully, we can be misled by their scales. For example, we should ask: "What would a change of scale in the vertical axis – e.g., reduction to 1/10, enlargement to 10/1 – do to this graph?" "Do the trends or irregularities in the graph look large because the vertical axis does not start at zero?" In order to avoid deceiving ourselves and others, even if the lowest quantity to be graphed is far above zero we should usually start the axis at zero. To save space we can introduce, in the axis between zero and the lowest quantity, a jagged segment, something like the Greek capital sigma, Σ.

Curve Fitting. Regarding curve fitting in general, the following quotation from Snedecor, a pioneer in the application of statistics in biology, is worth noting:

"A stupendous amount of time has been wasted in ill-advised curve fitting. Only when the end in view is clear should the task be undertaken. Often a graph of the data points is sufficient. Represent them by small circles or heavy dots. If desired, they may be connected by light line segments. Avoid drawing 'eye-fitted' curves. They are highly subjective and are apt to be misleading to both the perpetrator and the victim. Interpolation with these links stands a better chance of being good than does estimating by means of even the most artistic curves."

Running Averages.   Irregularities in a graph can be smoothed out by finding the average of the first three Y-values and plotting it against the average of the first three X-values, then dropping the lowest X and Y, plotting the averages of items 2, 3 and 4, and so on throughout the series. Two-point, four- or five-point running averages can also be used. Apart from showing that some irregularities are probably trivial, this method may help us to see what features should be sought in analysis, but it does not constitute a reliable analysis itself.

"Direct Inferences" from Graphs.   A clinical colleague took exception to the statements quoted above from Fisher and Hill, because, he said, some graphs had enabled him to draw conclusions. Such conclusions can only be of the most general kind — e.g., that the dots in a scatter diagram form an approximately rectilinear band — unless they are based on some information additional to what the graph provides. We may know that the observational error in a certain experiment could not conceivably account for the differences in levels of a series of dots. If, in a set of eight dots, each is at a higher level than its predecessor, we know that such an arrangement rarely occurs when dots are scattered at random. Such observations of graphs are analogous to the "eye tests" of actual figures.

Q IX – 24.   Are we going to be deceived by average trends?

A simple artificial example is probably the best way to demonstrate this danger. Let us suppose that measurements of some kind are made on four subjects at times 1, 2, 3, . . . , 9, with the following results in appropriate scale units, along with the average increases since the preceding observation:

Time	A	B	C	D	Average	Av. Increase
1	4	5	6	7	5.5	—
2	5	6	7	8	6.5	1.0
3	6	7	8	9	7.5	1.0
4	9	8	9	10	9.0	1.5
5	10	11	10	11	10.5	1.5
6	11	12	13	12	12.0	1.5
7	12	13	14	15	13.5	1.5
8	13	14	15	16	14.5	1.0
9	14	15	16	17	15.5	1.0

   The average rate of increase (the slope of the line on the graph) during the first two intervals is one unit of the variable per unit of time, then 1.5 units of the variable for the next four intervals, and thereafter one unit per unit of time. When we examine the individual subjects' records, however, we find that in each of them the rate of increase is one unit of the variable per unit of time, except over one interval when each shows a spurt of 3 units; but the spurt occurs at a different time in each subject. Consequently, the averages do not apply to any individual, nor to an "average" or most common individual, nor to the group as a whole, because all members of the group are alike in showing a 3-unit increase when the spurt occurs. Nor does the spurt of the averages, from Time 3 to Time 7, show what the group as a whole is doing; it merely reflects in diluted form a spurt by one subject in each interval.

   In real life we should expect to meet a counterpart of this scheme whenever we study phenomena in which there occurs a change in the rate of change (an acceleration or a deceleration), because different individuals put on a spurt, or slow down, at different distances from the starting point. The method of averaging can create false estimates of the time and size of growth spurts in children and of blood pressure changes in later life. The phenomenon is, however, not confined to time relationships. The independent variable may be drug dosage or temperature, and this calls to mind melting-point tests in chemistry. A pure chemical, having reached a certain temperature, melts suddenly, whereas if there is a mixture of chemicals the melting process is spread over a considerable temperature range. The biologic phenomenon also is due to heterogeneity — a mixture — but here none of the individuals are "impurities." The information from each of them is equally important.

   In the study of an individual, an average trend, represented for example by a straight line, may be adequate (see Chapter XV), and then a group of individuals will provide information about differences in these averages. If, however, we are studying spurts or slow-downs we have to determine (1) what proportion of individuals start to change their speed at different values of the independent variable, (2) the amount and (3) the duration of the altered speed.

   Actual figures need hardly be given to illustrate the problems that we run into when, instead of using a longitudinal method, we try to determine rates of change (e.g., in blood pressure) by a cross-sectional study of groups of persons at different values of the independent variable (e.g., age). The dependent variable might in reality have no trend up or down, or it might ascend (or descend) at the same rate in every subject; but the average trend (or lack of trend) that was found in the survey could give an entirely erroneous impression, because it would be influenced by the selection factors that determined which subjects (i.e., which values of the dependent variable) were in the survey at each value of the independent variable. This is a serious difficulty in the study of aging and in the establishment of "normal" values (see Chaper XIII).

Q IX – 25.   Are we going to confuse absolute and relative rates of change?

In the following example the independent variable can be time, temperature, or any other steadily changing variable. The dependent variable can be any measurement made on two individuals or on two groups, A and B.

Independent variable	1	2	3	4
A	20	15	10	5
B	4	3	2	1

In a graph of these figures the line for A would descend much more steeply than the line for B. This contrast has been seen when the mortality from pulmonary tuberculosis (A) has been compared with the mortality from nonpulmonary tuberculosis (B) over several decades. It would appear that, whatever was causing the decline in A, it was much less effective in B. If, however, we express the decrease in each period as a percentage of the level at the beginning of that period, we find the same percentages for A and B:

Independent variable	1-2	2-3	3-4
Change as per cent of initial level	25	33	50

A more useful form of presentation is by logarithms, thus:

Independent variable		1	2	3	4
Log. dep. variable	A	1.301	1.176	1.000	0.699
Log. dep. variable	B	0.602	0.477	0.301	0.000

If we now take the difference between the logarithms at the beginning and end of each period, we find that the differences are the same for A and B.

Independent variable	1-2	2-3	3-4
Difference of logarithms	0.125	0.176	0.301

This means that, if we plotted the original measurements of the two variables on semi-logarithmic paper, with the independent variable on the arithmetic scale and the dependent variable on the logarithmic scale, the corresponding segments of the A and B lines would be parallel. Such a graph is the quickest way to start exploring such problems.

Q IX – 26.   Are we going to be deceived by the "goodness of fit" of our data to a mathematical formula?

This question can be discussed in terms of two common types of graphs: (1) frequency graphs, with measurements on the horizontal (X) axis and frequencies on the vertical (Y) axis; (2) graphs that show concomitant variation or trends, with the independent variable on the X-axis and the dependent variable on the Y-axis. However, the question applies equally to data and formulae that are too complex to be graphed.

In terms of a graph containing dots that represent the data and a line derived from a mathematical formula, we can speak of a "good fit" when the discrepancies (commonly called "deviations" of the dots from the line) could be readily attributed to random processes. (Tests appropriate to various kinds of data have been devised, and the usual standards of "significance" are employed.) We can look at two approaches to formula fitting:

1. We have obtained the data in order to test a particular hypothesis. If this hypothesis is true the data should be well fitted by such and such a formula. If the fit is not good we reject the hypothesis. If it is good, the important point to remember is that the formula derived from some other hypothesis might also fit well. We must ask ourselves: "What other reasonable hypothesis might there be?"

2. We obtain the data and then look for a formula that will fit them. Here we may readily fool ourselves unless we remember three facts:

a. Mathematicians have produced numerous formulae representing frequency-distribution data and measurement-relationship data, and the number could be increased indefinitely. Sooner or later we could find a formula to fit our data.

b. When a formula fits our data this does not prove that the relationships used by the mathematician to produce the formula are structural or functional relationships in the material that produced our data. For example, the dots in our diagram may be well fitted by a parabola, containing X and X^2; but this does not mean that if the X in our data is some linear measurement, a surface area (X^2) has some biologic or chemical significance in our material.

Similarly, transformation of actual measurements into their logarithms is found useful in certain methods of data analysis, but this does not tell us anything about the process responsible for the actual measurements.

c. A good fit, well within the range of random variation, does not imply fit in all respects, particularly at the "edges" of the region of observation, where our data are scanty; and it is still more dangerous to trust extrapolation.

Two examples may illustrate these points, one from frequency distribution curves, the other from curves that represent relationships between measurements (trend curves).

Fallacies from Frequency Curves. The Gaussian frequency curve, a symmetrical bell-shaped curve discussed in Chapters XI and XIII, has been found to fit rather well the frequency distribution of statures of adults of the same sex and racial origin living in the same region; but if the curve represented exactly the factors responsible for differences in stature in such a group we would have to recognize the possibility of meeting a man a mile high and another man of stature *minus* one mile, because the curve never actually reaches the X-axis.

We know that this is nonsense, but we should beware of drawing nonsensical conclusions from less extreme extrapolation or from fallacious reasoning within the area of our actual observations. We may have obtained certain physiologic or biochemical data from diseased subjects and from persons whom we have so far classified as healthy, and we may find that a certain type of frequency curve fits the pooled data. A curve is essentially a continuous structure, but we must not imagine that the goodness of fit proves that our subjects constitute one population with respect to the variable that we are studying, or that the supposedly healthy harbor disease.

Fallacies from Trend Curves.   Some years ago, in studying the difference between the first and second readings, on a series of x-ray films, of the interspace between the tibia and femur in the human knee joint, I examined the relationship of the reading difference (Y) to the order in which the first readings were made (X). In the first part of the series (lower values of X) there was obviously a decrease in reading difference with increase in X. The relationship was curvilinear, but a parabola (open upward) was too strong a curve. Therefore X^3 was introduced into the equation. The effect of this is to produce a second curve farther along than the first and in the reverse direction, and hence the first curve is somewhat flattened. This maneuver still did not produce a good fit. Therefore X^4 was introduced and finally X^5. The fit improved progressively.

Now if X had been continued far above 50 (the number of films in the series) this formula would have produced a succession of waves in the following order: trough, crest, trough, crest; but there was in the dot diagram no obvious curve except the first. If the observer had examined a thousand films his reading difference would doubtless have fluctuated from time to time, but there was no reason to believe that his fluctuations would in any way have coincided with the waves derived from the equation. The formula was simply an empirically devised tool to fit the observed data, and it could have been used for estimation of a correction term, e.g., to reduce the influence of reading order in comparing films from different subjects. If we do not read too much into them, take too much out of them, or trust them too far, empirical formulae have important uses, as is indicated in Chapter XV.

Q IX – 27.   Are we going to reject observations that seem aberrant? If so, on what basis?

Unjustified Rejections.   I do not know whether any laboratory workers still practice the "best two out of three" habit, i.e., taking three readings but using only the two that are nearest together. This can be called an irresponsible habit because those who practiced it did not take the trouble to find out what it did to their results. It can, in fact, distort them greatly.

Equally unscientific was the proposal of a professor of biochemistry to discard a vitamin A determination from the liver of one fish out of a dozen of the same species because it was, in his opinion, far out of line. The graduate student who had made the determinations was not satisfied, because the proposal did not spring from any evidence of a fault in the technique, the observer or the fish. It apparently reflected simply the biochemist's chemical upbringing and lack of appreciation of the skewness of biologic frequency distributions — the asymmetry that causes one to find an individual measurement far above or below the rest of the measurements.

Rules Regarding Rejections. It is easy to criticize the more irresponsible rejections of outlying measurements, but no true scientist feels happy when he behaves like an automaton with his data, putting them through the process of analysis without regard to their possible defects. Like the graduate student with the fish livers, he would like some rational rules of behavior.

There is one definite rule: We ought never to discard a reading simply because it is an outlier. We must apply other information, but this should be very definite information. A physicist or chemist, well acquainted with the variable error of a particular method, may be justified in rejecting a reading because its magnitude shows that it was almost certainly due to a gross mistake. Sometimes, even in physics, such judgments have been subsequently proved wrong; and serious danger arises when this behavior is extended to physiologic and biochemical data which (1) are often obtained by techniques that have large and inadequately known variable errors, and (2) contain a large biological variation.

Certain numerical rules proposed for the rejection of outliers are based on the assumption of an approximately Gaussian distribution of readings, which is untenable for most biologic variables and questionable for most observational errors.

Outliers in Clinical Research. In clinical studies "exceptional cases" are often met. In a report on the treatment of breast abscesses with and without penicillin the mean duration of pus formation in 16 controls was 13.8 days; in 18 penicillin-treated women it was 6.3 days (Florey, Mac-Vine and Bigby). A statistical test (the t-test, discussed in Chapter XIV) showed that the difference was "significant" at the 5 per cent level. The report stated that one patient had been excluded from the calculation because pus formation had continued in her breast for 88 days, but as she was a control patient this did not affect the verdict in favor of penicillin.

If, however, the outlier had been in the penicillin-treated group, the investigators would have been in a difficult position. To exclude it, on the ground that it was only one case in 18 (about 5 per cent) might have led to a false or exaggerated verdict in favor of penicillin, because a hundred penicillin-treated cases might have provided a much greater proportion of resistant cases. At the time when this research was done, the problem would have been more difficult than it would be today, because the only test commonly known at that time, the "t" test, is derived from the Gaussian distribution, which is discussed in later chapters. Duration data, as in this case, often depart so far from the Gaussian distribution that a test derived from it can give a verdict of "nonsignificance" when in fact an appropriate test, not assuming a Gaussian distribution of measurements, shows a clear-cut difference between the effects of two treatments.

Today we are not faced with that problem, because a simple test, shown in Chapter XIV, is available. Therefore we can unhesitatingly adopt the following rule: Unless we are willing to report the results of clinical investigations merely as our impressions, we must not make selections among our data according to our notions of what is "typical" or "aberrant."

If, in the absence of a valid reason for rejecting an outlying observation, we include it in the analysis when we could have legitimately excluded it, we will increase the variation between sampling units within the treatment groups, and lower the sensitivity of our experiment. It is, however, preferable to obtain a verdict of "not proved" when in fact a difference exists, rather than obtain a false verdict of "significant."

Our concern with observations that appear aberrant should not cease with our decision to include or exclude them from analysis. If we are about to discard a value because it is "an obvious misreading," we should of course ask: "Is it *really* obvious?" Then, whatever we do with it, we should ask: "What is wrong with our system of immediate checking of readings?" A correct but unexpectedly large or small value should lead us to look carefully at our instruments, techniques, and sampling methods, to see whether any of these things introduce more heterogeneity than we desire. Aberrant values that actually stem from the nature of our material itself may provide useful clues to further research.

CHAPTER X

LOST INFORMATION

"Lost information" in this context means information that we planned to obtain and did not obtain. The losses can occur in any kind of research; here are half a dozen examples: (1) We have planned a cross-sectional survey of a certain group (previous patients, an occupational group or a healthy contrast-group for a clinical study), but we cannot find them all, or some refuse to cooperate. (2) In a forward-going study there is a progressive loss of subjects (attrition) as the study continues. (3) During a clinical trial patients drop out. (4) A piece of information is omitted from a record form in an experiment or survey, and the omission is discovered too late to rectify it. (5) If a patient appears for examination on a date other than the one required by the plan, the information that would have been obtained on the proper date is lost. (6) If a patient acquires another disease during a trial, his signs and symptoms may well be different from what they would have been without that occurrence; the desired information is missing.

Regarding completely missing subjects, the important thing to grasp is that the very fact of absence shows that there is something different about the absentee, and we must therefore ask: "Could this difference, or something associated with it, have any relation to the phenomena under study?" As later examples show, this is a much more difficult question to answer than many people think. Even if only one piece of information is missing, the suspicion of bias is present.

Q X – 1. Will large numbers compensate for lost information?

The answer is "Definitely not!" In a valuable discussion of the general principles of medical surveys, Hill (1951 a) pointed out the danger of trying to obtain information on a total population, such as an industrial group, and then failing to do so. He wrote as follows:

"We do not know whether those who choose to answer the questions, who choose to keep records or respond to the clarion call to a clinical examination, are representative of the population concerned — whether the refusals, the unknowns, the untraced have characteristics that differentiate them from those who are incorporated in the survey . . . The neurotic may be over-anxious to attend for clinical examination, the physically unfit in some circumstances may be anxious *not* to attend. The stupid may have more accidents and also be prone not to keep records. Those who do not return the questionnaire may include an unduly high proportion of negatives who conclude that they have nothing of interest to report, while the positives may include those who more freely respond. We record the successes but not the failures . . .

"I would therefore myself infinitely sooner have, say, a one in four sample of the population, of a size thereby which enabled me to pursue relentlessly, and complete the records for, all or nearly all the persons in it, than have to interpret figures derived from survey of the 'whole' population from which finally a quarter was missing. From the well-constructed sample we can at least infer the values that exist in the population, or, rather the limits between which they are most likely to lie. With the incomplete 'whole' population we are merely left with a spate of doubts and conclusions that should be, but too frequently are not, excessively tentative. Do not, therefore, think that the scientific aim is *necessarily* more likely to be achieved by approaching the population rather than a sample."

Hill's reference to estimates of population values shows the importance of strictly random samples. Having divided the population of 2000 by random numbers or an equivalent device into a sample of 500 to be investigated and 1500 not to be investigated, if we find out how many X's and not-X's there are in the 500, we can say: "Assuming that this random division was not one of those that happen rarely, how many and how few X's and not-X's may there be in the uninvestigated 1500?" (We can define "rarity" as less than 5 per cent, less than 1 per cent, or whatever percentage we choose.)

The phenomena that Hill mentioned have been abundantly illustrated when second and third attempts have been made to obtain responses to questionnaires. They were illustrated also in an analysis of the "order of coming up" in a population of 600 persons in a coal-mining district, all of whom volunteered to have their chests x-rayed (Cochrane). The observers persisted until all 600 had been examined, and divided the reports into three groups of 200, in the order of coming up for examination. It was then seen that "in general people with pneumoconiosis came up first and those with tuberculosis, particularly clinically significant tuberculosis, last."

Although Hill's remarks referred to large surveys, we must remember that the same factors can operate when we are trying to follow 50 patients over a period of time, or when we are studying a certain serum protein in 50 patients and try to obtain a contrast-sample from friends of the patients or from our colleagues.

Q X – 2. In a controlled trial what can be done about refusals to participate?

Usually nothing; and it is usually best not to induce an unwilling patient to participate, because he is likely to be uncooperative. The population is restricted to those who are willing to participate; but that does not vitiate the results as applicable to such persons.

Q X – 3. In a survey is it safe to make up for refusals and losses by enrolling more subjects?

In a proposal for a study of the attitudes and practices of parents with regard to the care of infants' health the following statement was made:

"If early results indicate that the sample of 400 is not large enough, because of too large an attrition rate, lack of cooperation, or sampling errors, another sample of 400 may be necessary."

The only interpretation that I can place on this statement is that the proposers of the plan believed that the uncooperative and the drop-outs would not differ, in any way that was relevant to the study, from those who cooperated fully all the time. In a properly conducted clinical trial of drugs, if a patient has to drop out because of removal to another city it is unsafe to treat even that event as an "act of God" irrelevant to the effects of the treatments under test. In a correct analysis we play the drop-outs in such a way as to avoid bias in favor of a new drug that is under test.

The project mentioned here was to be a study in attitudes to medical care, and we can be virtually certain that the uncooperative and the drop-outs would differ from the persons in the study in their attitudes, and consequent behavior, in the very thing that was to be studied. It is bad enough merely to disregard the uncooperative and the drop-outs; but the planners of this study proposed to compound the felony by adding to their sample more persons who *were* cooperative.

Q X – 4. What should be our maximum percentage of losses?

In a discussion of the no-response rate (lapse rate), Doll (1951) wrote that, from experience in a large number of surveys " . . . one can expect a refusal rate of 1 or 2 per cent however little is asked of those examined. Not everyone accepts this figure, and the Pneumoconiosis Research Unit [of the Medical Research Council of Great Britain] is not satisfied with any lapse rate at all. It is perhaps generally reasonable to allow a lapse rate of up to 5 per cent, but a lower one should always be aimed at and it must be realized that anything appreciably higher may materially bias the results."

In planning a piece of research we do not need to quote any authority on this matter, or take anyone else's word for the damage that can be done by nonresponses, drop-outs or failures to record the presence or absence of something that is under study. For example, if our answers are to be of the "Yes-No" type we can take a number representing our proposed sample size, and assume a certain number of nonresponders. We assume that 50 per cent of the responders said "Yes" and 50 per cent said "No." Then we assume (1) that all the nonresponders said "No," and (2) that they all said "Yes." By adding these answers to those obtained from the responders, we can see how much or how little information we would have regarding the true percentages of "Yes" and "No" reponses in our total sample. We can repeat the procedure with different numbers of nonresponders and different percentages of "Yes" answers from the responders. In planning a clinical trial we can adopt the same kind of procedure with assumed drop-outs and omissions of data.

In the planning of many research projects, if this simple arithmetic had been used, along with previous experience of response rates, drop-out rates and omissions of data, or with the aid of preliminary studies to explore these figures, much wasted research effort would have been avoided. Either the research would not have been started or steps would have been taken to minimize losses.

Q X – 5. How will we try to minimize losses?

The prescription for minimizing losses somewhat resembles advice to a graduating class. It contains four ingredients: forethought, imagination, ingenuity and persistence.

From the first thought of our research we must start planning in detail the prevention of losses. We must put ourselves in the place of the subjects whom we propose to study. We must invent a variety of ways to arouse their interest and to make the study as convenient as possible for them. Finally, indefatigable persistence is necessary in finding those who have failed to respond and in trying different methods to induce them to do so. The main difference between this prescription and most valedictory advice is that it has been acted upon and has achieved remarkable results in a number of studies of occupational groups and even general population samples.

In clinical studies an investigator starts with the advantage of the doctor-patient relationship, but he often has also a fatalistic attitude — some patients always disappear, and nothing can be done about it. Actually, a great deal can be done by applying the above prescription. The atmosphere of the clinic — the attitude of all personnel who may affect the patient — must be right. The concern about the study, and about the patient, must be genuine. There must be someone participating who has an interest in people, the proper approach to patients, a compulsive pride in maintaining contact with them, and ample time to exercise that compulsion.

One clinic, in a region where there were two ethnic groups, employed two secretaries for patient relationships and record keeping, one girl from each group. The clinic employed also the facilities of a credit bureau and of the police in the tracing of patients, but the secretaries proved more successful. Another device employed at the same clinic was the collection of the names and addresses, not only of relatives but of friends and acquaintances who came to visit patients while they were under hospital care. The result of the system, of which these are only a few details, was an unusual retention of contact with patients, even when they had moved to distant states.

To minimize the other type of lost information, i.e., omissions from data sheets, we require a regular routine of recording and checking (see Q IX – 12 and 13).

Q X – 6. Will we be able to retrieve bits of missing information?

Even if we cannot induce a person to participate as a subject in a survey we may be able to obtain some information about him; and even if a patient has moved to another city during a clinical trial it may be possible, through contact with a clinician in that city, to discover something about his condition. Even such fragmentary information may be of use when we are analyzing our results.

Q X – 7. How will we deal with the problem of lost information when analyzing our results?

Unless there is clear justification for some other action, the rule is: Play the losses both ways. For example, in an AB, X–not-X comparison, assume first that all the missing A's are X's and all the missing B's are not-X's and analyze the data. Then reverse the assumption and analyze again. Special cases, in which this rule may not apply, are of various types. Most of them can be illustrated from clinical drug trials, in which the causes of lost information, as defined at the beginning of this chapter, are numerous and very diverse. Even the simplest case often turns out not to be so simple when we think about it carefully.

General Rules in Drug Trials.   No detailed instructions can be formulated for the handling of problem cases, but five general rules are rather obvious:

1. We must decide what we are going to do about each problem case before our decision can be influenced by the outcome of the trial, i.e., before we break the code in a double-blind trial and much earlier when we are in a trial in which we are not blindfold.
2. If the completely observed patients show a "nonsignificant" difference between treatments, i.e., a verdict of "not proved," there is little need to incorporate the lost cases; but otherwise we should very rarely, and only for clearly defined reasons, ignore a lost case.
3. Unless there are very special reasons for counting the lost cases as "successes," they should all be counted as "failures." This will tend to lower the sensitivity of the experiment, but there is no safe way of avoiding this. (Occasionally, of course, it is possible to show in an A-B comparison that the verdict in favor of A persists even when we count all the missing A's as failures and all the missing B's as successes.)
4. Since any decision may introduce bias we should insure that the bias will not favor a new drug against a placebo or a standard drug. It would seem ludicrous to have to admit that our verdict in favor of a drug (perhaps with "P less than 0.01") was conditional on our having made the right decision regarding lost information; whereas if our decision creates a "nonsignificant" difference this simply means that we

have not enough evidence for a verdict in favor of the new drug, and this is indeed true.

5. Whenever we make a decision regarding a piece of lost information we must ask ourselves: "How will this decision affect the definition of the population to which the results of the trial will apply?"

These rules are applicable not only to complete losses, but also to cases in which information is missing on only one or two criteria of assessment. We cannot safely assume that omissions are random; e.g., a painful joint is less likely to be missed than a painless one. Moreover, if we are seeking verdicts on, say, five criteria, we must not assume that because a patient improved by criteria V, W, X and Y, he probably improved by criterion Z for which the data are missing.

One of the methods of treating the problem of drop-outs in some otherwise carefully conducted trials appears to stem from strange logic. The patients who dropped out and the patients who completed the trial are compared with respect to their characteristics at the beginning of the trial, or at some point during the trial if observations were made before drop-out occurred. If the two groups do not differ appreciably (or "significantly") the drop-outs are disregarded. Unless I misapprehend the procedure, it implies, in the first place, an acceptance of "no significant difference" as synonymous with "no real difference." More strikingly, however, it seems to confer on physicians a power of prophecy which, if they were directly questioned, they would firmly deny — the ability to forecast, from today's examination of a small group of patients with a very fluctuating disease, the status of that group 6 months hence.

Lost Information in a Drug Trial. In a 6-month double-blind trial conducted by the Cooperating Clinics Committee of the American Rheumatism Association (Mainland, 1961; Mainland and Sutcliffe, 1962), a certain drug (D) was compared with a placebo (P) in rheumatoid arthritis (with aspirin prescribed to all patients at the discretion of the individual physicians). The patients were classified, by various criteria, as improved or not improved (i.e. deteriorated or not detectably changed). Ten cases presented problems owing to loss of information. The data from the other 113 patients demonstrated a benefit that was clearly associated with the drug. Therefore the ten problem cases had to be scrutinized. The decisions do not claim infallibility, but illustrate an effort to avoid bias in favor of the drug without going to fantastic lengths in the attempt.

1. During the trial a patient was found to have cancer. By the protocol this would have barred him from the trial. Moreover, it was inconceivable that this disease could have been produced or accelerated by the trial; therefore the patient's data were omitted from the analysis. This was hardly a problem case; but when, in the course of a trial a disease develops that is not excluded by the protocol, the decision is not so automatic.

In the first place, we often cannot be sure that the intercurrent disease would have occurred if the patient had been on the other therapy in the trial. Secondly, let us suppose that the physician thinks that the new disease has set the patient back so much that he is not a fair test-object for either compound in the trial, and that therefore his data ought to be discarded. The definition of the population then becomes dependent on an individual clinician's judgment. Generally it is best to use the patient's data if he is kept in the trial, and to count him as a failure (not improved) if he is taken out of the trial because of the new disease. In this, as in all other problematical decisions, it is possible at the end to find out what the verdict of the trial would have been if a different decision had been made.

2. One patient had her medication (P) analyzed. She was dropped from the trial and her data was discarded. Therefore the definition of the population was implicitly modified to exclude patients who submitted their medicines for analysis. Quite probably she had been dissatisfied with her progress, and she might not have had the tablets analyzed if she had been on the drug; therefore, the decision may have biased the final results slightly against the drug.

3. One patient (P) received from a private physician the drug that was under test, and used it for some time before it was discovered by the physician in charge of the trial. The patient was assessed at the end of the trial as improved and was counted as an improved placebo patient.

4. In another placebo patient a similar incident occurred, but the drug received was another anti-rheumatic agent which was excluded by the protocol of the trial. This patient was judged to be unimproved at the end of the trial, and was so counted.

In Nos. 3 and 4, the actual disposal of the cases had to await the disclosure of the therapies that the patients had received in the trial; but the policy for handling such a case should be decided upon before this information is obtained. As an exercise, the reader might enumerate the various possibilities of bias in these cases, depending on the agent (P or D), on the observed outcome (improved or not improved), and on the analyst's decision — to omit the case, to count the patient as improved, or to count him as not improved.

5. One patient (D) moved to a distant city and was counted as not improved. It might be argued that such a move was quite independent of the effects of the therapy and that therefore the patient could have been dropped from the analysis. This is a dangerous line of argument. Even if we know that the plan for the move had been made before the trial, it would be almost impossible to know whether the move would have taken place if the patient had been in a different state of mind or body than he actually was; and the benefit (or failure of benefit) from the therapy might have been partly responsible for his condition.

6. One patient disappeared entirely, even from the police, and was counted as unimproved.

7. One patient (P) was one month late for the final visit, whereas the

maximum allowed departure from the schedule was 7 days. The actual assessment was disregarded and the patient was recorded as unimproved.

8. One patient had been dropped by the clinic concerned, because of lack of cooperation during the trial, and was counted as unimproved.

9. One patient (D) fractured her hip in the middle of the trial and was taken out of the trial permanently. It might be argued that this event was unconnected with the drug, which at best had a mild effect, but it certainly could not be so argued on patients treated by corticosteroids, because these drugs can create such a feeling of well-being that a patient may subject to excessive strain his bones and joints that have long been untaxed. Because this was an unusual event, the patient was omitted from the analysis and the definition of the population was restricted accordingly. The same decision could have been defended even if the patient had been continued on the trial therapy (either D or P).

10. The condition of one of the patients deteriorated so much that a more drastic treatment was considered necessary. This was clearly a failure of the therapy and the overall assessment (unimproved) presented no serious problem.

When these various decisions had been reached, the cases were pooled with the main data and it was found that they caused a negligible difference in the proportions of improved and unimproved patients.

In the handling of a problem case, different investigators might arrive at different decisions, and so might different users of the results. Therefore, in any detailed report of an investigation it is important to show what was decided about each case, and why. It is also important to present the tabulated results in such a way that any reader can insert the problem cases in different categories.

Some Other Problems. A few remarks on problems not exemplified by the foregoing ten patients may be useful.

1. Sometimes, in addition to the trial therapy, it is decided that some special therapy, not forbidden by the protocol, is desirable. In the trial of streptomycin in pulmonary tuberculosis (Medical Research Council, 1948) previously mentioned, several patients were treated by pneumoperitoneum, i.e., introduction of air into the peritoneal cavity to cause elevation of the diaphragm and partial collapse of the lung. If this had been a double-blind trial, the comparison of incidence of pneumoperitoneum in the streptomycin and bed-rest group might have been a measure of the effect of therapy. Sometimes it might turn out that an A-treated group, with special therapy to certain patients, did as well as the B-treated group, few of whom required the special therapy; and this also would be useful information. In general, after analysis of the whole data it is desirable to look separately at the outcome in the patients who received the special therapy.

2. Temporary interruption of therapy, or lowering of dosage, because of undesirable effects attributable to the therapy, does not pose a serious

problem in analysis, because it reflects the circumstances of ordinary practice. When the trial protocol has prescribed a particular dose, however, we can compare the responses of the underdosed and fully dosed groups.

3. When patients are actually taken out of a placebo-drug trial because of such undesirable signs or symptoms, we are left with a sample of a drug-treated population that can tolerate the drug, and we can imagine ourselves saying silently, as we prescribe for a future patient: "If you can tolerate the drug you are likely to do better than on a placebo." We should not forget, however, that a patient who is doing well may not be taken out of a trial on account of undesirable effects as readily as a patient who shows the same effects but is not doing well.

4. Sometimes a patient cannot perform one of the tests that is to be used as a measure of change under therapy, e.g., a person who is completely bedridden with rheumatoid arthritis cannot demonstrate how long it takes him to walk 50 feet. The results of this particular measure can apply only to those who can perform the function, and this is one objection to composite indices for which some patients cannot provide all the components.

5. Death in some trials is a measure of difference between two treatments, but in most trials it is rare, and the often difficult question arises: "Was it in any way attributable to the disease, and therefore perhaps to the failure of the therapy?" It is probably best to consider the deaths separately, and to define the population under study as one that would not die under the conditions of the trial.

Q X – 8. What are we to do about lost information in an experiment on nonhuman material?

The best answer to that question is often: "Jettison the experiment and start afresh with a plan that will prevent the losses." However, there are sometimes inevitable occurrences, such as intercurrent infection and death of animals, and a great variety of odd accidents that occur in all kinds of experiments, and then the principles discussed above with reference to human data are applicable.

It is true that in rather complicated agricultural and other experiments methods are used for estimating "missing values" by using the data that are present, on the assumption that the losses are random. If we assume that a gap means a bias, this device does not help, and that is generally the safer assumption. At all events, an experimenter is hardly likely to share the exultation of an electronic-computer expert who announced that he had trained his machine to "plug all the holes in a mass of data that was full of them."

CHAPTER XI

ESTIMATING POPULATION PERCENTAGES FROM SAMPLES OF FREQUENCY DATA–AN INTRODUCTION TO RANDOM PROCESSES

This chapter is a continuation of the discussion started under Q VI – 21 — "How will we estimate what our results really tell us, numerically, about the population represented by our sample?" In reviewing that discussion we should note why, in trying to answer the question, we go into the world of "pure chance," the artificial world of disk sampling, and bring out some information that is useful in the real world. In most medical research our samples are not strictly random samples of their parent populations; therefore our estimate of error, pure random sampling error, is a minimum estimate. However, random processes affect considerably the composition of our samples, and so it is often safe to act *as if* a sample were a random sample, provided that we are always on the lookout for more reliable information.

Experiences with Random Processes

We will look at the details of a random sampling experiment, not only for its use in the present problem but because such experience enables us to start at the right place in dealing with more complicated problems — and in dealing with statisticians. It is lamentable that very intelligent people say, sometimes apologetically and sometimes defiantly: "I don't know anything about statistics." By performing two sets of simple experiments they would have the foundations of statistics at their finger tips, both physically and intellectually. One set of experiments would be sampling from a barrel containing well mixed disks. The other set would be the shuffling of, say, 40 playing cards, 10 marked "F" and 30 marked "S," and dividing them into two samples of various sizes. Nowadays, of course, we do not need to take the time to prepare and mix disks or to shuffle cards, because we can use random numbers, as is shown later.

In performing such experiments we must continually think about their relationship to, and distance from, the real world; and that is where, in more complex situations, a statistician can do much for scientific investigation, if he is the right kind of statistician. If we have thus watched random processes at work in simple cases, we can say to a statistician who is prescribing for us a research design or analysis: "Please explain this in terms of disk sampling or card shuffling, whichever is more appropriate." Then, if we are willing to describe to him, and if possible show him, slowly, in detail and with repetition, our bit of the real world (our purposes, investigational material, conditions and methods), we can say to him: "Please show the connection between your prescribed method and the facts, difficulties and doubts in this bit of the real world." By his response to these two requests we will soon know whether we have got hold of the right kind of statistician. But we do not deserve the right kind of statistician if we are not willing to think hard along with him.

The Sample

After a properly conducted clinical trial containing 20 A-treated and 20 B-treated patients, we have decided that drug B was more effective than drug A when the effects were measured by numbers of improved cases. We decide to use drug B until something more promising appears, but we would like to know what our sample of 20 B-treated patients can tell us about the percentages of improved cases that we can expect. Of the 20 patients, 17 (85 per cent) were classified as improved, and 3 (15 per cent) were classified as not improved (deteriorated or not appreciably changed). The nearest that we can come to the prediction that we desire is an answer to the following question: "If this were a strictly random sample from a very large population, what would we know about the percentage of improved patients in that population?"

Analogous Problems

The same kind of question can be asked about any sample of individuals, animate or inanimate, that are classed as X's and not-X's (a binomial system). If a surgeon, having listened to a paper about a new operation that was successful in 17 out of 20 patients, would like to tell the speaker how little his figures really showed, he could use the answer that we will find for the B-treated patients. When a certain chemical is injected into 20 animals, 3 die and 17 survive. The pharmacologist wishes to know what percentage might die if he injected the same chemical in the same dose into a very large number of animals of the same kind and under the same conditions. A certain diagnostic test has been applied to 20 patients who are shown by other methods to have a certain disease. The test result was positive in 17 and negative in 3. What percentage of false negatives might the test give if we continued to use it on similar patients?

Approaches to Population Values

We will look first at an experimental approach, and then at the equivalent mathematical approach — an experiment on paper. Finally we will see how the answer can be obtained from Table I (see Appendix).

The Experimental Approach

The experiment described here was performed for another purpose, but we can use it to answer the question: "If a sample of 20 patients, containing 3 F's (failures) and 17 S's (successes), were a strictly random sample from some population or other, would it be unlikely that the population percentage of F's was 30? In other words, would 3 F's out of 20 be a rare kind of random sample from a population containing 30 per cent F's?" To avoid being influenced by the results of the experiment, we adopt in advance a definition of "rare." In this instance, for a reason given later, we depart from the customary "5 per cent rarity," and define the "rare" class as the group of samples lying farthest below the population value (30 per cent F's) and comprising not more than 2.5 per cent of the total random samples of all kinds obtainable from that population.

In the experiment 1000 circular metal-rimmed cardboard disks (labeling tags), one inch in diameter, were used. Three hundred disks were marked "F" and 700 were marked "S." Then all were placed in a box and mixed thoroughly by taking handfuls and allowing the disks to dribble through the fingers. From time to time the disks were poured from one box to another, and the mixing by hand was repeated.

This first mixing was continued for about half an hour, and then, to obtain a sample, a handful was taken and 20 of the disks were laid on the table without previous inspection of the markings on them. The remainder of the handful was returned to the box, as was the sample after its composition (number of F's and S's) had been recorded. The thousand disks were then mixed as before nine or ten times, poured into the other box, remixed, and sampled again, until 1000 samples of 20 were obtained.

If this experiment were to be repeated today, I would use random numbers, letting any three digits (say 1, 2 and 3) represent F's, and the remaining seven digits represent S's. As each successive set of 20 digits was met, the numbers of F's and S's would be recorded.

An "Infinite" Population. Even in such a simple procedure as disk sampling we must try to avoid being tricked by our technique. Let us picture what must have happened toward the end of each individual shuffling just before a sample was taken. One disk after another would come into a position such that it would be removed by the sampler's hand. As each disk came into position it would leave one less of its kind (F or S) to be moved from the general mass into what can be called the "sampling area." Therefore only the first disk to move into the area would be strictly from the 30:70 population; but we stipulated samples from exactly that population. We could have obtained such samples if we had taken one disk at a time, recorded its mark, returned it to the box and reshuffled before taking the next disk, thus making up each sample of 20 by single-disk samples. Our thousand disks would then have become an "infinite" population, which can be defined as one whose structure is not affected by sampling. When we have previously used the term "very large population" we have side-stepped the phrase "large enough to be effectively infinite in comparison with our sample."

Since each sample of 20 in the actual experiment was small relative to the total population, the effect of the bias was considered negligible in a demonstration performance. In actual sampling from a finite population, when we wish to estimate the contents of that population, the effect of removal of a sample should never be assumed negligible. Chapter XII mentions a technique for making such an estimate. The methods of the present chapter are of more general use in medical research, because we are commonly concerned with populations that we would create by continuing to do the same thing (e.g., apply a medical treatment) to more and more subjects of the same kind.

Results of the Sampling Experiment. The results of the disk experiment are shown in Table 2. Two features should be observed:

Table 2. Frequency Distribution of 1000 Random Samples of "Failure" and "Success" Disks

Population: 30 per cent F disks.
No. of disks in each sample = 20.

F's in Sample No.	Per Cent	No. of Samples	Relative Frequency	Percentage Frequency
0	0	0	0.000	0.0
1	5	7	0.007	0.7
2	10	28	0.028	2.8
3	15	68	0.068	6.8
4	20	129	0.129	12.9
5	25	157	0.157	15.7
6	30	206	0.206	20.6
7	35	166	0.166	16.6
8	40	123	0.123	12.3
9	45	68	0.068	6.8
10	50	31	0.031	3.1
11	55	15	0.015	1.5
12	60	2	0.002	0.2
13	65	0	0.000	0.0
..	..	..	....	...
..	..	..	....	...
20	100	0	0.000	0.0
Total		1000	1.000	100.0

1. Some classes of sample, such as zero F's, were not met in this experiment, but from much larger sampling experiments we know that if we had continued the sampling we would sooner or later have found a few samples in those classes. We know also that the percentages in some of the other classes would have changed slightly; but the thousand samples are quite adequate to use with the clinical-trial sample.

2. The peak of the frequency distribution is, as we would expect, at 6 F's, i.e., 30 per cent F's as in the parent population. That percentage is the *mode* or *modal value* — the most fashionable value (French, *la mode*, the fashion). It is important to note, however, that the modal class contains only one fifth of the total samples. A sample value was more likely to differ from the "true" (population) value than to represent it exactly, and this is true of most sampling distributions.

"Rare" Samples. The tails (end-parts) of the distribution contain the rarest classes of samples. Having adopted the 2.5 per cent standard, we make the cut-off between 1 F and 2 F's. It is true that this excludes only 0.7 per cent of the samples, but if we made the cut-off between 2 F's and 3 F's we would classify as "rare" too many samples, 3.5 per cent of the total. The difference from 2.5 per cent seems trivial, but it is generally safer to err by setting too high a standard than too low. On the 2.5 per cent standard, the clinical-trial sample would not be classified as rare.

We could also make a 2.5 per cent cut-off in the opposite tail, which we would use if we were working with a sample containing more than 30 per cent F's, e.g., 11 F's. Using both tails in this way, we would classify less than 5 per cent of all the samples as rare. However, in the present type of problem we are always concerned with one tail of the postulated distribution. In this instance we are asking: "Is the observed sample percentage so far *below* 30 per cent F's that it would lie in the *lower* tail of a frequency distribution of random samples obtained from a population containing 30 per cent F's?"

We could, of course, cut off a tail containing not more than 5 per cent of the samples by making the cut-off between 2 F's and 3 F's. This was not chosen because the techniques and formulae used in constructing Table I (see Appendix) were based on 2.5 per cent cut-off points. If samples like our observed sample would be in the lower 2.5 per cent class of a random distribution we can say that at least 97.5 per cent of the random samples would have higher percentages of F's than did our observed sample, instead of saying "at least 95 per cent" as with a 5 per cent cut-off.

A Mathematical Shortcut

We did not actually need to perform the disk-sampling experiment because in the late seventeenth century, a period of great interest in games of chance, it was shown that the binomial expansion would give us the information that we desired. Readers who, like myself, are unsophisticated in gambling and mathematics, can gain insight and assurance

regarding the mathematical shortcut by considering the simplest mathematical example. If we mix thoroughly the individuals of a population
containing 1000 disks (500 F's and 500 S's) and take 1000 random samples,
each containing two disks, we know what will happen. In approximately
half of our samples the first disk that we draw will be F and in the
other half it will be S. In approximately half the samples in which the
first disk was F the second disk will be F also, and in the other half it
will be S; and the same will be true for the samples in which the first
disk was S. Therefore, for every contribution to the FF (or SS) class
there will be two contributions to the FS class. (In this connection it is
immaterial whether F was first or second in the pair.) Our overall
results will therefore be approximately the following:

Contents of Sample	Proportion
2 F's, 0 S's	0.25 (25 per cent)
1 F, 1 S	0.50 (50 per cent)
0 F's, 2 S's	0.25 (25 per cent)

We know that the more nearly uniform in shape, texture and weight
are the disks that we use, and the larger our number of samples, the
nearer we will approach to these proportions. As we proceed, our experience will not be quite the same as in many mathematical processes, which
lead us steadily toward some limiting value. Our "interim" totals will
sometimes approach those that are given above, and then move a little
away from them. This is the way in which random processes act; but
as we continue, these fluctuations will become less and less in proportion
to our total number of samples.

We can now express the same step-by-step process more briefly by
letting p = the proportion of F's in the population (0.5) and q = the
proportion of S's (also 0.5). Then we have:

Contents of Sample	Proportion
2 F's	$p \times p = p^2 = 0.25$
1 F, 1 S	$2 \times p \times q = 2p^1q^1 = 0.50$
2 S's	$q \times q = q^2 = 0.25$

The above series of symbols represent the expansion of the expression
$(p + q)^2$, in which the superscript 2 represents the sample size, while
in the individual terms the superscripts represent the numbers of F's and
S's, e.g., p^1q^1 indicates 1 F and 1 S.

To obtain the percentage frequencies of random samples of 20 from
a population containing 30 per cent F's, we can expand $(p + q)^{20}$ and
then substitute 0.3 (the proportion of F's) for p, and 0.7 (the proportion
of S's) for q. When this was done, the results were very like those of our
disk-sampling experiment (Table 3).

Table 3. Frequency Distribution of 1000 Random Samples of "Failure" and "Success" Disks — Comparison of Results of Experiment and Binomial Expansion

Population: 30 per cent F disks.
No. of disks in each sample = 20.

| F's in Sample | | Relative Frequency | |
No.	Per cent	Experiment (Table 2)	Binomial Expansion
0	0	0.000	0.001
1	5	0.007	0.007
2	10	0.028	0.028
3	15	0.068	0.072
4	20	0.129	0.130
5	25	0.157	0.179
6	30	0.206	0.192
7	35	0.166	0.164
8	40	0.123	0.114
9	45	0.068	0.066
10	50	0.031	0.031
11	55	0.015	0.012
12	60	0.002	0.004
13	65	0.000	0.001
14	70	0.000	0.000
..	..	...	...
..	..	...	...
20	100	0.000	0.000
	Total	1.000	1.001

A Second Sampling Experiment

We have accepted a population containing 30 per cent F's as a possible parent of our clinical-trial sample because, in a world of random sampling, a sample of 20 containing 3 F's does not meet our standard of rarity. Now we may ask: "Would we, on the same standard, accept or reject a population containing 40 per cent F's?" By using the binomial expansion we can perform the experiment on paper. The expansion of $(p + q)^{20}$, when 0.4 is substituted for p and 0.6 for q, shows the following frequencies in the tail that contains 3 F's:

No. of F's	Percentage Frequency
0	0.00
1	0.05
2	0.31
3	1.24
4	3.50

The 2.5 per cent cut-off point is between 3 F's and 4 F's. Therefore our clinical-trial sample is in the "rare" class and we reject a population containing 40 per cent F's as an unlikely parent.

The Boundary between Acceptance and Rejection

We next ask: "What is the boundary or limit between population percentages that we accept as compatible with our sample and those that we reject as unlikely?" We could answer the question by working up from 30 per cent and down from 40 per cent, displaying all the frequency distributions for each percentage of F's, until we found a population that would provide the required frequency distribution. This would be a distribution in which (1) the cut-off point would exclude exactly 2.5 per cent of the total random samples, (2) the samples containing 3 F's would lie at the cut-off point.

Actually, of course, the group of samples containing 3 F's could not lie *on* the cut-off point, with some of them counted as "rare" and some as "not rare." Therefore, we choose a population such that the percentage frequencies of zero F's, 1 F, 2 F's and 3 F's would total 2.5 per cent of the total samples. That is, samples containing 3 F's lie in the 2.5 per cent area immediately adjacent to the cut-off point. When this condition is met, the population percentage of F's is called the *upper limit* (UL) of the population value for the observed sample.

The Meaning of the Upper Limit. As will be shown later, for our sample of 3 F's the upper limit (UL) of the population value, correct to the nearest whole number, is 38 per cent F's. We therefore try to visualize a frequency distribution of samples of 20 with its peak at about 38 per cent F's. We cannot visualize it exactly, because 38 per cent of 20 is not a whole number; but we are not concerned with this. The important part to visualize is the lower (left-hand) 2.5 per cent tail, with samples containing 3 F's immediately adjacent to the cut-off point. The actual tail, found from the binomial expansion with $p = 0.38$, $q = 0.62$ and N (the sample size) $= 20$, is as follows:

No. of F's	0	1	2	3	4
Per Cent Frequency	0.007	0.086	0.503	1.849	4.816

The total from zero through 3 F's is 2.445 per cent. By using a population value of 37.9 per cent F's we can come closer to 2.5 per cent, and 37.93 brings us still closer, but for our purpose 38 per cent is adequate.

We must try to see as clearly as possible what is implied by the rule of procedure that has given us this result. All our rules of procedure in testing samples and in making estimates are designed so that our frequency of erroneous judgments shall not exceed some specified amount. Remembering that we are in the world of strictly random samples — a refined form of the gambler's world — we visualize all the various binomial populations from which we would take random samples during a lifetime in that world. We do not know what the population percentage frequencies of X's (F's in our clinical-trial example) really are, and we do not know whether we are sampling the same population or different populations all the time. From every sample we estimate the upper limit of its parent population value.

Let us suppose that we meet a sample of 20 individuals containing 1 X and 19 not-X's. Unknown to us, it is really a random sample from a population containing 38 per cent X's. Therefore, as is seen from the figures just given for the population containing 38 per cent F's, it really belongs to the middle of the 2.5 per cent tail. We apply our 2.5 per cent rule and find the upper limit, UL per cent X's. That is, we say in effect: "We do not believe that the population percentage is greater than UL." Our belief would be wrong, because if UL were the true value, our sample would lie immediately adjacent to the cut-off point, and that would mean that UL per cent would be less than 38 per cent. (As will be seen from Table I later, it would be 25 per cent X's.)

To see how often we would make such a mistake, we must remember that the very act of random sampling insures that when we take a large number of random samples, either from the same or different populations, not more than 2.5 per cent of them will belong to the left-hand (lower) 2.5 per cent area of rarity; that is what "area of rarity" means. More exactly, if we took more and more samples we would come closer and closer to the 2.5 per cent frequency. Our rule of procedure for estimating limits therefore insures that our error of judgment (rejection of population values) in the world of random sampling would in the long run not exceed 2.5 per cent. That is our Type I error (Q VI – 11). Actually, we would do better than this, because some binomial sampling distributions have, at one or both ends, no tail as small as 2.5 per cent. Therefore we could not commit a Type I error with samples from these populations.

Statements of Estimated Limits

Having made an estimate such as 38 per cent F's as the upper limit for a population percentage, how are we going to report it to others? This question introduces the very important topic of statistical jargon. If we try to make our meaning clear, our verbosity is likely to be rejected by journal editors, or at least by their statistical referees, who will point out that concise technical terms are available. If we use such terms, many readers will not understand them, even if they think they do. To this argument the statistical referees would probably reply that readers ought to learn the meanings of the terms.

The attitude of the statistical referee may be all very well for professional statisticians talking to each other, although even they have had disputes about terms — "confidence limits" versus "fiducial limits," for example. An important point is that a professional of any kind, being familiar with the concepts and usages in his field, is at least likely to know what his jargon does *not* mean, much more so than workers in other fields, even when they have learned the terms that he uses. For example, "confidence limits" and "fiducial limits" have recently started to appear in medical literature. Sometimes they refer, as they should, to population

values, but sometimes they are applied to estimates of the range of variation between individual measurements in a frequency distribution. The
medical specialists who use statistical terms wrongly would be horrified
if the rest of us did the same with their own jargon; but such mistakes
are quite understandable. They indicate that we must strive for communication between different specialties with minimal jargon.

In the past I have applied the term "confidence limits" to population estimates such as those under discussion, but it is desirable to seek for a more
self-explanatory expression. The important first step is to make our statement conditional. We could say: "*If* this sample were a strictly random
sample from a very large population, the estimated upper limit of the
population value *would be* 38 per cent F's." If we now added that the
maximum risk of underestimation would be 2.5 per cent, we might cause
confusion. Although the idea of risk (a percentage or per thousand frequency of some undesirable occurrence) is familiar, the close apposition
of 38 per cent and 2.5 per cent would almost certainly cause some readers
to conclude that the maximum possible upper limit was 40.5 per cent F's!
It would be better to say something like this: "The maximum frequency
of underestimation by this method would be 2.5 of all upper limit
estimates."

Estimating Lower Limits

Starting again with our sample of 20 patients containing 3 F's, we
could go through the same kind of performance (disk-sampling experiments or binomial expansions) in estimating the lower limit (LL) of its
population percentage. As will be shown later, we would arrive at the
value, correct to the first decimal figure, 3.2 per cent F's. In trying to
visualize the sampling distribution from this population we cannot imagine
a peak at "3.2 per cent of 20." It must be high at zero and at 1 F; but
what it really looks like we do not care, because again it is the tail that
concerns us. In the right-hand tail, starting at the 2.5 per cent cut-off
point, we visualize, in succession, samples that contain 3 F's, 4 F's, . . .,
20 F's. Then we can express the results just as for the upper limit, with
appropriate changes of wording, e.g., we can say that the maximum frequency of *over*estimation would be 2.5 per cent. Combining the two
estimates, we could say: "If this sample were a strictly random sample
. . ., the estimated lower and upper limits of the population value would
be respectively 3.2 and 38 per cent F's. The maximum frequency of
overestimation of lower limits, and of underestimation of upper limits,
would be 2.5 per cent of all such estimates."

Interval between Limits

With the lower limit at 3.2 per cent F's, the upper limit at 38 per cent,
and the sample value, 15 per cent, between the two, we have an arrangement that looks something like the beginning of a frequency distribution,
and some students have tried to represent it as such, with a peak at the
observed sample and tailing off to the upper and lower limits. This is of
course a complete misconception. If we were given a sample of 20 con-

taining 3 F's and were told that it was a strictly random sample of some population or other, we could say that, by our 2.5 per cent standard, it was "unlikely" to have come from a population containing 3.2 per cent F's or less, and "unlikely" to have come from a population containing 38 per cent F's or more.

The interval between the lower limit and the upper limit has been called the "confidence interval" or "confidence band," but it is really our zone of ignorance, and would be so even in a world of random sampling — the zone in which we would accept any population as a possible parent of our sample. We would not know, unless from some other source of information, what populations might exist in that interval. There might even be none at all, and our sample might really be a rare sample from a population at or beyond the upper or lower limits that we have estimated.

It is often very desirable to indicate our ignorance in a report. Thus, after stating our estimates of the limits, and their risk of error, we could say: "The population value might lie anywhere between those limits; but it would be impossible to estimate its value more closely without increasing our frequency of error above 2.5 per cent."

Returning now to the real world, we find that the primary, and very great, value of these estimates lies in the revelation of our ignorance. Even in a world of random samples, and even if we knew that a wide range of population percentages existed, 3 F's in a sample of 20 should not be seriously taken to mean 15 per cent F's or something very near it, but "probably somewhere between 3 per cent and 38 per cent F's." In the real world, the interval ought perhaps to be wider, but the range of 35 percentage points should suffice to keep us from overconfidence.

Tables of Binomial Population Limits

The figures 3.2 per cent and 38 per cent were obtained by taking the observed sample (3 F's out of 20) to Table I (see Appendix) and proceeding as follows:

1. We look for X = 3, i.e., the F's in the sample are X's in the table; the S's are not-X's.

2. We move horizontally until we find the entry "**20** 3.2; 38." The bold-faced figures are sample sizes (N) and the lower and upper limits (LL and UL) are separated by semicolons.

To save printing, no sample values of X greater than half of N are shown, but this causes no trouble. For example, with N = 20 and S = 17, to find the population limits for S we take the opposite class (3 F's) and find the limits for percentage of F's. Then we subtract them from 100 per cent, thus:

LL of F = 3.2 per cent; therefore UL of S = 96.8 per cent.
UL of F = 38 per cent; therefore LL of S = 62 per cent.

Table I ends at $X = 50$ and $N = 100$. Thereafter, Table II carries on, with some initial overlap on Table I. (Table II is entered by using the sample percentage of X's, not the absolute numbers.)

Preparation of Tables I and II. Both tables were prepared, by rounding and interpolation, from larger tables first published in 1948 (Mainland) and later revised and extended (Mainland, Herrera and Sutcliffe).[*] The larger tables were prepared from formulae in Table VIII.I of Fisher and Yates' *Statistical Tables* (1948 edition), and the resulting estimates were extensively checked by graphic methods and by testing against binomial expansions.

Reliability of Tables I and II. The rounding and interpolation, used in the preparation of these tables, made the 2.5 per cent tail frequencies less exact than in the original tables. In a few instances the tail frequencies corresponding to the tabulated population estimates are 1 per cent or nearly 5 per cent. However, for most purposes in medical research, the estimates appear to be sufficiently accurate. One hundred of them, especially those in which rounding would have caused most damage, were tested by binomial expansions obtained from the Harvard Computation Laboratory's *Table of the Cumulative Binomial Probability Distribution;* and it appears that the entries in Tables I and II can be safely used with the following precautions:

If a population percentage is expressed to the nearest whole number, the estimate that would give exactly 2.5 per cent in the tail of the distribution will be within ± 0.5 of the tabulated value (e.g., 38 per cent indicates between 37.5 and 38.5 per cent).

If one decimal place appears in the tabulated value, the allowance should be ± 0.1; e.g., 3.2 per cent X's indicates between 3.1 and 3.3 per cent.

The entries in the tables have been spaced close enough to make linear interpolation, by eye, easy and sufficiently accurate.

Sample Size and Precision

Inspection of Tables I and II helps us to grasp relationships between sample size and the precision of our observations. Compare, for instance, the intervals between lower and upper limits for various samples in which the X's constitute 20 per cent of the sample: 2 X's out of 10, 4 X's out of 20, 20 X's out of 100, 40 X's out of 200 (Table II), and so on.

A useful relationship may be noted in Table II. The interval between LL and UL at $N = 400$ is half the interval at 100. This suggests a square-root relationship, which does in fact hold true here and elsewhere. For example, at $X = 20$ per cent the interval is 7 percentage points at $N =$

---

[*] In the larger tables, the limits discussed in this chapter and presented in Tables I and II are called "95 per cent confidence limits" — a common custom. There are also tables of 99 per cent and 80 per cent limits, which provide error risks, as defined in this chapter, of 0.5 per cent and 10 per cent respectively.

500, and 5 percentage points at N = 1000. The ratio of N's is 1:2, and dividing 7 by $\sqrt{2}$, i.e., 1.414, we find 4.95, almost exactly 5 percentage points. Hence, from the intervals at N = 1000 we can estimate fairly accurately the intervals at N's greater than 1000.

Zero and 100 Per Cent Frequencies

Estimated upper limits show how little we may safely infer from the absence of a phenomenon, or the non-occurrence of an event, when our samples are small. If X is an event and there are no X's in a sample of 20, the event might never occur, even if we took an infinitely large sample — our lower limit for X is zero. Table I, at X = 0 and N = 20, shows, however, that the upper limit is 17 per cent X's. That is, unless we are willing to risk being wrong in more than 2.5 per cent of our upper limit estimates, we must not infer that our sample's parent population would be unlikely to contain fewer than 17 per cent X's. Similarly, if all individuals in a sample of 20 are X's, the lower limit is 100 − 17 = 83 per cent X's.

To understand rather more clearly what the estimate 17 per cent X's tells us, let us use, for a little more precision, the value 16.84 per cent X's, from which 17 was obtained by rounding. We visualize a frequency distribution of random samples, each containing 20 individuals, with its peak about 16.84 per cent X's. In its left-hand tail are samples containing no X's, and they constitute exactly 2.5 per cent of all the samples. Now let us visualize a distribution with its peak at 15 per cent X's. We have, as it were, pushed the distribution more to the left, and samples with no X's will therefore be commoner than before; they will constitute more than 2.5 per cent of the total samples.

Small Samples in Drug Screening

Under Q VII – 8 there was mentioned the number 14, a sample size recently popular in a certain anti-cancer drug testing organization. Some clinicians have expressed great satisfaction because "a statistician had shown them that they need use only 14 patients, without controls, to test a compound." One may wonder whether the satisfaction would have been as great if they had understood more fully what the statement implied. The statistician cannot be criticized for this lack of understanding; he merely gave some binomial-distribution information that he was asked for. But if we are going to act on the basis of statistical information we ought to try very hard to understand what it means — unless we are content to accept the status of junior technician.

We are not concerned here with the fact that 14 cancer patients, however minutely categorized, may be far from randomly representative of the whole country's patients in the same category. Nor have we in mind observational error or the lack of objectivity, specificity or sensitivity of the criteria of assessment. Let us imagine that all patients with a certain cancer were as alike as disks in a sampling experiment, and that information about their condition was as definite as "X" and "not-X" marked on the disks. Then let us see what Table I tells us about random samples of 14 patients from such a population.

At $X = 0$ and $N = 14$ we find that the estimated upper limit is 23 per cent X's. That is, if none of the patients treated by the drug showed improvement, the investigator, speaking rather colloquially, could say that it was "unlikely" that as many as 23 per cent of such patients would show improvement. More technically, if the population contained 23 per cent of improved cases, approximately 97.5 per cent of samples of 14 patients would contain one or more who showed improvement. (Another binomial expansion, with $p = 0.20$ (20 per cent population frequency of improved cases) showed that 95 per cent of random samples would contain one or more improved cases.)

However, the upper limit 23 per cent (or 20 per cent) also means that the investigator cannot, with the same degree of confidence, rule out a lower population percentage of improved cases. For example, a binomial expansion with $p = 0.15$ showed that, if the population frequency were 15 per cent, 10 per cent of random samples of 14 individuals would contain no improved cases.

A clinician, or the drug-testing organization for which he is working, may consider that such a coarse screening is all that can be aimed at when there are many drugs to test; but the further implications of $N = 14$ should be faced.

In the organization that favored $N = 14$ as a sample size, it was stated that if a drug showed "promising results" a large-scale trial of the drug, with a contrast-group deprived of the drug, would be conducted. But what are "promising results" in a sample of 14 patients? Table I gives some pertinent information:

No. of Improved Cases out of 14	Population Per Cent LL	UL
1	0.18	34
2	1.8	43
3	4.7	51
4	8.4	58

This is the kind of information on which a decision to conduct, or not conduct, a large trial would have to be based, as least in part. There would probably be other information, such as the effects of the drug on animal tumors, perhaps the effects of related drugs on human beings, perhaps the degree of apparent effect on the patients who were improved in the sample of 14. However, if an investigator, testing a certain agent on 14 patients, saw improvement in only one patient, he would have to face the fact that this low value might be due to sampling variation, and that, if he discarded the drug, he might be withholding benefit from about 30 per cent of patients.

Let us imagine, also, the attitude of an investigator who had obtained 4 "successes," believed to be real, in 14 patients. How willingly would he agree to a large trial that would deprive half the patients of the drug when he had seen it "successful" in nearly 30 per cent of his patients? After his faith in samples of 14 had been built up, it would be something of a shock for him to learn that, even if his "successes" were real, and even if his sample were strictly random, he ought not to expect with confidence a success rate of much more than 9 per cent in a population of similar patients.

Admittedly, the plethora of new drugs places the administrators of drug-testing organizations in a predicament; but this hardly excuses their failure to learn, and announce to investigators, the full consequences of using small samples in screening. The proponents of samples of 14 appear to have formed only half a plan. The other half of the plan might have been presented in terms such as the following: "We propose to use samples of 14 patients; and before a drug can qualify for a large-scale trial it must have been followed by improvement in at least 10 out of the 14, because then we would expect benefit in at least 42 per cent of a population randomly represented by the sample." (Four X's [failures] out of 14 give an upper limit of 58 per cent; i.e., a lower limit of 42 per cent successes.)

Another area of drug research in which the absence of X's in a very small sample seems to create surprising conviction is the testing of new drugs for undesirable (including toxic) effects. An investigator tests the drug on 4 patients, and if he does not find toxic effects he gives it to 20 patients. But the upper limit, estimated from zero X's in a sample of 4, is 60 per cent X's. Therefore he will have learned very little about the risk to which he will expose the 20 patients. The procedure seems to be based on the belief that a drug is either toxic to nearly everyone or toxic to hardly anyone; and this is not borne out by experience. Incidentally, in the search for quickly developing toxicity a sequential design (Q VI –18) can be a useful method of reducing the number of subjects exposed to risk.

Majorities and Minorities

Among 10 patients, treated by a certain method, 9 (the majority) recovered and 1 did not. In 81 right lower limbs of American Negro cadavers 46 limbs (56.8 per cent, the majority) contained what was called "Pattern 4" of femoral artery branches, and 35 limbs contained one or other of the remaining eight patterns.

The occurrence of a majority in one class in a binomial sample tells us nothing unless it gives evidence that this is likely to be true in the parent population. In order to use the tables of estimated population limits, we look at the minority in the sample. If 9 patients out of 10 recover, and one fails to do so, we ask: "Is the proportion of failures in the population unlikely to be as high as 50 per cent?" Table I shows that the upper limit estimated from one X in a sample of 10 is 44.5 per cent X's, and we can report as follows: Among strictly random samples of 10 subjects from a population containing 44.5 per cent failures, 97.5 per cent of the subjects would contain more than one failure. Therefore it would be even more unlikely for such a sample to be a random sample from a population containing equal numbers of successes and failures.

In considering majorities and minorities we must of course beware of wrong denominators $(Q V - 6)$. Among 8 bubonic plague patients who had meningitis, 6 were males and 2 were females. The observer stated that therefore males seemed more susceptible to this complication, and his statement was allowed publication in one of the foremost medical journals. Even if the figures were 600 males and 200 females the denominator would still be wrong. (When some medical students were asked to criticize the inference regarding meningitis in plague, one of them said that he believed that it was true, because the professor of pathology [who was a clever purveyor of facts] had told the class that males were more susceptible than females to all diseases except three.)

Paired Comparisons

In an animal experiment two animals from each litter may be used, one receiving treatment A and the other treatment B. In the comparison of two diagnostic tests, e.g., to detect the presence of a certain "factor" in the blood, both tests should be applied to each patient and, whenever possible, to the same sample of blood. In a series of patients a certain infection may have attacked the right arm, eye, ear or kidney, more often than the left; and a certain paralysis may have affected the lower limb more often than the upper. In all these examples the minority-majority analysis can be used. Intrasubject cross-over comparisons of treatments require special consideration (see Chapter XII).

In the comparison of blood tests on 80 patients who had a particular disease the following results were obtained:

> Both positive: 60
> Both negative: 2
> A positive, B negative: 12
> A negative, B positive: 6

The question to be answered was: "Which test was the better one, in the sense of producing fewer false negatives?"

We must take great care in setting up such figures for comparison $(Q V - 1)$. If we were to set up a contingency table —

	Positive	Negative	Total
A	72	8	80
B	66	14	80

— we would be handling the data as if we had two separate sets of 80 patients. If we took the 22 negatives and asked if the difference, 8 versus 14, was big enough to make us believe that it was a "real" (population) difference, we would be counting some people twice and others only once.

The only patients who gave evidence regarding the difference between the tests when used under the same conditions (applied to bloods of the same patients) were 18. The 6 cases in which A was negative and B was positive we call "X's." We take them to Table I and at $N = 18$ we find that the upper limit is 59 per cent X's. We can therefore report as follows:

"If these 18 cases were a strictly random sample from a very large population of patients in whom the tests differed in their verdicts, the estimated upper limit of the population frequency of patients showing A negative and B positive would be 59 per cent (maximum frequency of underestimation $=$ approximately 2.5 per cent of all such estimates). Therefore it is very possible that test B is actually superior to test A."

In this comparison we have disregarded the patients in whom the verdicts of the test agreed, but this might be our chief concern. If one test required more technical skill than the other, we might choose the simpler one, provided that the agreement was sufficiently frequent, even if the more complicated test gave a lower percentage of false negatives. To help us in our decision we could take the total sample of 80 (18 disagreements and 62 agreements) to Table I and find that the limits for the population percentages of disagreements are 14 and 33, i.e., the limits for agreements are 67 and 86 per cent.

Diversity of Applications. Statistics textbooks often give the impression that in order to analyze data we must learn numerous different principles and an abundance of tests. Actually, the principles are few and the same analytical methods are appropriate in widely separated fields. To illustrate, the following figures from a fictitious anatomy laboratory can be analyzed by the same procedure as were the data from the diagnostic tests. They represent the presence and absence of a muscle, such as the palmaris longus.

Muscle Present	No. of Cadavers
On both sides	80
On right side only	11
On left side only	1
On neither side	8
Total	100

Do these figures indicate a tendency for the muscle to be more often present on the right side than on the left side?

Genetic Ratios

Let us suppose that an animal breeding experiment or a collection of human pedigrees shows that a certain characteristic (C) is present in 92 out of 200 individuals but absent from the remaining 108. In a preliminary examination of the data we wish to consider five possible Mendelian ratios (C:not-C), namely 1:2, 7:9, 9:7 and 2:1. In order to use the estimated limits of population frequencies we must convert the ratios to percentage frequencies of C, namely 33.3, 43.75, 50, 56.25 and 66.7 per cent.

The estimated population limits for 92 out of 200, i.e., 46 per cent C's, are given in Table II (see Appendix): 39 per cent and 53 per cent. In the interval between these two limits are 43.75 per cent (ratio 7:9) and 50 per cent (1:1). Therefore we accept them as possible values, compatible with our sample. The others we exclude as unlikely in the sense already defined. In fact, more extensive tables (Mainland, Herrera and Sutcliffe) show that we can exclude these ratios with even greater assurance than Table II permits; our risk of error is less than 0.5 per cent.

Paired Measurements — The Sign Test

Many paired comparisons are made by measurements — for example, a measured response of litter mates, one on treatment A, the other on treatment B; weights of right and left kidneys in the same human cadaver. In many cases, apparently, all that the investigator wishes to know is whether there is sufficient evidence that treatment A and B differ in effectiveness, or that the right kidney "has a tendency" to be heavier (or lighter) than the left kidney. And yet, after finding the A-minus-B difference for each pair of readings and the average difference, he may go through the whole process of calculating the squares and square roots necessary for a t-test of the mean difference, although the answer to his actual question is staring him in the face, or can be easily found from a table of population limits estimated from binomial samples. All that he requires is the *sign* of each difference.

For instance, with 2 plus signs and 38 minus signs in a sample of 40 paired measurements, Table I shows that the upper limit of the proportion of plus signs is 17 per cent. Having met such a sample, an investigator could be virtually certain that it was not a random sample from a population containing anywhere near 50 per cent of each sign.

If the 40 pairs had contained 2 plus signs, 35 minus signs and 3 zeros, the zeros would represent a difference too small to be detected by the method of measurement, and would not show the direction of the difference. Therefore the investigator's question would be concerned with detectable differences, and he would enter Table I with 2 minus signs out of 37 pairs.

It can often happen, of course, that the sign test does not give convincing evidence of a difference between treatment effects whereas analysis that uses the actual measurements (by methods shown in Chapter XIV) will show convincing evidence of a difference. This is because measurements are more sensitive than counts. We should realize, however, that the sign test and a measurement test are asking somewhat different questions; and we ought to decide early on whether we are going to analyze measurements as measurement data or as enumeration data (Q V – 2). Perhaps we will decide to look at both aspects of the data.

The Parent Population in Matched-pair Experiments

We can use the foregoing example in an effort to see how the random assignment of treatments A and B within each pair justifies a sign test, or for that matter, a test that utilizes the measured A-minus-B differences. We have repeatedly used the phrase, "If this sample were a strictly random sample"; and what we must try to see is that, if there were no difference in the effects of A and B, we would have a random sample of plus and minus signs from a population in which 50 per cent of the signs are positive and 50 per cent are negative.

At the beginning of the experiment we take up one member of a pair of animals and look at a list of treatment assignments derived from odd and even random digits. We find that the animal first taken up in the first pair is to receive treatment B; therefore the other animal will receive treatment A. We do likewise with the whole series of 40 pairs. For convenience, let us call the first animal in each pair "V" and the second animal "W."

Let us even imagine that for some unknown reason all the V's will show greater change in the variable under test than the corresponding W's. If we took V-minus-W differences all would be positive. But some V's are A-treated and others are B-treated. Therefore, if the treatment difference lies only in the letter A or B, some of the A-minus-B differences will be positive and some will be negative. Which shall be positive and which negative has been decided by the odd and even random digits. But we have used a random sample of odd and even digits from a table which contains 50 per cent of each. (Even if the total odds and evens in the whole table are not quite equal, the difference from 50 per cent is negligible.) And so, if the treatments do not differ in their effects we will at the end have a random sample from a population containing 50 per cent positive signs and 50 per cent negative signs.

This is an example of the way in which random assignment leads to a valid inference within an experiment; but we must continually remind ourselves of two facts:

1. We have no assurance that the sample of litter mates itself was a random sample of any well defined population of litter mates.

2. In a survey, e.g., of human kidney weights, we cannot picture random assignment of kidneys to right and left sides, but all organs are subject to a number of mutually independent factors influencing their weight; i.e., they are to some extent influenced by random processes, and if these were the only cause of differences in weight between right and left kidneys the result would be equivalent to a random assignment of heavier and lighter kidneys to the two sides on a 50:50 basis. If we found that right kidneys were heavier than left kidneys in more autopsy subjects than could be adequately attributed to such assignment, we would have to ask many questions, beginning with: "What conceivable factors could bring into our autopsy survey a preponderance of subjects with heavier right kidneys if this difference did not exist in the population?"

From the Binomial to the Gaussian Distribution

The binomial expansion makes it possible to find the frequency distribution of random samples of any size from any binomial population; but it is a laborious task with any except the smallest samples. Tables I and II, and their previously published larger parents, would have been impossible to produce, with the available facilities, directly from binomial expansions. Books containing a considerable number of expansions have been published, and electronic computers nowadays could quickly produce more of them; but small-scale investigators need, if possible, a more direct way of testing their results than by means of a reference library containing statistical tables, perhaps in another town.

In this instance what the mathematicians invented (or some of them might say "discovered") is illustrated by Figure 1, which shows binomial frequency distributions with increasing size of sample, N. Where

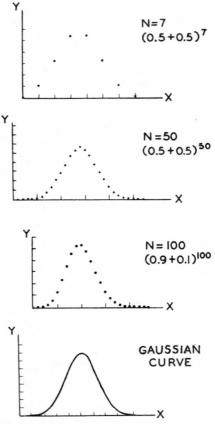

Figure 1. Genesis of Gaussian curve from binomial distributions with increasing size of sample (N). The X axis represents the class of sample (e.g., No. of F's). The Y axis represents the percentage frequencies of occurrence in random sampling.

$p = q = \frac{1}{2}$, the distribution is symmetrical from the start, but even when p and q are unequal the graphs become more and more symmetrical as N is increased. Also, if we use the same total area for all the graphs, the dots come closer and closer together. In effect they become a continuous curve. This is the "Gaussian" curve, but it may be mentioned that the title gives excessive credit to one man, albeit a man who deserves much honor in mathematics. A more accurate title would be "the curve of De Moivre, Bernouilli, Laplace and Gauss."

The Gaussian curve was often called "the normal curve of error" because it was believed to represent the variation among instrument readings, but "error" has quite rightly been dropped, and now the terms "normal curve" and "normal frequency distribution" are commonly used. This would be safe enough if everyone would always remember that "normal" in this connection means simply "standard" (Latin, *norma*, a carpenter's square). Unfortunately, many people either forget or never know this limited implication of "normal"; and there is already so much confusion regarding this word in medicine that I have in recent years decided that it is best to avoid increasing the confusion by the use of the same term in two senses.

By taking larger and larger binomial samples we could come on graph paper as close as we wished to the Gaussian curve. Then, starting at the center, which we could call 0, we could move along the X-axis in the negative and positive directions and at each point we could measure the height (Y). It is essentially this building-up process that the mathematician pursues in developing the formula for the Gaussian curve. Hardly anyone in medicine need ever see the formula, even if he frequently uses information derived from it, because such information has been published in tables.

Some medical workers use the term "Gaussian" as if it meant any bell-shaped frequency curve. This is not correct; strictly speaking, there is only one Gaussian curve. And yet, if we draw the same Gaussian curve with a different X-scale and retain the same Y-scale, the graphs appear different. We need something more specific to define the curve than simply the relationship between height and distance from the center. We need some kind of standard yardstick to measure the distances from the center. These distances are called "deviations" and the yardstick is the "standard deviation."

The Standard Deviation

To whatever scale it is drawn, the side of a Gaussian curve looks like a straight line over a considerable stretch; but if we look at the details of its height we find that just after leaving the summit it descends with increasing rapidity and then the slope changes and thereafter the speed is progressively slower. We can drop to the X-axis a vertical from the point where the slope changes (the point of inflection, i.e., "bending"), and then the distance from the center, so marked, is given the name "standard deviation."

The standard deviation is often symbolized by the Greek small letter "sigma" (σ), but here the abbreviation "SD" will be used. In some contexts a standard deviation is called a "standard error," but "error" in this connection has the same meaning as "deviation" or "difference" or "variation" (Latin, *errare*, to wander). In all contexts the term "standard deviation" can be used. Chapter XIV shows how to calculate the standard deviation of a set of measurements, but here we are concerned not with its structure but with its function as a yardstick.

By using the standard deviation, we can refine our statement about heights at different parts of the Gaussian curve. Whatever scale units are employed, if we take any points on the X-axis and express their distances from the center as fractions or multiples of the standard deviation, e.g., k times SD, we find that the height of the curve at each point (each value of k) has its own particular relationship to the height at the center. Since the curve is symmetrical, this ratio is the same at −k (SD) as at +k (SD).

Multiples of SD as Cut-off Points

The most important common use of the standard deviation is not to determine the frequency of items at different points on the X-axis, but to tell us what proportion of the total items in the frequency distribution lie beyond certain points. This information could be found from a large-scale graph of the curve, but it has been derived from the formula for the curve and has been published in various tables. Thus (Fig. 2) outside the range 1 SD on each side of the center lie approximately one third of the total items, one sixth on the left and one sixth on the right. A familiar percentage of exclusion is seen in the lower part of the figure. To obtain our 2.5 per cent rarity class at each end of the distribution, we mark the cut-off point at a distance of 1.96 SD from the center — for most purposes, 2 SD is adequate.

A few more relationships between SD and exclusions are in the following list:

Range on Each Side of Center	Excluded Per Cent of Total
± 0.6745 SD	50.00
± 1 SD	31.73
± 1.282 SD	20.00
± 1.645 SD	10.00
± 1.96 SD	5.00
± 2 SD	4.55
± 2.576 SD	1.00
± 3 SD	0.27

Further information is shown in Table VII (see Appendix).

The "Probable" Error. The first item in the above list, approximately 2/3 SD, is the "probable error" or "probable deviation." It was formerly much used, although its users would have had some difficulty in saying what was "probable" about it, except that the "probability" of an item being found within its range was equal to the "probability" of an item

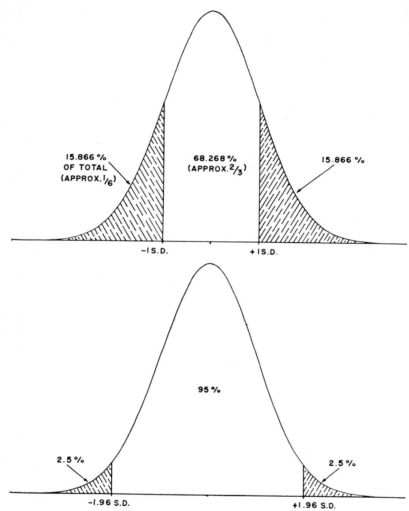

15.866 %
OF TOTAL
(APPROX. 1/6)

68.268 %
(APPROX. 2/3)

15.866 %

−1 S.D.

+1 S.D.

95 %

2.5 %

2.5 %

−1.96 S.D.

+1.96 S.D.

Figure 2.   Gaussian distributions to show proportions excluded
by multiples of the standard deviation.

being found outside its range. This information, however, is seldom
of much use, because it does not tell us how far beyond the probable
error the distribution may extend. Therefore in the days when we calculated the probable error (because a prominent statistician had set the
custom and we felt that we had to do so), we used to multiply it by 3
to obtain the equivalent of 2 SD.

The habit lingered long after its foolishness had been pointed out;
and one biologist defended it by saying that a probable error meant
more to physicists than a standard deviation or standard error (perhaps
by some association with the "half-life" measure of radioactivity). It

would not have been mentioned here, except that it illustrates something that we should remember when looking at current habits of statistical analysis. The persistence of a habit is no proof of its utility or even of its safety.

The Binomial Standard Deviation

We can now look at this instrument, the Gaussian curve, that is offered to lighten our labor with binomial distributions. First, a suitable standard deviation must be calculated. Little direct use of it is made in the techniques prescribed in this book; therefore more detailed discussion is postponed until Chapter XVI. However, we must look at it here, because it is common in medical literature and is often used without knowledge of the risk.

If N is the total number of individuals in a binomial sample, and p and q are population frequencies (e.g., 0.3 for F's and 0.7 for S's), the standard deviation is $\sqrt{Npq}$. This is a curious-looking structure; but it can be shown to be exactly equivalent to the standard deviation of a set of measurements (Chapter XVI, sect. 1).

Applying this formula to our binomial sample of 20 disks from a population containing 30 per cent F's, we have:

$$\sqrt{Npq} = \sqrt{20 \times 0.3 \times 0.7} = \sqrt{4.10} = 2.025 \text{ F's per sample of 20.}$$

We now imagine that the binomial distribution is a Gaussian curve with its mode at the population percentage, 30 per cent F's, i.e., 6 F's per sample of 20. To cut off the 2.5 per cent tails, we write:

$$6 \pm 1.96 \times 2.025 = 6 \pm 3.969 = 2.031 \text{ F's and } 9.969 \text{ F's.}$$

This means that the lower cut-off point would be between 2 F's and 3 F's, and the upper would be between 9 F's and 10 F's.

Returning to Table 3 (p. 193) we see that the proper cut-off points lie between 1 F and 2 F's and between 10 F's and 11 F's. The Gaussian method has excluded more than 2.5 per cent of the samples at each end, although not much more. By taking 2 SD ($\pm$ 4.05 F's) instead of 1.96 SD, we reach the proper location for the cut-off points. Indeed, with samples even smaller than 20, and with population percentages far more unequal than 30 and 70, the Gaussian approximation (with $\pm$ 2 SD) often does very well, *provided that we start from the population percentages.*

Risks of the Gaussian Approximation

The italicized clause in the last sentence had the following implication. In our actual research we do not start with a population but with a sample, and we wish to estimate population limits (with maximum error frequency of 2.5 per cent). If we would take the trouble to try a number of population percentages and, using $2\sqrt{Npq}$, go through the procedure shown above, we would approach the binomially estimated limits as close as we would need in many cases. However, this would be time-consuming, and the method commonly shown in textbooks, and applied in journal articles, starts with the frequencies found in the sample. If we have a sample of 20 containing 3 F's (i.e., 0.15 of 20) the SD is calculated as $\sqrt{20 \times 0.15 \times 0.85} = \sqrt{2.55} = 1.597$ disks per sample of 20.

Then the sample value, 3 F's, is used instead of any population value (which is unknown) and the limits are written as:

$$3 \pm 2 \times 1.597 = 3 \pm 3.194 = -0.194 \text{ and } +6.194 \text{ F's per sample of 20.}$$

As percentages these limits would be -0.970 per cent F's and 30.970 per cent F's. The multiplier 1.96 does not mend matters, and comparison of these estimates (especially the minus value!) with those in Table I (3.2 per cent and 38 per cent) shows why Tables I and II were prepared. Indeed, it shows why the formulae used in making these tables were produced in the first place, namely, the formulae in Table VIII.I of Fisher and Yates' *Statistical Tables*.

With larger samples and with sample frequencies nearer 50 per cent, the errors are not so glaring, but they are still too great in many of the samples that are met in small-scale medical research.

This criticism of the simple use of the Gaussian curve does not imply, however, that it played no part in the production of Tables I and II. On the contrary, a large part of the Fisher and Yates table consists of correction terms to be used along with the Gaussian multipliers of SD, namely, 1.96 and 2.576.

Attitude to Labor-saving Approximations

It appears that two principles should underlie our attitude to this matter of the Gaussian-curve approximation to the binomial distribution, and they are applicable to all other labor-saving approximations that statistical mathematicians offer us:

1. Whatever mathematical "proofs" may have been used in the development of a technique, they are best looked upon as methods of inventing the technique. They are not proofs that the technique will give us the correct answers with our kind of data. That can be shown only by extensive comparisons of their answers with the answers given by the exact method, in this instance the binomial distribution.

2. If an approximation is found to give answers that are near enough, for our purposes, to the exact answers, we need not be greatly concerned with how the approximation was invented. Thus, if $2\sqrt{Npq}$ had worked well when p and q were taken from the observed sample instead of from a series of hypothetical populations, we need not have worried about the apparent illogicality of the substitution.

Multinomial Samples

So far, we have been discussing binomial samples, but many types of material can be divided into three or more classes — multinomial classification. We will look at three examples: (1) genetic ratios, (2) assessment of clinical change, and (3) frequency of location of a disease.

Genetic Ratios.   In animal or plant breeding experiments, or in observations on human beings, we know that if certain characteristics are inherited according to a certain Mendelian law the animals, plants or persons should be distributed in the ratio 9:3:3:1. This is the hypothesis that is to be tested by the data.

In the binomial case, say a 3:1 ratio, we can, and often do, use a binomial distribution with population ratio 3:1 (75 per cent versus 25 per cent) and N equal to the size of our sample. That is, we display the consequences of the hypothesis and compare our sample with them. If the sample would lie in a predetermined "rare" class we reject the hypothesis. If we meet many such problems we can buy a book of binomial expansions ("binomial probabilities") to save our labor; but we have seen that estimated population limits, as in Tables I and II, give us the answer more directly.

For the multinomial problem, with sample size N, we would display the expansion of $(p + q + r + s)^N$, where $p = 9/16, q = 3/16, r = 3/16$ and $s = 1/16$. However, this is even more laborious than a binomial expansion, and there are no widely available or comprehensive tables to help us. Therefore an approximation called the "chi-square goodness of fit" test is commonly used. It is derived from the Gaussian distribution but with certain precautions it is reliable. The arithmetic, which is shown in many textbooks, is similar to, but not quite the same as, that of the "chi-square contingency test" shown in Chapter XII.

Assessment of Clinical Change.   In the assessment of patients' change after treatment, a fivefold classification may be used, ranging from "much worse" through "no appreciable change" to "much better." This differs considerably from the genetic example. Even if the classification is based on actual measurements such as amounts of increase or decrease in the width of the x-ray shadow of the heart, the divisions beyond the central class are arbitrary; and when the changes are not measured the scheme is largely subjective. This is no real impediment in a double-blind comparison of treatments when the same observer assesses all patients; but in communicating the results of any particular treatment to other people the finer distinctions, e.g., between "moderate" and "severe," are of doubtful value, because other observers, assessing the same patients, would probably assign some borderline cases differently. Therefore, the "population" that any one observer would build up, even if his criteria remained perfectly constant, would probably differ from those of other observers. The second difference from the genetic-ratio example is that there is here no predetermined hypothesis, giving certain numbers that would be expected in each class.

For these reasons it appears sensible to group the data and see what information can be obtained from it by simple methods. Even the "worse, no change, better" classification can be criticized for subjectivity; but it is surely desirable for every observer to ask a question like this:

"If my criteria and my future patients did not differ systematically from those that produced the results in this sample, what would this sample tell me about the results to be expected in my long-run use of this treatment?" Since there are three classes in the group, there is an extensive variety of ratios that could be tested (by chi-square as in the genetic example), and the test seems rather pointless.

On the other hand, simpler questions, dividing the data binomially, lead to specific answers that can be found directly from Tables I or II. In many situations the most appropriate division is between "better" and "not better." In others, mere arrest of the disease is important, and then the division is between "worse" and "not worse." In either case, the pooled classes can be separated again; e.g., one could ask: "Of those classified as 'not worse,' what percentage might be in the improved class?"

Frequency of Location of a Disease. A surgeon, reviewing his experience of tumors of the large intestine, showed the unequal frequencies with which they occurred in different parts (cecum, ascending colon, transverse colon, and so on), apparently believing that these differences indicated a tendency for the tumors to occur unequally in different locations.

A clinician can hardly be expected to apply statistical tests to every set of figures that he presents, because sometimes he merely mentions them to show the source or type of material studied. But all figures create impressions, and it is wise for him to warn his audience against untested figures. If, however, he proposes to draw some conclusions from his figures, he is in effect setting up a hypothesis and stating his belief that it is true or not true. There seems to be no escape from testing the hypothesis, or at least no escape from a presentation of the figures in such a way that others could use them in testing it.

In the present example the appropriate "null" hypothesis would probably not be an equal incidence of tumors in all segments (a 1:1:1 . . . . ratio), but perhaps a ratio based on the relative areas of mucosa in the different segments, or perhaps even their relative lengths. If that hypothesis were disproved, there would arise some much more difficult questions regarding selection factors. If all points in the intestine developed tumors with equal frequency, what factors might prevent a particular surgeon from seeing them with equal frequency during a period of X years? For example, would rapidity of development, or type of effect, produced by tumors in different parts be selection factors? If this kind of question were thought of at the very beginning, it would probably reduce the number of hypotheses, opinions or speculations announced at medical meetings.

"Probability" and "Significance"

We have come through this chapter rather well, without depending on these troublesome words for help in the exposition, and we could do the same in succeeding chapters; but this would not be fair to medical readers because they can hardly open a medical journal without meeting this pair of words or their close relatives. Moreover, the binomial and Gaussian-curve data in this chapter give us an opportunity to see more clearly than in Chapter VI the numerical concepts that underlie the use of these words. If we grasp these concepts now, we can carry them through all subsequent chapters.

Probabilities, Chances and Odds. Starting with 300 F-disks and 700 S-disks, if we knew that we could take strictly random samples, one disk per sample, replacing each disk after recording its letter, we would know at the outset that the total of all samples would, as we continued, approach 30 per cent F's and 70 per cent S's. Therefore we could say that the "probability" of picking an F-disk in any one sampling was 30 per cent or 0.3. "Probability" in this connection refers to events that are due to random processes and is defined as the *relative frequency* of an event, i.e., the frequency of that kind of event divided by the frequency of all the kinds of events possible in the particular situation.

Under these conditions the implication of prophecy in the word "probability" is justified. Although we do not know which kind of disk will come up next, we know what will be found in the long run. The same idea is expressed in phrases like, "We have 7 chances out of 10 of picking an S-disk" and "The odds against picking an F-disk are 7 to 3."

The Tail Probability, P. Looking at the lower tail-region of the binomial distribution in Table 3 (p. 193) from a population containing 30 per cent F's, we find the following:

No. of F's	0	1	2	3
Percentage frequency	0.1	0.7	2.8	7.2
Probability (p)	0.001	0.007	0.028	0.072

In classifying a sample-type as "rare" we have to watch the implications of our verdict. If we classified 2 F's as "rare" we would have to classify likewise 1 F and zero F's, a total of 3.6 per cent of all the random samples. That is, the probability of meeting a sample in this group (No. of F's $= 0$ or 1 or 2) would be 0.036. This is the probability that is commonly indicated by the capital letter "P" to distinguish it from the probability of any individual kind of event (e.g., samples containing 2 F's), which is indicated by the small (lower case) "p." (When one sees "p" instead of "P" in a medical journal one may well wonder whether it is due to praiseworthy disregard of convention or to ignorance of what the "probability" indicates.)

Reporting P Values and "Significance." We have seen that a sample of 20 containing 1 F would be "rare" in this distribution by our 2.5 per cent standard. If we wish to use P in expressing this, we should be very careful to make our meaning clear. One may read in a report that a sample of 20 individuals contained 1 F, and that this was "significantly different from a true (population) frequency of 30 per cent F's (P less than 0.05)"; or ". . . (P in one tail less than 0.025)." One would think that a person who could write that must know what it means; but remarks made by some of those who write such things induce the question: "How often are such statements merely transcriptions of ill-understood jargon from another field of specialization?"

One hears, for example, phrases like "a 95 per cent probability that the population percentage lies between X per cent and Y per cent" and "a greater than 5 per cent chance that the sample came from a population containing 30 per cent F's." Having experienced confusion in this area myself, I am convinced that our only hope to reduce it is to hold fast to the idea that numerical (as distinct from colloquial) "probability" refers to the results of random sampling experiments such as the sampling of disks in a barrel, or that, in other contexts, it refers to the results of card-shuffling experiments. Probability tells us the frequency of events (samples of specified composition) which are produced in such experiments.

With that idea in mind, if we look at a statement about the "probability" that a population lies within a certain range, we try to visualize a barrel of disks, each disk bearing a population value, some of them being inside the specified range and some of them outside it — a "population of population values." We recognize immediately that this is not the basis of our estimation of population values, as in Table I. Or again, if we hear about "a greater than 5 per cent chance that a particular sample came from a certain population," we try to visualize a barrel of disks, some of which came from that population and some did not. We see again that this is not at all the kind of information by which we classify a population as a possible (or unlikely) parent of an observed sample.

In view of this, if we wish to use P in stating our conclusions about a sample or a population, how are we going to make it clear to ourselves and others what we mean by "P"? Let us imagine that we have obtained a sample of 20 individuals containing one F. We test it by Table 3 and find that the corresponding P in the tail where the sample would lie is less than 0.025. The P does not tell us anything about the probability of *this sample* or of other samples from its actual but unknown parent population. We have to know a population before we can tell anything about the p's or P's of samples from it. Our statement must therefore be conditional, and it could read as follows: "In a random sampling experiment, where samples of 20 individuals were taken from a population containing 30 per cent F's, samples containing 1 F *would have* a probability P of less than 0.025; that is, samples containing 1 F or zero F's would together comprise less than 2.5 per cent of the total samples. Therefore it was considered unlikely that a population, randomly represented by the observed sample, would contain as many as 30 per cent F's."

This statement would indicate our definition of "unlikely," and our conclusion would, correctly, be based on a random sampling experiment. However, the conclusion would not be of much interest unless it meant something in the world from which the sample had actually come. This meaning could be shown by a statement such as the following: "If the same form of treatment were applied to many more individuals, unless the subjects and conditions were systematically different from those affecting the sample of 20, it is unlikely that the overall percentage of F's would be as high as 30." This is an attempt to describe the real-world equivalent of random sampling conditions by using the concept of a "systematic" difference in contrast to variable or fluctuating differences (see under Q VI – 21). In any particular case the "conditions" that might change could be exemplified – for instance, types of patients or animals, techniques, and so on.

To consider the translation of a "nonsignificant" difference we can take the sample of 20 containing 2 F's, which might be reported thus: "The difference from a true (population) value of 30 per cent F's was not significant at the 5 per cent level (P greater than 0.05)" or ". . . (P in one tail greater than 0.025)." We would refer to the random sampling experiment as before, state that samples containing 2 or fewer F's would comprise more than 2.5 per cent of the total samples, and then continue thus: "Therefore it was considered quite possible that a population, randomly represented by the observed sample, would contain 30 per cent F's or more." Or we could say that the sample was not considered "incompatible" with a population value of 30 per cent F's or more.

The practical implication of this conclusion could be expressed as follows: "If the same treatment were applied to many more individuals, even if the subjects and conditions remained essentially the same as when this sample was obtained, the sample did not give adequate evidence that the overall incidence of F's would be less than 30 per cent."

The Problem of P from Both Tails. Unless it is stated that P is "from one tail," i.e., the tail where the observed sample would lie if it were in a random sampling distribution, it is usually implied that P from the opposite tail is included, and this presents a certain problem.

If in a random sampling experiment we decide to adopt a certain standard of rarity (e.g., 5 per cent or 1 per cent) and if we are sampling from a symmetrical (50:50) binomial distribution, we can place our cut-off points (2.5 per cent or 0.5 per cent) at equal distances to left and right of the center. But if the distribution is not symmetrical (e.g., Table 3, p. 193) the cut-off points will not be at equal distances from the center; a particular distance "means more" in terms of rarity on one side than on the other side. Moreover, the frequencies of the various classes of sample beyond the cut-off points do not correspond in the two tails.

In many distributions there are not enough rare samples at one end to enable us to mark the 2.5 per cent cut-off point in that tail. However, in order to save the labor of exploring both ends of every distribution, it is customary to mark the cut-off point in the tail where the observed sample would lie, and then to allow for the fact that it might be possible to do the same at the opposite end. The effect can be shown by two examples:

1. If it is stated that for a sample of 20 containing 1 F from a population of 30 per cent F's the P value (from both tails) is less than 0.05, this has the following implications:

a. Samples containing 1 F and zero F's together comprise less than 2.5 per cent of the total samples.

b. Even if there were samples of equal rarity forming the other tail of the distribution, the two tails together would comprise less than 5 per cent of the total samples.

2. If, on the other hand, the P value (both tails) for a sample containing 2 F's is said to be greater than 0.05, the implications are as follows:

a. Samples containing 2 F's, 1 F and zero F's comprise more than 2.5 per cent of the total samples.

b. If the other tail were composed of samples of equal rarity, the two tails together would comprise more than 5 per cent of the total samples.

Now it could happen that P (one tail) corresponding to the observed sample was, say, 0.035, but that there was no tail of rare samples (no 2.5 per cent cut-off point) at the other end of the distribution. Therefore, by this practice we sometimes conclude that samples are somewhat less rare than they really are: but this is a safer error than to exaggerate their rarity.

CHAPTER XII

COMPARISON OF SAMPLES
OF FREQUENCY DATA

The main topic of this chapter was first discussed in Chapter II and it has been met again at many points thereafter. Here we can look at techniques, without discussing again in detail the implications and dangers of such technical terms as "significance" and "P." The primary example is taken from an experiment, but the techniques are equally applicable to survey data, provided that we keep always in mind the limitations of the inferences that can be drawn from such data.

The presentation is intended to serve a double purpose: (1) to show how to perform a test that is very widely applicable in medical research, and (2) to show how we should try to understand the basis of any tests that we perform.

Data from a Clinical Trial

The figures in this example were obtained from a report on the comparison of two drugs in rheumatoid arthritis. The assessments were made at the beginning and end of the trial by means of a standard scheme of classification of the patient's capacity to perform the tasks of his usual occupation; and the results were reported as "improved" or "not improved" (unchanged or deteriorated). The figures could equally well have come from an experiment on animals or any other sampling units for which the outcome was recorded as X and not-X. They are arranged in a fourfold contingency table thus:

Treatment	Patients Improved	Patients Not Improved	Total
A	8	8	16
B	4	12	16
Total	12	20	32

The proportion of improved cases *after* treatment A was 50 per cent; *after* treatment B, 25 per cent. The experimenters wished to know

218

whether the difference, 25 percentage points, was, at least in part, *caused by* the difference in treatment. The patients had been assigned to the treatments by random numbers and the trial was stated to have been completely double-blind. Therefore, although the description of procedures and precautions was not as detailed as it ought to have been, we will assume for the purpose of illustration that the randomization was responsible for any bias between the two groups.

Rationale of the Tests — Randomization

To start on the road toward answering the experimenters' question, we visualize 32 index cards, 12 marked "I" (Improved) and 20 marked "NI" (Not Improved), and imagine that we arrange them in random order, divide them into two equal groups of 16, count the I's and NI's in each group and then repeat the process many times. In the light of this we can express the experimenters' question thus: "In such a series of randomizations would the difference of 8 I's in one group of 16 patients and 4 I's in the other group of 16 be large enough to be classifiable as 'rare'?" The investigators themselves adopted the customary definition of rarity — the most extreme 5 per cent of randomly produced differences — and we will follow them. We could now answer the question by any one of four methods:

1. A physical experiment — the randomization of cards by actual shuffling or by random numbers.
2. An experiment on paper — the working out of all the possible ways of dividing 12 I's between two groups of 16.
3. A mathematical shortcut of Method (2).
4. A quick mathematical test (chi-square) which has been shown to give a close approximation to Method (3).

Method (1) has just been described, and of course it is far too long if a shorter method is available. Method (2) is even longer, but we must examine it, for it is the foundation of the methods that are actually used, namely, Methods (3) and (4).

Display of All Possible Arrangements

Here is a very simple example:

Treatment	I	NI	Total
A	2	1	3
B	0	3	3
Total	2	4	6

Let us distinguish the individual patients: I_a, I_b, NI_a, NI_b, NI_c, NI_d. There are 20 possible arrangements of 6 items in two groups of 3, and we can discover them by confining ourselves to the A-group, since the remaining 3 items will be in the B-group. The arrangements in the A-group are:

2 I's and 1 NI:
    $I_aI_bNI_a$ $I_aI_bNI_b$ $I_aI_bNI_c$ $I_aI_bNI_d$
1 I and 2 NI's:
    $I_aNI_aNI_b$ $I_aNI_aNI_c$ $I_aNI_aNI_d$ $I_aNI_bNI_c$ $I_aNI_bNI_d$ $I_aNI_cNI_d$
    $I_bNI_aNI_b$ $I_bNI_aNI_c$ $I_bNI_aNI_d$ $I_bNI_bNI_c$ $I_bNI_bNI_d$ $I_bNI_cNI_d$
Zero I's and 3 NI's:
    $NI_aNI_bNI_c$ $NI_aNI_bNI_d$ $NI_aNI_cNI_d$ $NI_bNI_cNI_d$

In summary, we have:

Treatment	I	NI	Frequency out of 20
A	2	1	4 (0.2 = 20 per cent)
B	0	3	
A	1	2	12 (0.6 = 60 per cent)
B	1	2	
A	0	3	4 (0.2 = 20 per cent)
B	2	1	

At this point we must stop and ask ourselves: "How do we know that this experiment on paper represents what would happen in card shuffling?" The answer is: "In the same way as we know about coin-tossing — through long experience and special experiments." We have displayed what we would approach by continued trials; the more uniform the cards the nearer would we approach to it.

In the clinical-trial problem (equal division of 32 patients) the possible arrangements are more than 600 million. Obviously, a shortcut is necessary.

Mathematical Shortcut to Complete Display

This method, called the "exact treatment of 2×2 tables," was published by R. A. Fisher in the fifth (1934) edition of his *Statistical Methods for Research Workers,* and is in all subsequent editions. The formula is based on our knowledge of permutations and combinations, and not on any assumptions of particular population percentages, Gaussian distributions or the like. Applied to the present problem, it produced the frequency distribution in Table 4. That distribution corresponds to the one that was obtained stepwise for samples of 3 and 3, because the shortcut is a condensation of the step-by-step method, just as the binomial expansion is a condensation of the step-by-step method of discovering the frequency distribution of single samples from a binomial population (p. 192). The table shows the frequency of occurrence of sample-pairs that would be found by display of all possible arrangements when 32 patients (12 I's and 20 NI's) were divided into two samples of 16, labeled "A" and "B";

Table 4. Results of Application of Fisher's "Exact" Test
to a Fourfold Contingency Table

Repeated random division of 32 patients (12 "improved" and 20 "not improved") into two samples of 16, labeled "A" and "B," would lead toward this distribution.

Improved Cases

A	B	Relative Frequency	Percentage Frequency
12	0	0.0000	0.00*
11	1	0.0003	0.03
10	2	0.0043	0.43
9	3	0.0283	2.83
8	4	0.1038	10.38
7	5	0.2213	22.13
6	6	0.2840	28.40
5	7	0.2213	22.13
4	8	0.1038	10.38
3	9	0.0283	2.83
2	10	0.0043	0.43
1	11	0.0003	0.03
0	12	0.0000	0.00*
	Total	1.0000	100.00

*less than 1 in 10,000

and, as stated in the table itself, this is the distribution that we would approach by repeated randomization.*

The 2.5 Per Cent Cut-off Points. In order to apply the 5 per cent standard of rarity (the 5 per cent level of "significance") we place a cut-off point in each tail so that it will exclude not more than 2.5 per cent of the total distribution of sample-pairs. It lies between the 9-versus-3 and the 10-versus-2 differences in each tail, because the distribution is symmetrical, as always happens when samples are equal in size or when the total X's and not-X's are equal. At first sight, this location of the cut-off point might seem as if we were following the 2.5 per cent rule too slavishly. These points actually exclude, at each end, 0.46 per cent of the total sample-pairs, whereas if we brought the points nearer the center of the distribution by one class of sample-pair they would exclude

---

* The term "exact" was applied by Fisher in contrast to the approximation obtained by the chi-square test; but it may be mentioned that the resulting "exact" distribution (e.g., in Table 4) is called the "hypergeometric distribution," which, a statistical dictionary informs us, "derives its name from the fact that the probability generating function may be put in the form of a hypergeometric series"; and Webster's Dictionary tells us that a hypergeometric series is one that "transcends an ordinary geometric series." For many of us this is not very illuminating, but if a person has a large number of "exact" tests to do and wishes to obtain a book of tables that gives the answers for many different sizes of samples he should know what to ask for — *Tables of the Hypergeometric Probability Distribution* by Lieberman and Owen.

3.29 per cent in each tail, a total of 6.58 per cent, which is not much greater than 5 per cent.

We must remember, however, that the 5 per cent standard (1 in 20) is a rather low standard if taken literally; and in this connection it is worth while to recall the statement made by R. A. Fisher when he introduced the 5 per cent level (P = 0.05) in connection with the chi-square test (*Statistical Methods*, sect. 20):

"In preparing this table we have borne in mind that in practice we do not want to know the exact value of P for any observed χ^2, but, in the first place, whether or not the observed value is open to suspicion. If P is between .1 and .9 there is certainly no reason to suspect the hypothesis tested. If it is below .02 it is strongly indicated that the hypothesis fails to account for the whole of the facts. We shall not often be astray if we draw a conventional line at .05, and consider that higher values of χ^2 indicate a real discrepancy." (The hypothesis here referred to was of course the "null" hypothesis.)

We can say that we use the 5 per cent standard in order to insure that our real risk of being led astray when random processes alone are responsible for a phenomenon (our Type I error) will seldom be more than 2 or 3 per cent.

The One-tailed Test. Placing a cut-off point in each tail implies that we would accept a verdict in favor of either A or B. If one agent is a placebo and the other is a drug it is sometimes asserted that only the tail in favor of the drug should be marked off, on the grounds that a placebo, being a no-drug treatment, cannot do better than a drug. Those who act on this belief place a 5 per cent cut-off point in the tail that shows better results associated with the drug; i.e., they apply a "one-tailed test." This implies that, however much the result of a trial seemed to favor a placebo, the investigators would say that they knew that it was due to the randomization; but one wonders what would happen if such an extreme result were actually encountered. The method may be suitable in some experiments; but many drugs are so potent that patients are better off on a placebo. In any kind of experiment we should beware of the temptation to lower our standards by giving ourselves a better chance of obtaining a "positive" result.

Location of the Observed Sample-pair. In our present example the exact location of the cut-off point need not disturb us, because the observed inequality (A:B, 8:4 or 4:8) would itself be found in more than 20 per cent of a series of card shufflings without addition of any more extreme differences. Therefore, if we were so impressed by the 25 percentage points difference in improvement rate between the A and B groups that we attributed it to the difference in treatment, our risk of Type I error would be high. If we called an inequality of 8:4 (and 4:8) "significant" we would obviously have to apply the same verdict to more extreme inequalities also (9:3, and so on). Hence, our real risk of error in each tail of the distribution would be $10.38 + 2.83 + 0.43 + 0.03 = 13.67$ per cent, and our total risk of error would be $2 \times 13.67 = 27.34$ per cent.

Expression of the Verdict. An orthodox way of stating the verdict from this test would be: "The difference was very far from significant at the 5 per cent level, because P (both tails) from Fisher's 'exact' test was 0.2734." Another orthodox expression would be: "The apparent association between the difference in outcome and difference in treatment was very far from significant at the 5 per cent level."

A more explanatory statement is longer and clumsier, but it gives more assurance that our readers, and we ourselves, will know what we are talking about. We might use the following: "P (one tail) from Fisher's 'exact' test was 0.1367. This means that, if there were no treatment difference at all, but if the random assignment used in this trial were repeatedly applied to 32 patients of whom 12 were improved and 20 not improved, 13.67 per cent of the randomizations would produce as great or greater differences, in favor of drug A, as was observed in this trial. An equal number of the assignments would produce the same evidence in favor of drug B. It was therefore concluded that this trial, by itself, did not produce adequate evidence of an association between difference in treatment and difference in improvement rate."

In the last sentence of the above verdict, the phrase "by itself" is worth noting. Trials of the same drugs by other workers showed differences in outcome that were in the same direction, i.e., in favor of drug A. This is an example of the way in which evidence can be built up.

Expressing a Verdict of "Significance." Let us suppose that in this trial 10 improved cases had been in the A-group and 2 in the B-group. Such sample-pairs would be beyond the 0.5 per cent cut-off point in each tail of the randomization distribution; and an orthodox expression of the verdict would have been: "The difference was significant at the 1 per cent level." Trying to make a more explanatory statement, we could follow the pattern suggested above, but begin with the fact that P (one tail) in Fisher's "exact" test was 0.0046. We could translate this in terms of repeated randomization, and state that if there were no association of any kind between treatment difference and outcome difference, only 0.46 per cent of the random assignments would cause as great or greater differences in favor of drug A, with an equal number in favor of B. This would be accepted as proof of association, and then the question of causal interpretation would have to be discussed, with detailed evidence regarding the way in which the trial was conducted.

Let us suppose, now, that we were reporting on a survey of some kind, with the independent variable recorded as A or B, and the dependent variable recorded as X or not-X. We could report the verdict as follows: "P (one tail) from Fisher's 'exact' test was 0.0046. That means that if there were no association of any kind between the dependent and independent variables the observed inequality in the assignment of X's to the A- and B-group would be very rare. In a long series of repeated random assignments, as by card shuffling, only 0.92 per cent of them would show as large and larger differences in either direction (excess of X's in A or in B)." The inference would be that an association existed — either spurious, i.e., in the sample only; or real, i.e., in the population.

The Quick Test — Chi-square

Fisher's "exact" test is not very complicated, because it consists largely in the addition and subtraction of logarithms of factorials, and it is not very time-consuming in many of the small samples in which it is most often desirable. However, it is unnecessary in the vast majority of cases, because the fourfold contingency table chi-square (χ^2) is an adequate substitute. First, we will display the test in true cookbook fashion as a formula without showing its justification. We repeat the clinical-trial data for reference:

Treatment	Patients Improved	Patients Not Improved	Total
A	8	8	16
B	4	12	16
Total	12	20	32

$$\text{Chi-square (with Yates' correction)} = \frac{(8 \times 12 - 8 \times 4 - 32/2)^2 \times 32}{12 \times 20 \times 16 \times 16} = 1.20$$

The procedure can be described in five stages as follows:

1. Cross-multiply the numbers in the "cells" (the four spaces inside the table), and subtract the smaller product from the larger.
2. Reduce the difference of the products by half the grand total. This is called "Yates' correction." Sometimes the correction term is larger than the difference between the products, but this causes no difficulty. It indicates that chi-square would be so small that there is no evidence at all of an association between the treatment difference and the outcome difference. Therefore we stop the calculation.
3. Square the corrected difference of products, and multiply by the grand total. The result is the numerator of chi-square.
4. To find the denominator, multiply together the four subtotals.
5. Divide the numerator by the denominator.

We now take the chi-square that we have calculated to Fisher's Table of the Distribution of Chi-Square, first published in his *Statistical Methods for Research Workers,* later in Fisher and Yates' *Statistical Tables for Biological, Agricultural and Medical Research,* and reproduced in many statistical textbooks. The first line of chi-square values in the table is what we use in evaluating a fourfold contingency table, and here are some of the items in it:

Probability (P)	Chi-square
0.90	0.0158
0.80	0.0642
0.70	0.148
0.50	0.455
0.30	1.074
0.20	1.642
0.10	2.706
0.05	3.841
0.02	5.412
0.01	6.635
0.001	10.827

This is simply a display of a random sampling distribution of chi-square values. Let us imagine that we had a barrel of disks, with a certain percentage marked "Improved" — any percentage other than zero or 100 per cent — and the rest marked "Not Improved." Let us then suppose that we took random samples in pairs (equal or unequal samples), called one sample "A" and the other sample "B," recorded the numbers of "Improved" and "Not Improved" in each sample, and calculated chi-square for each pair of samples. The table tells us how often we would find various values of chi-square if we did a large experiment of this kind. More accurately, it tells us the chi-square frequencies that we would approach if we not only continued sampling indefinitely, but if we used larger and larger samples in the experiment.

The values of chi-square in the table are simply cut-off points, and the P values are, as elsewhere, simply relative frequencies (proportions) of items found beyond the cut-off points in a frequency distribution produced by a random process. For example, 0.1 (10 per cent) of the chi-square values would be greater than 2.706, and 0.05 (5 per cent) of them would be greater than 3.841.

Chi-square can be described as a way of finding the rarity of differences produced by random processes, and we now take to this table of chi-squares our clinical-trial chi-square to find its rarity. Obviously, the P value corresponding to 1.20 would lie between 0.30 and 0.20, presumably nearer to 0.30, and by no stretch of the word "rarity" could we call such a chi-square "rare." Therefore in this instance the chi-square verdict agrees with the verdict from the exact test, and if such agreement were found to be very common we would be justified in using chi-square instead of the exact test.

Justification of Chi-square with Fourfold Tables
The chi-square distribution is fundamentally a display of the differences found within pairs (and other multiples) of random samples of *measurement* data from Gaussian distributions; but then it was shown that it could be used with binomial data, provided that the samples

were large enough, just as the Gaussian distribution itself can be used instead of the binomial distribution to display single samples. This was long before the invention of the exact test for fourfold tables, and when that test was invented it became possible to answer the question: "How accurately does chi-square represent the differences in fourfold tables when the samples are created, not by random sampling from a barrel containing an indefinitely large number of disks, but by random shuffling of a finite number of cards?" In numerical terms we ask: "How close does P from chi-square come to the exact P? Does the difference seriously affect our verdict on fourfold tables?"

As soon as the exact test was invented, it was found by Frank Yates, a collaborator of R. A. Fisher, that a correction term, introduced into the formula for the fourfold-table chi-square, greatly improved the agreement of its P with the exact P. This is called Yates' "correction for continuity" because it makes an adjustment for the fact that tables of the chi-square distribution are derived from continuous (Gaussian) distributions, whereas the data in fourfold tables come from discontinuous (binomial) distributions. Hereafter, when we refer to the fourfold-table chi-square the qualification "with Yates' correction" will be implied even if it is not mentioned.

The comparison of chi-square with the exact test must, of course, be done empirically; and, as an illustration, we can start with our clinical-trial result. The exact P (both tails) was 0.2734. For chi-square = 1.20; P from Fisher's chi-square table was between 0.2 and 0.3, presumably nearer to the latter. This is close enough for practical purposes, but it is interesting to find the chi-square P more precisely. This was done by using another table (Yule and Kendall), and the answer was P = 0.2733, identical with the exact P to the third decimal place. It might be suspected that this was an example specially chosen to boost the credit of chi-square, but in fact it was not, and very close agreement is often found, even with very small samples when they are equal in size.

Practice with Chi-square

Readers might find it useful to work through other combinations in the series of sample-pairs derived from the clinical-trial data, imagining in each case that they have obtained a single pair of samples from a different experiment or survey. The chi-square values shown below have four decimal places because they were used to obtain rather detailed values of P for comparison with the exact P's; but in practice one decimal place is often sufficient.

A slide rule or four-figure logarithm table can be used; and in some instances rough cancellation of items in the numerator and denominator will suffice to show whether the value is far above or below the 5 per cent or 1 per cent standard.

The "interval" P's are from Fisher's list, quoted above; the P's in parentheses are from the table of Yule and Kendall. The ½P's are also shown, for a special reason. They are a close approximation to the exact P's for one tail, and it is desirable to get used to thinking in terms of separate tails because it helps us to solve the problem of unequal tails discussed later.

No. of X's		Chi-square	P from	½P from	Exact P
A	B	(Yates' Correction)	Chi-square	Chi-square	(One Tail)
(1) 9	3	3.3333	0.05–0.10	0.025–0.05	
			(0.0679)	(0.0339)	0.0328
(2) 10	2	6.5333	approx. 0.01	approx. 0.005	
			(0.0106)	(0.0053)	0.0046
(3) 11	1	10.8000	approx. 0.001	approx. 0.0005	
			(0.00101)	(0.0005)	0.0003

In trying to formulate a more explanatory verdict than the automatic "significant (or not significant) at the such-and-such level of significance," one should start by stating that chi-square (with Yates' correction) was considered to be a sufficiently reliable substitute for the "exact" method in estimating the frequency of differences produced by randomization alone. (The limits of chi-square's reliability are discussed below.) Then one should take the ½P from chi-square (the "interval" value, because the detailed value is very seldom needed), and indicate its meaning in terms of randomization as was done for the exact P.

If a number of verdicts of this kind are to be given in the same report, one need not repeat the story with each verdict. It can be given at the outset. To avoid the reader's losing sight of the meaning of the exact P (and its approximate equivalent, obtained by chi-square), it is useful to call it the "frequency in randomization experiments," or "randomization frequency"; and then to bring in that phrase whenever P is mentioned.

The Problem of Unequal Tails

Let us suppose that an investigation has produced the following four-fold table:

Treatment	X	Not-X	Total
A	1	9	10
B	4	2	6
Total	5	11	16

Chi-square (with Yates' correction) $= 3.278$. Therefore P from Fisher's table (p. 225) is between 0.10 and 0.05. We could give a verdict "not significant at the 5 per cent level"; but what exactly would it mean? What does the P represent? We are facing the same problem as the one discussed in Chapter XI — the problem of P from both tails when binomial distributions are nonsymmetrical. Chi-square, being developed from the Gaussian distribution, pictures equal tails; but we know that the exact distribution for this sample-pair would not be symmetrical, because the samples are not equal, and neither are the total X's and not-X's.

It has been shown that, even in these cases, ½P from chi-square (with Yates' correction) is very close to the exact P from the tail in which the sample-pair lies. In this instance, with chi-square = 3.278, ½P is between 0.05 and 0.025. That is, if we randomly divided 5 X's between A (containing 10 individuals) and B (containing 6 individuals) and repeated the randomization many times, we would in the long run find that something between 2.5 and 5 per cent of the sample-pairs contained A-B differences as great as in the original (observed) sample-pair or greater, and in the same direction.

If there were no equally rare or rarer samples at the opposite end of the distribution, we would feel justified in calling the difference "significant at the 5 per cent level." In fact, in this instance there were no such rare sample-pairs — the opposite tail of the distribution was "blunt" because a sample-pair with 5 X's in A and none in B comprised more than 5 per cent of the total distribution. However, unless we are prepared in such cases to find exact P's, our only way to be sure of keeping our Type I error below 5 per cent is to make a statement such as the following: "Chi-square = 3.278. Therefore ½P is between 0.025 and 0.05. This shows that randomization alone would produce, in more than 2.5 per cent of sample-pairs, differences as great as, and greater than, the observed difference, and in the same direction (a higher proportion of X's in B than in A). Therefore the observed difference was not considered large enough to prove an association between the variables under test." In some cases we will thereby unwittingly set a 2.5 per cent standard of "significance" instead of a 5 per cent standard, as in the example discussed here; but this is an error on the "safe" side.

Reliability of Chi-square Verdicts

In all the instances shown above, ½P from chi-square has been very close to the exact P (one tail); but the examples were not selected for that reason. The chi-square and exact tests have been extensively compared with respect to their verdicts at the 5 per cent and 1 per cent levels of significance. In one survey more than 500 such comparisons were made (Mainland, 1948). Many of the individual samples contained from 4 to 20 individuals, but many larger samples were also studied. The survey included equal as well as unequal samples, while the other subtotals (X and not-X) were sometimes equal and sometimes differed greatly. From this experience and from later, less systematic explorations it became clear that a few simple precautions or rules make it possible to use chi-square (with Yates' correction) confidently in the vast majority of fourfold contingency tables.

The safety of chi-square is not related very directly to sample size or to the equality of adjacent subtotals, but to a quantity which can be quickly calculated by multiplying together the smaller subtotal in the two rows by the smaller subtotal in the two columns, and then dividing the product by the grand total. The result is often labeled "m." For example, in the table containing samples of 6 and 10, with 5 X's and 11 not-X's, $m = (5 \times 6)/16$. It is sufficient to note that this is approximately 2.

If m is not greater than 1, chi-square should not be used, but the exact test. Such cases are very rare.

The following interpretation of chi-square will tend, if anything, to produce some verdicts of "nonsignificance" which the exact test would reverse, but in research this is generally less serious than an error in the opposite direction.

Chi-square (with Yates' Correction)	P	½P
below 4	greater than 0.05	greater than 0.025
4 or more	less than 0.05	less than 0.025
7 or more	less than 0.01	less than 0.005

The chief exceptions to these relationships are as follows:

If m is not greater than 5, and chi-square is between 3.5 and 4, the exact P (one tail) is sometimes greater and sometimes less than 0.025.

If m is greater than 5 but not greater than 20, and chi-square is 3.8 or 3.9, the exact P (one tail) is sometimes greater and sometimes less than 0.025.

In these doubtful cases the exact test can be used. Table VIII of Fisher and Yates gives an almost equally reliable verdict with less calculation, but many workers would probably find it easier to perform the exact test.

However, before seeking a more definite numerical answer than chi-square can give, we must remember that these are borderline cases. We can say that very likely 2 or 3 per cent of the appropriate randomization trials would produce differences as great as, or greater than, our observed difference in the same direction, and might also produce differences of almost equal frequency in the opposite direction (at the other end of the distribution). The shorthand expression would be "on the borderline of significance at the 5 per cent level." Then we can make up our minds in view of the particular circumstances of the problem under study.

The chi-square P values of 0.10 and greater have not been as thoroughly compared with exact P's as have those around $P = 0.05$. When m is between 1 and 10 the ½P values from chi-square indicate the exact P (one tail) only roughly; but they appear to be close enough for most purposes, because their chief value lies in showing us how unconvincing is our evidence of an association. If P from chi-square is between 0.20 and 0.30, we can say that differences as great as, and greater than, the observed difference in the same direction would be produced in at least 10 per cent of the randomization trials.

Tables for Testing Equal Samples

If we have two binomial samples, each containing N individuals up to N = 200, and we wish to test for "significance" at the 5 per cent and 1 per cent levels, chi-square is unnecessary, because Tables III and IV give information equivalent to that obtainable by the exact test (see Appendix).

The use of the tables can be illustrated by examples from the clinical-trial data used earlier in this chapter.

Treatment	Improved	Not Improved	Total
A	8	8	16
B	4	12	16
Total	12	20	32

The simplest procedure is to turn the contingency table around until the smallest of the four values in its cells (here 4) is at the top left hand corner, thus:

Treatment	Improved	Not Improved
B	4	12
A	8	8

The B-sample is now Sample (1), the A-sample is Sample (2). Improved patients are X's, and we write:

$$\text{No. of X's in } (1)/\text{No. of X's in } (2) = 4/8.$$

Then we look in Table III along the entries at N = 16 until we find 4/11. This means that with 4 X's in Sample (1) we need at least 11 X's in Sample (2) for a verdict of "significant at the 5 per cent level." The observed difference does not nearly reach the standard. That is, with 4/8 we know that the randomization frequency (P in both tails) would be considerably greater than 0.05. As we have seen, it would be 0.2734.

As another example, let us consider a table with the following contents:

Treatment	Improved	Not Improved	Total
A	10	6	16
B	2	14	16

We take to Table III the quantity 2/10 and we find that 2/9 is sufficient for "significance at the 5 per cent level." Therefore we take it to Table IV and find that it qualifies even for significance at the 1 per cent level. As we saw previously (p. 227) the exact P (one tail) would be 0.0046.

The spacing of the N's in the tables is sufficiently close for linear interpolation. To illustrate interpolation between the ratios we can take

$N = 80$ in Table III, starting at $16/29$. The next entry is $23/36$. We note that 29 is 13 more than 16 and that 36 is 13 more than 23. This indicates that the intermediate values are $17/30$, $18/31$, $19/32$ and so on. The next entry beyond $23/36$ is $24/38$, which starts a difference of 14, and this continues to $40/54$.

Preparation of Tables III and IV. These tables have been extracted from previously published tables (Mainland, 1948; Mainland and Murray; Mainland, Herrera and Sutcliffe) which were prepared by the "exact" method through $N = 20$, and beyond that mostly by chi-square (with Yates' correction), the chi-square values being tested for "significance" by Table VIII of Fisher and Yates. Where there was any doubt, however, the exact method was applied. In many parts of the series it was found, as indicated above, that differences between adjacent entries were constant over such long ranges that chi-square or exact-test calculations were required only at intervals. Many entries that are omitted from the tables were, however, actually calculated, and interpolation can be considered safe.

Step-by-step Calculation of Chi-square

We have seen that a mysterious formula can be used, without removal of its mystery, to tell us how often various things happen when we divide a set of items into two groups by a strictly random process. Our confidence in the formula depends on comparisons that have been made between (a) the frequencies (P's) that we obtain by its use and (b) the frequencies from the exact test, which is based on our knowledge of random sorting such as card shuffling. We do not need to know the step-by-step procedure of which the formula is a condensation, or why that particular procedure was invented, or the nature of the proof (or discovery) of the frequency of occurrence of various values of chi-square. If it were found tomorrow that this proof (or discovery) had been based on a mistake, it would not shake our confidence in the use of chi-square (with precautions specified above) in the testing of fourfold tables.

However, it seems a pity to use condensed formulae and not try to remove some of their mystery, especially when the step-by-step procedure makes considerable sense, even to a nonmathematician. In the case of chi-square, moreover, we need to know the step-by-step method if we are going to test contingency tables that contain more than two columns and more than two rows.

The following ideas are presented by one who has looked at the development of statistical techniques from the outside. The ideas have helped to remove some of the mystery for him, and they may help others also. They do not pretend to represent the lines of reasoning followed by the mathematicians who devised the chi-square technique, but show how an experimenter might try to devise a fourfold-table test, the difficulties that he would meet, and the general lines along which mathematicians tackle such difficulties.

An Imaginary Experimenter's Attempts. Let us imagine the experimenter living before the "exact" test for fourfold contingency tables was dreamed of, and that one of his experiments had resulted in the sample-pair already discussed:

	Outcome		
Treatment	X	Not-X	Total
A	1	9	10
B	4	2	6
Total	5	11	16

He wished to find out how often such differences would occur if there were no difference between the two treatments, i.e., if both samples had come from the same population of treated subjects. He knew about random sampling, but did not know about statistical tests; so he proposed to construct a population of disks and take random samples of 10 and 6 until he had a large number of sample-pairs. But what should he choose as the proportions of X's and not-X's in the population?

The experimenter might argue thus: If there were no difference between the treatments, the A and B labels would mean nothing. The two samples together would then be equivalent to one random sample of 16 subjects, and its proportion of X's (5 out of 16) would be more likely to be near the proportion in the population than far away from it. Following this line of reasoning he would mark his disks in the proportion of 5 X's to 11 not-X's.

By such a sampling experiment he could certainly obtain an answer to his question about the frequency of the difference in his fourfold table; but he would probably feel he ought to introduce somewhat different population proportions of X's and not-X's, and repeat the experiment. If he did so, he would find that the answers differed from one experiment to another. Moreover, he would realize that by this method he would have to perform a series of sampling experiments for every contingency table that he produced in his researches.

He might attempt to get around this difficulty by expressing all his sample-differences as percentages (e.g., X's in B minus X's in A = 66.7 − 10.0 = 56.7 per cent X's) in order to see if one sampling experiment, or a small series of them, would produce information adequate for all time. He would soon find that the series of experiments would have to be extremely large, because big percentage differences would be much commoner when samples were small than when they were large. He would then visualize a series of sampling experiments for a wide range of sample sizes. He would be still more appalled by the thought of contingency tables larger than fourfold. At this stage, we may suppose, he would turn to a mathematician.

The Mathematician's Approach.   Our experimenter may be imaginary, but his difficulties are real. In trying to overcome them, both in frequency data and in measurement data, the statistical mathematician adopts the following general line of approach. He tries to express, and test, the differences between contents of samples in a form that will have the following characteristics: (1) It will in itself make allowance for the effects of sample sizes. (2) It will not need to be changed for every different parent population. (3) It will be usable with more than one form of data (e.g., with contingency tables containing any number of cells). (4) It will enable the mathematician to make use of a random sampling distribution that he already knows.

For such purposes, the most widely used distribution is the Gaussian. In Chapter XI it was seen that the Gaussian curve, although developed by enlarging binomial samples indefinitely, can be used, with certain precautions, to give information about the variation among individual binomial samples that are relatively small. It would be reasonable to suppose, therefore, that it could give information about differences between two or more such samples; and this is what it does by way of chi-square. The mathematician invents a formula that can be filled in from the observed data to give a numerical quantity (chi-square, for instance); but it is not necessary that random samples of this quantity (e.g., from a disk-sampling experiment) shall actually form a Gaussian distribution. All that the mathematician needs is a quantity whose sampling distribution can be derived from the Gaussian distribution; and chi-square is an example of this.

By this general line of approach, statistical mathematicians have produced a number of extremely useful formulae. We should never forget, however, that the Gaussian distribution is a limit approached by taking larger and larger binomial samples. Therefore the general rule is that the bigger the sample, the better is a formula invented from the Gaussian distribution. By a "good" formula here, we mean one that gives results close enough, for our particular purpose, to the results that we would obtain by actual random sampling, as shown, for example, in the binomial distribution or in the "exact" test for fourfold tables. The formulae must always be tested empirically, as exemplified in Chapter XI and in this present chapter.

Steps in the Fourfold-table Chi-square. We illustrate the seven steps by using the imaginary experimenter's table:

	Outcome		
Treatment	X	Not-X	Total
A	1	9	10
B	4	2	6
Total	5	11	16

1. We start, as did the imaginary experimenter, by finding the proportion of X's and not-X's in the total 16 subjects, i.e., 5/16 and 11/16 respectively. We are not disturbed by the fact that these may not be the actual population values, because chi-square utilizes the sample estimates in this way.

2. We then say: "If 5/16 of the population were X's, the average

numbers of X's in sets of random samples of 10 subjects would be 5/16 of 10 = 3.125 X's. This is called the "expected" (E) number of X's for the A-sample. For each of the other three cells in the table the E's are calculated, or can be found by subtracting 3.125 from the subtotals. The four E's are then: AX, 3.125; A–not-X, 6.875; BX, 1.875; B–not-X, 4.125. (Incidentally, we can see now why the product of 6 and 5, divided by 16, is given the letter m; it is the minimum expected value.)

3. We find the difference between the observed (O) and expected (E) values, and this appears, even to a nonmathematician, like a sensible way to measure the pull of the two treatments (A and B) away from the center or average value. The (O − E)'s are, of course, the same in each cell (2.125), two of them negative and two positive, but we disregard the signs.

4. We introduce Yates' correction which, as previously mentioned, makes the chi-square P's, derived from a continuous (Gaussian) curve, much more like the P's from the exact distribution which is discontinuous. We apply the correction by reducing each (O − E) by half a unit, i.e., $(O − E)_c = 2.125 − 0.5 = 1.625$. The ultimate effect is exactly the same as in the chi-square condensed formula, although there we subtract half the grand total. (It is important to remember that the correction is not to be used with tables larger than fourfold.)

5. The next step looks strange. We square the $(O − E)_c$ in each cell: $1.625^2 = 2.6406$. Perhaps we can get an inkling of the reason if we remember that the mathematician is aiming at an expression that gives him a path to the Gaussian distribution or a distribution derived from it. The yardstick in that distribution is the standard deviation (Chapter XI) and, as is shown in Chapter XIII, the first step in calculating a standard deviation is to square the individual deviations, i.e., differences, between the average and the individual measurements.

6. We now divide each $(O − E)_c^2$ by its corresponding E. This does not appear unreasonable when we reflect that if an average value (here represented by E) is small, a particular difference from it should have more weight than if the average value is large. (A centimeter difference in length means much more in mice than in elephants.) The values of $(O − E)_c^2/E$ are 0.845, 0.384, 1.408 and 0.640.

7. We add these four contributions to produce chi-square (with Yates' correction) = 3.277, which is identical, except for a rounding effect in the last digit, with the value obtained by the condensed formula.

This last step illustrates the general, and quite simple, formula for chi-square. If S stands for "the sum of all quantities of the following type," then:

$$\text{chi-square} = S\{(O − E)^2/E\}$$

Contingency Tables Larger than Fourfold

If we have more than two samples of frequency data to compare, or if the samples (two or more) contain more than two classes, the contingency table is larger than fourfold, but a chi-square test is again appropriate. Except that Yates' correction is not used, the arithmetic is the same as in the step-by-step method for fourfold tables.

Extensive comparisons with exact distributions have not been made, but it is commonly accepted that the chi-square method is reliable unless the expected (E) value in one of the cells is less than 5. It is customary to get around this difficulty by pooling adjacent rows or columns and calculating chi-square for the resulting smaller table. However, it appears that smaller E's than 5 are safe if special treatment is applied (Haldane).

"Degrees of Freedom."   P values for all sizes of contingency tables are to be obtained from Fisher's table of the chi-square distribution from which the P's for fourfold tables were quoted earlier. One must, however, enter the table with the proper "*n*" value, which is called the "number of degrees of freedom." The following example may elucidate the term. If there are 5 columns and 3 rows of cells in a table, the contents of any four of the cells in a row may vary independently of each other, but the content of the remaining cell, whichever it may be, is fixed by the rest, because the row total is constant. Similarly, with 3 rows, the contents of only two cells in each column can vary independently. The total number of possibilities for independent variation is therefore $(5-1) \times (3-1) = 8$ degrees of freedom. It has been shown that P for chi-square does not depend on the number of rows or columns as such, but on the number of degrees of freedom. Thus in Fisher's table, at $n = 8$ the chi-square under $P = 0.05$ is 15.507, and this would hold true whether the contingency table had 9 columns and 2 rows or 3 columns and 5 rows. (Obviously, a fourfold table has only one degree of freedom.)

Conversion to Fourfold Tables.   A clinical trial may produce a contingency table consisting of two rows (treatments) and several columns representing graded changes, from "much worse" to "much better." These are two samples of "multinomial" data, and should be considered in the same way as the clinical multinomial data discussed in Chapter XI. There is usually little to be gained from 5×2 table analysis of such data, or even from a 3×2 analysis. The kinds of questions that we wish to ask are:

1. Was there an A-B difference in the incidence of improvement versus no improvement (no change plus deterioration)?

2. Among the unimproved cases was there an A-B difference in the incidence of no change versus deterioration?

Two fourfold tables will answer those questions.

Either or both variables in a contingency table can, of course, be measurement classes. For example, if the rows contain treatments, the columns can contain changes in the size of the x-ray shadow of the heart or in an antibody titer. Even here a fourfold-table analysis may be all that is needed. We might, for example, decide that a change of less than ± 0.5 cm. in the transverse diameter of the heart shadow was of no consequence and then the two columns would represent respectively increase and decrease of more than 0.5 cm.

Analysis of Cross-over Data

Before this section is studied, earlier discussions of cross-over experiments should be reviewed (pp. 49 and 84). The following data were selected from an A-versus-B double-blind cross-over trial in which the extent of a skin rash was assessed, and the changes were classified as either improvement or no improvement (deterioration or no change):

Patients Who Showed Improvement	AB Sequence	BA Sequence
In both periods	3	2
In period (1), not in (2)	3	0
In period (2), not in (1)	0	4
In neither period	0	0

Although the rash was not actually measured, estimates of its extent were made and expressed as percentages of total skin area. These measurement data are analyzed in Chapter XIV. Here the frequency data are analyzed as if they had been produced by clinical impression or by patients' responses, in an alternate-week therapy trial, to such questions as: "Do you feel better this week than last week, or worse, or about the same?"

An Incorrect Presentation. Data of this kind are too often presented in the following form: Treatment A — Improved, 12; Not improved, 0. Treatment B — Improved, 5; Not improved, 7. This makes it appear that there were 24 independent sampling units, whereas there were only 12 patients. It would be wrong to analyze these figures in a fourfold contingency table. Even if an author has analyzed the original figures correctly, if he presents them in this form he hides from his readers the very information that the cross-over design was intended to elicit — the behavior of the same patients under different drugs and in relation to sequence of treatment.

Relation of Analysis to Design. The patients who provide an answer to the primary question, regarding possible difference in drug effect, are 7 in number and all of them showed improvement after treatment A. It might therefore be thought sufficient to point out that "seven of a kind" is a rather rare occurrence when there is an equal chance for two kinds to occur. That would have been the proper form of analysis if periods (1) and (2) in each patient had been looked upon as a pair of twins, and the drugs A and B had been assigned to the periods in each patient by the toss of a coin or by odd and even random numbers. This method of assignment would have pooled the possible bias due to differences between periods (1) and (2) with other biases, and would have made the randomization responsible for the resultant bias. The essence of the cross-over design is that it separates the difference between the periods — the sequence effect — from other factors, enables us to measure it and make allowance for it in seeking for a difference between A and B treatments. To give ourselves the best chance of detecting such a difference we must have AB and BA sequence groups that are equal or nearly equal in size, and patients must be randomly assigned to them. The coin-tossing method does not insure equality; therefore we assign sequences to equal numbers as by card shuffling, and we must analyze the data accordingly. In fact, the sequences are now, as it were, "treatments." We proceed as follows:

Sequence	Improved in (1), not (2)	Improved in (2), not (1)	Total
AB	3	0	3
BA	0	4	4
Total	3	4	7

The design of the experiment has taken into account the fact that, regardless of therapy, patients might very well differ from each other in the amount, or even the direction, of the differences between the first and second periods. It has randomly assigned these interpatient differences to the sequence groups, and has left only one systematic difference — the fact that in the AB sequence the first therapy is A, while in the BA sequence it is B. Therefore, if the difference in outcome was greater than we were prepared to attribute to randomization alone, and if we were confident that the experiment had been carried out properly, we would attribute the difference in outcome to the difference between the therapies.

This small sample, which was taken merely for illustration from an experiment that was still to continue, could not produce sufficient evidence of anything but randomization effects, because although the difference was maximal, chi-square (with Yates' correction) was only 3.44.

Further Analyses. In a cross-over experiment the subjects that show no interperiod difference in outcome are not wasted. They help to answer the question: "Does the sequence matter?" First, using all the subjects, we make the following comparison:

Sequence	Outcome in Periods (1) and (2) Same	Different
AB	3	3
BA	2	4

There is no suggestion of a difference in relation to sequences, but with larger numbers there might have been a demonstrable difference, from various causes, including the following:

1. A carry-over of A's effect into B's period in the AB sequence. This

might, as it were, remove some patients from the upper right cell into the upper left cell but it would not affect the two lower cells.

2. A delayed effect of A, so that it did not start to act until B's period in the AB sequence. This might move some patients from the upper left cell to the upper right cell, and also some from the lower right cell to the lower left cell because A would not be effective until after the second period.

3. A trend toward improvement, independent of therapy. This might make B in period (2) appear as good as A had been in period (1), although B was actually inferior to A. Therefore it would move patients from the upper right cell to the upper left cell, and perhaps also move some from the lower left to the lower right cell.

Even if, with fair sizes of samples, no difference is detected by the foregoing analysis, it is desirable to examine separately the subjects in whom the outcome was alike in both periods:

Sequence	Improved	Not Improved
AB	. .	. .
BA	. .	. .

These two outcome-groups can be considered respectively more amenable, and more resistant, to therapy. In the interpretation of the results the same interplay of factors, such as carry-over, should be considered.

Such analyses are specially useful when no therapy difference has been demonstrated by the first analysis. Although we may try to prevent carry-over by inserting an interval during which neither A nor B is permitted, in the study of a new drug we may make this interval too short, or we may be unaware of the delayed action of the drug. These additional analyses can thus lead to a more satisfactory trial.

Sample Sizes Required for Fourfold Tables

The subject of sample sizes has been discussed rather fully in Chapter VIII. Here, we can be more technical about Table V, which shows the sizes necessary in equal samples, each containing up to 100 individuals (see Appendix).

Let us suppose that we have reason to believe that treatment A, applied to a very large number (an indefinitely large population) of subjects of any kind, would produce a certain effect, X, in about 50 per cent of them. If treatment B would, under the same conditions, produce the same effect in 75 per cent of such a population, we wish to have strong assurance that a forthcoming experiment, comparing A-treated and B-treated subjects, will not fail to demonstrate a difference between the effects of the treatments. By "demonstrate a difference" we mean that a fourfold contingency table test will show that the difference in the numbers of X's in the A and B samples will be large enough to reach the 5 per cent level of "significance." By "strong assurance" we mean that we must know that 95 per cent of such experiments would be "successful" in this sense, i.e., that the experiment would have a "power" of 0.95.

In Table V at A:50 per cent X's, B:75 per cent X's, and N = 100, we find 94.5 per cent S (successful experiments). That is, the A and B samples must each contain at least 100 subjects to give us the necessary assurance. The table is applicable to any experiments or surveys in which the independent variable is divided into two classes (A and B) and the dependent variable is recorded as X or not-X (an all-or-none assessment).

Above population values of 15 per cent X's the intervals may appear arbitrarily irregular, but they were chosen to correspond to the estimates or guesses that we commonly make in practice — about a quarter, a third, a half, two thirds, and so on.

Preparation of Table V. This table (Mainland and Sutcliffe, 1953; Mainland, Herrera and Sutcliffe) was prepared by a method equivalent to the simultaneous sampling of well mixed disks in two barrels, one barrel containing A per cent X's, the other containing B per cent X's, and then applying an exact fourfold contingency table test to each sample-pair. In actuality, for each population percentage and sample size, a binomial distribution (as in Chapter XI) was obtained from published tables. Then, for each pair of populations, A and B, all possible combinations were found.

For instance, let us suppose that samples of 20 containing 4 X's would be found in 0.1 (10 per cent) of all random samples of that size from a population containing A per cent X's, and that samples of 20 containing 12 X's would be found in 0.2 (20 per cent) of all random samples from a population containing B per cent X's. Then these two samples would be found in $0.1 \times 0.2 = 0.02$ (2 per cent) of all combinations of samples of 20 from those two populations. Reference to Table III shows that this difference (4 versus 12) would be "significant at the 5 per cent level" (see Appendix). That is, if we set our Type I error at 5 per cent, we would accept this difference as evidence of an association between treatment difference and difference in outcome. Therefore an experiment that produced such a sample-pair would be "successful" by definition, and we have already seen that such sample-pairs would be met in 2 per cent of all experiments with that pair of populations. When all possible combinations of samples of 20 had thus been tested, the total percentage of successful experiments would be entered in Table V.

Estimation of Percentages in Finite Populations

Chapter XI showed how to estimate binomial population percentages when the population is indefinitely large, or "infinite." For many purposes we can say that a population is infinite in comparison with a sample when the sample comprises 1 per cent of the population or less, because removal of the sample has a negligible effect on the population percentage of X's. If, however, we have a population such as 2000 persons in a certain industry and we take a one-fourth random sample, the remaining three fourths may contain a very different percentage of X's

than did the population before the sample was removed. To estimate
how many X's the unexamined group may contain (upper and lower
limits) we can use a fourfold contingency table, with columns headed
"X" and "Not-X," and rows headed "Examined" (500) and "Not Examined" (1500).

Let us suppose that the sample of 500 contains 50 X's and 450 not-X's.
These are inserted in the first row. In the second row we write x in the
X-column and $(1500 - x)$ in the Not-X column. Then, unless something
unusual has happened — something that would occur in less than 5 per
cent of random selections — x will not be greater than a certain value
or less than some other value. To find these values we can calculate chi-
square from the fourfold table and equate it to 3.841 (for $P = 0.05$).
The result will be an equation containing x^2, and by solving it we will
find the required upper and lower limits of x. If we add them to the 50
X's observed in the sample, we will obtain the estimated upper and lower
limits of the number of X's in the total 2000 with an error risk of
5 per cent.

To simplify the calculation we can use 4 instead of 3.841, and we can
omit Yates' correction term. This omission will cause too small a difference between the observed number of X's (50) and the estimates
of x; but these estimates can then be tried, along with the correction
terms (in this case 2000/2), and x can be altered until the required
chi-square (4) is reached. For smaller risk of error, larger values of
chi-square can be used. (There is a formula that leads more directly
to the population limits than does this chi-square method, but I prefer
the longer route because I can see more clearly why it is leading to the
objective.)

Other Topics
Under the heading of this chapter a number of other topics could be
discussed. Some of them are mentioned elsewhere.

1. Estimation of population differences from the difference between
a pair of binomial samples, one from each population, is discussed in
Chapter XVI, sect. 2.

2. The sequential design was introduced in Chapter VI under
Q VI – 18. An example is given in Chapter XVI, sect. 3.

3. Analysis of frequencies by measurement-data methods. Many of
the observations that we make by counting, such as pulse rates, leukocyte counts (per cubic mm.) and differential leukocyte counts (expressed
as percentages) are functionally measurements, and are appropriately
analyzed by methods shown in Chapters XIII and XIV.

CHAPTER XIII

VARIATION BETWEEN
MEASUREMENTS

This chapter is concerned with measurements made in what may be called "single-variable" surveys, which set out to discover how many subjects have such and such measurements. That is, they are frequency distribution studies, even if each value of the variable is represented by only one subject. The purposes of such surveys are very diverse, as may be seen from the following examples:

1. Male students' statures (Table 5, p. 247). These will be used to illustrate common methods of displaying and describing frequency distributions, and of expressing variation for the purpose of assessing individuals.
2. Total and differential leukocyte counts.
3. Numbers of valves in the left cephalic vein (Table 6, p. 266).
4. Duration of life after appearance of symptoms in tuberculous meningitis.
5. Clearance of diphtheria bacilli from the throats of carriers.
6. Changes in the symptoms and signs in patients with rheumatoid arthritis during a drug trial.
7. Differences between 100 glucose determinations made on the same specimen of urine.

Since the purpose of many collections of measurements on human beings is the establishment of clinical "norms," this is an appropriate place to look at that problem.

"Normal" Values
Of all the decisions that a medical practitioner has to make, probably the commonest is the decision whether some feature in a patient, such as blood pressure, basal metabolic rate, or the size of the subcutaneous inguinal ring, is to be considered "normal" or not. Here we are using

"normal" in the medical, not in the statistical (Gaussian) sense, but it will be readily seen that the judgment is fundamentally statistical.

No definition of "normal" meets all theoretical objections, or can be applied under all circumstances; and yet some such word is essential. To find a generally useful definition, we must first see what the word should not imply, and then observe how measurements or other features, commonly called normal, are arrived at.

"Normal" should not be taken as equivalent to "ideal" or "perfect," because then it ceases to be applicable to actual beings or things. "The most commonly occurring" is vague and sometimes untrue; for example, dental caries is very common, but is a disease. "Normal" is not equivalent to "average," and a practitioner should be able to explain the distinction to a mother who is worried because her child's weight is a little below the average that is shown in a weight table. Variation is an essential feature of life, and instead of saying "normal" we should say "within normal limits." We shall then not be victims of a confusion of terms that led a famous obstetrician to declare that normal pelves are rarely seen!

In medicine, as in statistics, "normal" indicates a standard, and it would be much less confusing if we used that word, as is done in some "standard weight tables." The best of such tables illustrate the ordinary way of setting up a standard. Healthy persons are weighed and divided into stature classes. Then within each stature class certain limits of weight are set, but not by taking the highest and lowest weight in each class. The location of the limits will be discussed later, but the method already suggests a definition. A feature is called "normal" — or better, "within standard limits" — if it falls within a certain range of variation derived from the examination of healthy people. (The phrase "derived from" is better than "found in," which might imply that we used the observed extreme values.)

This definition leads to another question: What is "healthy"? Here again, every definition is criticized, but we need some kind of definition, not only in setting up norms, but for everyday use. Health has been defined as adaptation to one's environment, i.e., fitness for survival. In application to human beings this implies also "fitness to perform the functions expected of one." For example, an old man's heart may be suitable for his mode of life, although it would not be considered healthy in a young man. Despite their flaws, such definitions help us in establishing standards, if we remember that "healthy" implies:

1. Healthy according to current conceptions.

2. Healthy in all respects relevant to the feature concerned. In forming weight standards we do not exclude persons because they have bunions.

Abnormal (Aberrant) Features

On the above basis we can form a working definition of abnormal or aberrant or "substandard" features as belonging to one or other of two classes:

1. Features that are diseased or associated with disease, as cause or effect, or in some indirect way.

2. Features that are found in healthy persons, but beyond the range adopted as standard.

Limitations of Definitions

Some limitation of the foregoing definitions can be illustrated by two rather special cases:

1. A person may have eyesight that is within standard limits for general purposes, but is unsuitable for certain occupations, as in certain branches of the armed services.

2. There is so much variation in the relationships of the teeth to each other in the same jaw, and of upper-jaw teeth to lower-jaw teeth, that it is difficult to decide what are satisfactory limits. If the arrangement obviously interferes with function, there is no problem in classification. Some lesser deformities may be compensated for physically by the chewing mechanism, but can still, by their psychologic effect, render their possessors less well adapted to life; and by reducing their prospects of mating, can reduce the chances of survival of their stock. Such conditions could, if their effects were clearly established, be classified as substandard.

There are, however, many irregularities of children's teeth that parents and dentists feel should be corrected, although they probably have no adverse effect on health or survival. Here, apparently, is a transition from biologic or clinical standards to esthetic, cosmetic, or "Hollywood" standards, and if the term "normal" is still used its definition has to be changed.

General Principles in Establishing Standard Values

Anyone who is acquainted with correct sampling methods can see what general principles ought to be observed in collecting data for the establishment of standard values. With these principles in mind he will know what to look for before using a supposed standard. When he has to use values that have unknown or questionable validity he will be skeptical, even if he has found them in a very valuable reference book (Sunderman and Boerner). If such skepticism became general, the impetus to provide sound values would increase.

Disregard of Principles.   The principles are not quite so flagrantly disregarded as they were forty years ago, when students were taught that the normal red cell counts were 5 million per cubic mm. for men and 4.5 million for women — figures originally based on the blood counts of only four persons (Osgood). In 1932, sixty years after physicians started studying gastric acidity in the sick, a study of values from healthy subjects was published (Vanzant, Alvarez and others).

Such studies are, however, still too rare. Supposedly normal weights of internal organs are passed from textbook to textbook, frequently without reference to the source of information. The source is often a collection of weights obtained at hospital autopsies, although sound criteria of selection have been clearly established — organs from healthy persons killed in accidents and dead within 24 hours of the accident; with exclusion, for vascular organs (spleen, liver, kidney) of subjects who have lost much blood. (Examples from the Minnesota work in this field, with references, are given elsewhere — Mainland, 1945.)

When such simple data as organ weights are improperly collected and used, one wonders what are the criteria of a physician who states that, on examining a patient's abdominal wall, he found the liver "slightly enlarged." Of much greater importance is the unreliability of physiologic and biochemical standards, which purport to be precise. Nutritional needs of young children have been deduced from those of older children and adults. Statements of vitamin requirements have been authoritatively given to the public, although the figures may hardly be more than orders of magnitude.

One of the commonest faults in establishing standard limits is to make the interval between them too narrow. For qualitative features little or no allowance for variation may be made at all. When the calyces of the kidney pelvis were first shown by x-rays, many patterns were considered abnormal, until the breadth of variation, unassociated with disease, was shown; and yet this lesson, and many others like it, had not been learned by some of the physicians who started using the system of bronchial segmentation of the lungs immediately after its discovery. Probably owing to the way in which they themselves had been taught anatomy, they used and taught one pattern of segmentation, instead of remembering that further exploration would almost certainly reveal variations, as it soon did in profusion.

Selection of Standard Limits

As we learn more about the borderlines of health and disease we will be more able to detect, in apparently healthy persons, measurements or other features that foretell disease. Such features will then be classified as abnormal, substandard or undesirable. A step in this direction was seen in the publication of weight tables in which the standards for older persons were the same as for those aged 30 (Gray, 1940). The reason was that insurance records and other long-term studies had shown that persons whose weight after age 30 rises above those standards have, on the average, higher disease incidence and lower life expectancy than persons whose weight does not rise (Reed and Love; Dublin and Marks).

Difficulties in Obtaining Criteria

The difficulties in obtaining such criteria can be seen if we consider blood pressures, ignoring for the purposes of this discussion the results of various surveys that have actually been made. A cross-sectional survey entails all the risks of error discussed in Chapter VII and elsewhere. Three in particular may be noted here:

1. The difficulty of getting large comparable groups at different ages. Young and middle-aged people of all economic classes are fairly easy

to obtain. For old people the survey might be largely restricted to those in institutions.

2. The prevalence-incidence fallacy (Q V – 8). Let us suppose that the average blood pressure were found to be the same at all ages. This might be due to actual stability or to a higher mortality of those whose pressures went up (or down). If the observed average were higher in the older groups, this might not indicate a rise in individuals, but merely the absence, from the older groups surveyed, of those with low pressures.

3. The difficulty of interpreting an association, if found, between high pressure and disease. Such an association would not indicate that high pressure would foretell disease.

It is difficult to believe that any contributors to a journal of gerontology would be unaware of these difficulties; and yet some of them write as if age *differences,* found in a cross-sectional survey, were synonymous with age *changes.*

A longitudinal study is clearly preferable to a cross-sectional one, but it has its own difficulties, such as the biased loss of subjects, differences in techniques of different observers at different periods, and the unwillingness of bright research workers to continue, year after year, collecting information in the hope that they or their successors 20 or 30 years later will be able to draw some conclusions from them. The best solution of the problem seems to be a combination of cross-sectional studies with short-term longitudinal studies, i.e., studies that begin simultaneously on different groups and are conducted, by the same observers, for a limited period, perhaps 5 years at most. Overlap is often desirable; e.g., one group might be studied from age 20 to 25, another from age 24 to 29, and so on.

Intersubject Variation

However far we progress in the selection of criteria of "health," there will still remain variation among the subjects chosen as healthy or "standard," and we will have to set arbitrary limits within the standard group. The problem is statistical, and we run risks of Type I and Type II errors. If, in a "standard" group of women of a certain stature, we place a cut-off point so as to exclude the 10 per cent that have the lowest weights, that will lead us to "view with suspicion" the weight of a woman patient of that stature if it falls below the cut-off point. We may call her "underweight" when in fact her weight may not be associated with disease, either present or future. In other words, so far as weight is concerned, she may really belong to the population of "standard" women — her weight may be the proper weight for her. If so, our verdict of "underweight," implying a suspicion that she belongs to a population whose weights are low through association with present or future disease, is the same as a verdict of "significance" when there is in fact no real difference. If we were, unknown to ourselves, examining the weights of the standard women, we would pronounce 10 per cent of them "underweight"; therefore that is our risk of a Type I error at that end of the distribution of weights.

In the assessment of weight it matters little if we classify too many persons, for the time being, as "underweight," because that constitutes only a small part of our evaluation of a patient. But in many circumstances a misclassification is not so innocuous. For instance, if an ophthalmologist classifies a person's intra-ocular pressure as "abnormally high," even if he finds nothing wrong with the field of vision he will consider his verdict as pointing toward glaucoma. Therefore he ought to act, by prescription and by continued follow-up. Too many Type I errors would thus load him with unnecessary work and, what is much worse, they would needlessly alarm many people who would know, or would discover, that glaucoma often leads to blindness.

If, on the other hand, the ophthalmologist commits a Type II error, i.e., disregards an intra-ocular pressure because it is within the accepted "normal" range when it is in fact a precursor of glaucoma, the result can be disastrous. Unfortunately, the Type II error, here as in many other statistical judgments, is an important concept rather than a useful tool. We know very little about "norms of disease" — the frequency distributions of measurements (typified in our discussion by weight) in the various diseases. That is, we do not know what proportion of the measurements of a certain variable in various diseases actually overlap into the region that we accept as within the standard range. In other words, we can seldom affix a numerical value to our risk of a Type II error.

"Individual Norms"

In the foregoing discussion there slipped in a phrase: "the proper weight for her." That introduces an important concept. In assessing an individual we have commonly to use, as a first step, the characteristics of a group; but as soon as possible we try to assess an individual by himself. A particular value of a certain variable may be "abnormal" for the group but "normal" for the individual, or vice versa. We may be able to discover this by reference to past information, but usually we have to depend on repeated examination of the individual.

We ought to remember this possibility also in assessing change in an individual. For example, basal metabolic rates are expressed in percentages, and the range of intersubject variation for healthy persons has been given as -12 to $+12$ per cent. Let us suppose that a certain man has a BMR of -7 on one occasion and $+8$ a month later. Both readings are within the standard range. Are we to conclude that the change indicates nothing of any consequence? If a certain man, who had no deformity or injury, was reported to have a stature of $5'7''$ on one occasion and $5'10''$ a month (or even many years) later, we would infer that either an error in reading (or recording) had occurred or that something biologically very strange had happened. This, of course, indicates what variation we need to know in assessing change — not intersubject variation of absolute readings but intersubject variation in the difference between readings made on the same subjects on different occasions.

Standards in Qualitative Data

When any anatomic pattern, such as the scheme of branches of the femoral artery or the roots of origin of the splanchnic nerves, is examined in several hundred cadavers, great intersubject variation is discovered. Some of the patterns are fairly common, although the commonest (which may be the one that anatomists teach as *the* pattern) may occur in much less than 50 per cent of the cadavers. Some patterns, on the other hand, are very rare. This kind of variation occurs with anything, structural or functional, whose components (or multiple causal factors) can vary more or less independently of each other, e.g., nerve plexuses, lungs, and behavior patterns. Expression by measurement is usually very difficult; therefore qualitative classification is used.

If a rare structure or function impairs fitness for survival, its classification as "abnormal" is easy. But many rarities show no evidence of effect on survival. Classification of "abnormalities" (or the less strong term "anomalies") may then be desired on a basis of frequency. If so, it should be systematic. We should arrange the classes in order of frequency (a single-tailed distribution) and label the end of the tail containing 5 per cent (or some other stated fraction) of the total as "abnormal" or "anomalous."

Such precise numerical labeling is, however, seldom very useful. In research the actual frequencies in the various classes must be considered. For clinical purposes, high precision of relative frequencies is unnecessary, because in a difficult diagnosis even rare possibilities must be considered, and a competent surgeon will be aware of all anatomic possibilities that may affect the success of an operation.

Table 5. Frequency Distribution of Statures of 1000 Dalhousie University Male Students

(These figures are for illustration only, not for anthropometric purposes.)

Stature ft. in.	Frequency (No. of Students)	Stature ft. in.	Frequency (No. of Students)
5 0	0	5 10	150
5 1	3	5 11	99
5 2	1	6 0	84
5 3	9	6 1	40
5 4	30	6 2	13
5 5	44	6 3	4
5 6	84	6 4	3
5 7	111	6 5	1
5 8	171	6 6	0
5 9	153		
		Total	1000

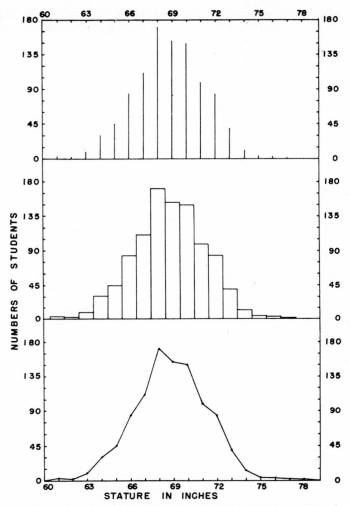

Figure 3.   Frequency distribution of statures in Table 5. Upper: line diagram.
Middle: histogram. Lower: polygon.

Frequency Distributions of Measurements

Table 5 was derived from the records made at a university health
service during the annual examination of students, and the data are
used here only for demonstration purposes. For ease in computation the
number was limited to 1000.

Grouped Frequency Classes. If the data were to be used for the
setting up of stature standards or for the calculation of averages or other
quantities, the original measurements would be used. However, when
certain of the measurements in a series are represented by few individuals there are often irregularities (ups and downs) which disappear

if more individuals are collected. With any particular series, in order to obtain a clearer picture, without being overimpressed by irregularities that may well be fortuitous, we customarily group adjacent measurements. Many of the measurements in this series were expressed to the nearest quarter-inch, but in Table 5 inch-classes were used. Each stature in the table represents the midvalue of a class, e.g., 5'5" indicates all measurements between 5'4.5" and 5'5.5". The *class width* or *interval* is 1", and so, necessarily, is the distance from one midvalue to the next. If the widths were not uniform the picture would be distorted.

For the mere demonstration of the shape of the distribution the number of classes depends on the sample size; it may be 10 or less. If calculations are to be made on the grouped data the grouping should not be too coarse. Many statistical textbooks contain instructions for such calculation, which lightens the arithmetical burden; but nowadays when adding machines and calculating machines are common, there is less need for such devices than formerly. The figures can be put into the machine without grouping.

In constructing Table 5, when a measurement fell exactly on a boundary, e.g., 5'5.5", half a unit was contributed to each of the adjacent classes. (For simplicity, a few such fractions were eliminated, but this did not essentially change the picture.)

Graphic Representation.   As shown in Figure 3, such a frequency distribution can be represented by a graph containing vertical lines or bars, or by vertical rectangles — *a histogram.* (The Greek *histos* means "web" or "tissue" as in "histology"; and the name "histogram" is suggested by the appearance of the group of rectangles.) These two forms of graph can be used also for distributions such as the binominal, which are discontinuous (discrete). For many types of measurement data, however, a third type of graph is often used, the *frequency polygon,* shown in the lower part of Figure 3. This is based on the conception of measurement distributions as continuous. We visualize finer and finer measurement scales being used and the occurrence of individuals at each point, on even the finest scale, with the result that the dots on a frequency graph would have narrower and narrower intervals between them. All actual measurement distributions are, of course, discontinuous, but it is commonly found that if a polygon is drawn from relatively coarse-scaled measurements (e.g., inches of stature) it does not differ greatly from a polygon drawn from the same measurements recorded on a finer scale (quarter-inches).

Shapes of Distributions

The distribution in Figure 3 is almost symmetrical and in other respects, also, it is not unlike a Gaussian curve produced mathematically or graphically from a frequency distribution of large binomial samples, as described in Chapter XI. In fact, frequency distributions of statures of adults of the same sex and of fairly similar racial origin are among the nearest approaches among biologic material to the Gaussian distribution. Most biologic and other real distributions are narrower or flatter than the Gaussian, and most of them are nonsymmetrical, i.e., *skewed,* with a longer tail at one end than the other. If the longer tail is in the region of the higher values of the variable the skewness is called *positive*; if the longer tail is in the region of the lower values the distribution is *negatively* skewed. All such distributions, however, if they have only one peak but two tails, can be described as "bell-shaped."

Causes of Bell-shaped Distributions

We can think of various reasons why a frequency distribution of statures should be bell-shaped. We recall the way in which a distribution of that shape is quickly created by random sampling from a binomial population of disks, the reason being that the differences in the composition of the samples are due to a number of *independent factors,* the motions imparted by our fingers to each individual disk. Stature is built up of segments — head, neck, trunk, thigh, leg and foot — all partly independent of each other in size.

Even if all segments are affected together in the direction of largeness (or smallness), so that a group of persons is, on the average, tall (or short), the factors (genetic, endocrine and dietary) that affect all the segments in a particular individual are nevertheless partly independent of each other. Some of these factors tend to tallness, others to shortness.

To express the effect in a simplified form, it is as if many people receive about equal numbers of tallness and shortness factors; some receive more tallness factors, a few receive many, and so on, thus producing the right-hand side of the frequency distribution. A similar disproportion of shortness factors produces the left-hand side of the distribution. *To some extent,* therefore, each person is like a sample in a binomial distribution.

There is, however, a still simpler and more general phenomenon that can create a bell-shaped distribution. Let us suppose that for an individual measurement, of any kind, to be large in comparison with others, two "plus" factors must contribute to it, that for a measurement to be small two "minus" factors must contribute, and that the combination "plus minus" results in a medium-sized measurement. Then let us suppose that at the beginning there are equal numbers of pluses and minuses, and that there is completely random combination. The result, as in tossing two coins, will be: ++, 25 per cent; +—, 50 per cent; ——, 25 per cent. This is the embryonic beginning of a bell-shaped curve.

It appears that the inheritance of bodily dimensions and other biologic measurements follows this kind of pattern, although with many complications. Certainly it is a basic pattern in observational variation. Let us suppose that at each step in a series of readings (of burets, pipets, syringes, and so on) we tend to err sometimes on the plus side and sometimes on the minus side, and that the direction (plus or minus) of the error at any one step is independent of the direction at the preceding or succeeding steps. Each experiment of the same type produces a final reading which is the end-product of a series of such steps. Then, under the conditions described, a few final readings will be high, others will be low, many will be in between, and the commonest will be those in which the pluses and minuses have been fairly evenly balanced. Even three steps of such a process would produce the following distribution: $1(++++)$, $4(+++-)$, $6(++--)$, $4(+---)$, $1(----)$.

By continuing to play with plus and minus errors in this way, we could approach as near as we wished to a Gaussian curve; but we must beware of falling into the same trap as did the mathematicians who proposed the Gaussian curve as the exact frequency distribution of variable (random) errors in physical measurements. The factors that actually produce observational variation do not behave in this simple fashion. They often produce a bell-shaped distribution, but "bell-shaped" is not synonymous with Gaussian.

In this connection we may recall the remark that has been attributed, in various forms, to several different authors: "Everybody believes in the Gaussian law — the experimenters because they think that it can be proved by mathematics, the mathematicians because they think that it has been proved by observation." Apparently in all instances in which large bodies of data on observational variation have been tested against the Gaussian curve they have shown disagreement with it.

In Chapters XI and XII we have seen examples of the great value of the Gaussian curve, and more examples will be met later; but in every instance its value has had to be established empirically.

Averages and Individual Variation

If we wish to grasp the salient features of frequency distributions, especially bell-shaped ones, we can do so by noting two features:

1. The position of the center or central region, numerically expressed by an "average."
2. The amount of scatter, i.e., the variation among individuals.

The word "average" often refers to the arithmetic average (arithmetic mean). More broadly, it includes also the mode and the median.

The Mode

From its definition ("the most fashionable class") we see that the modal class in the stature distribution in Table 5 is 5'8". The mode in a symmetrical bell-shaped distribution is the same as the mean and the median. In skew distributions of measurements the longer tail, as it were, pulls out the mean, without altering the mode or median very much.

For most purposes the mode is not a very useful measure. Even in large samples its numerical value depends on the class values chosen in the grouping of the measurements.

Distributions with More than One Mode

Some frequency distributions have two modes and are called *bimodal*. Others have still more modes. Extra modes always suggest a mixing of two or more populations, but figures and graphs must not be taken at their face value. In many instances the smaller peaks are fortuitous occurrences and would be smoothed out by enlarging the sample. To test this possibility we can fit a smooth unimodal curve of some kind to the data, and find out whether the peaks and troughs depart more from the curve than could be adequately explained by random sampling variation; but we seldom know what curve would be appropriate, and the procedure is complicated. If any attention at all is to be paid to the irregularities a simpler method is usually sufficient.

First, we must look at the method of observation and of grouping the data. For example, when the heartbeats of a number of persons are counted for a quarter-minute and the frequency distribution shows beats per minute, there are inevitably peaks at multiples of four, e.g., at 64, 68, 72, and so on, with gaps between. The commonest cause of irregularity is the choice of classes that are too narrow. If the sample is large enough this can be corrected by broader grouping.

After eliminating such technical factors, if two or more modes remain we should examine the material investigated and see if there is any obvious reason for them, e.g., age differences or sex differences. Then we can divide the total series into groups according to the suspected variable and test for intergroup differences in the variable under study. However, if we throw suspicion on many different variables, one after another, we are likely to find, by chance alone, one that produces a "statistically significant" intergroup difference. This is a solitary finding which is only a hint for research on new material.

Investigators of human gastric hydrochloric acid did better than this (Vanzant, Alvarez, and others). In the fluid drawn from the stomachs of healthy subjects the concentration of the acid was determined, and frequency distributions were prepared, with acid concentration as X and numbers of subjects as Y. Each sex-age group provided a separate series and the majority of the distributions showed bimodality. In seeking for a cause, the investigators separated the records of persons with no free acid from the records of those with free and combined acid (i.e., united with mucin and protein). The resulting frequency distributions for total acid were all unimodal. The special feature here was that the hypothesis was tested not on one but on all the subgroups.

Finally, it should be noted that two or more populations may be mixed, and yet show only one mode in the resulting (combined) frequency distribution. This was demonstrated, for example, by combining fictitious stature data of 1000 men (mean = 5'9") and of 500 women (mean = 5'4"), each group having the intersubject variation in stature that is commonly present. Even if 1000 men's statures were mixed with 1000 women's statures the resulting frequency distribution, although rather flat-topped, would not be bimodal. To produce bimodality, either the means would have to be farther apart or the intersubject variation would have to be smaller.

The Median

For any series of measurements arranged in ascending order of magnitude, the median (50 per cent point) is the value that would cut the series in two parts, with 50 per cent of the measurements below it and

50 per cent above it. If the number of measurements is even, the median lies between the middle of two items, and to obtain a numerical value we define it as midway between them. If the number of measurements is odd, the actual middle item is taken as the median. We are, of course, generally implying that the actual cut-off point would lie within a certain range of the middle item. Thus, if the middle measurement were 3.7 units and measurements were made to the first decimal place, the cut-off point would lie between 3.65 and 3.75 units. Even so, the choice of the middle item seems a little strange, because although it cuts the series into two equal parts, each of them contains less than half the measurements.

A little thought may make the choice seem more rational. Let us suppose that the actual middle value in a series is 3.7 units. Whatever the total may be, the number of measurements up to and including 3.7 units comprises "at least" 50 per cent of the total, and so do the measurements counted from the other end down to and including 3.7 units. The larger the series the closer does the middle value approach to a 50 per cent cut-off point. Or again, if we consider our series of measurements a random sample of a population of such measurements, the observed middle value is an "unbiased" estimate of the population median. That is, if we took larger and larger samples the successive middle items would lead progressively toward the population median, although of course with random fluctuations on the way.

A Simple Method. A simple rule for finding the median, whether the number of items (N) is odd or even, is to calculate $(N + 1)/2$. For example, with 20 items arranged in ascending order, e.g., on index cards, the median is the value of the $21/2 = 10.5$th item (midway between the 10th and 11th). With 21 items it is taken as the value of the 11th item.

The Problem of Identical Measurements. If the middle item and several around it have the same value, we may take that value as the median, but often a more precise estimate is desirable. We can illustrate the method of finding it by use of the coarsely grouped items in the stature distribution. The median in Table 5 obviously lies in the 5'9" class, i.e., between 5'8.5" and 5'9.5", because somewhere in that class we would meet the 500th and 501st students. The numbers of students from the shortest up to and including those in the 5'8" class (the "cumulative sum") is 453. To make up 500 we require 47 from the 5'9" class. We then visualize the measurements of the 153 students in that class as spread evenly over its one-inch width, each occupying the center of a space $1/153$ inch in width. The boundary between the 47th and 48th students would be $47/153 = 0.31$ inch above 5'8.5", and the median can be taken as 5'8.81". This is an arbitrary procedure but it is found to give estimates that are close to those obtained from the same original measurements when they are less coarsely grouped.

Value of the Median

The median has not been found as useful as the arithmetic mean in the methods of analysis that have been developed for the comparison of samples of measurements; but it has much to recommend it as an easily found and understandable indicator of the numerical center of any series of measurements, *whatever the shape of the frequency distribution.* Where distributions are very skew it is specially valuable. Many economic data are of this kind. Thus, in deciding whether the cost of living is high we compare it with incomes. In a certain city it may not be exorbitant to a person with "average" income in the sense of "mean" income. It may, nevertheless, be very high for more than 50 per cent of the people, because the mean is raised by a few very large incomes. The cost of medical care in a community should likewise be compared, not with mean income, but with median income.

The Mean

The word "mean," by itself, stands for "arithmetic mean," i.e., the sum of a series of measurements divided by the total number of measurements. The other means, geometric and harmonic, do not require discussion here.

A Critical Look at the Mean. We are so used to taking the mean of a set of readings that we seldom ask ourselves why we do so, or what it tells us, or whether it is, in a particular instance, useless or misleading. The mean is very extensively employed in the comparison of samples of measurements, and in Chapter XIV we will consider it in that connection. Here we are looking at it as the expression of the central region of frequency distributions.

Whatever the form of the distribution of measurements, the mean lies between the extremes, but very seldom midway between them. It is true that it has two rather neat relationships with its component measurements:

1. Most obviously, when the deviations of all the measurements from their mean are added, with plus and minus signs included, the sum of the deviations must be zero.

2. The sum of the squares of the deviations from the mean is less than the sum of squares of deviations from any other quantity.

The second property has been very helpful in developing a great many statistical maneuvers, some of which are useful to investigators; but neither of these properties appears specially valuable in discovering or presenting information about standard body weights or the time required to clear diphtheria bacilli from the throats of carriers or, for that matter, any of the examples of measurement data given at the beginning of this chapter.

The mean is not necessarily a more typical value than any of the individual measurements; nor does it necessarily indicate what we are most likely to meet if we continue measuring. If we make a graph of the ages at which people die, with age on the X-axis and frequency on the Y-axis, we find a U-shaped or J-shaped distribution. Starting fairly high with children under one year, it descends in early childhood, runs fairly horizontally for a decade or so, then ascends from adolescence to old age.

The mean age at death is therefore far different from the ages at which deaths most commonly occur, i.e., early childhood and old age.

This is a fairly obvious example of a misleading mean, which would not deceive anyone who thought about his data; but when we calculate the means of bell-shaped distributions or of samples therefrom, we appear to have authoritative precedent and logic on our side. The mere fact that the mean makes use of all the actual measurements, instead of merely counting them and picking the middle one, makes it seem so much more informative than the median.

Again, in bell-shaped distributions like those of statures and weights, which are often used for teaching purposes, the mean gives, more or less, an indication of the value of the median and of the mode. For the stature distribution in Table 5, the mean is 5'8.82", and the estimated median, as we have seen, was 5'8.81". The mode is in the 5'7.5" to 5'8.5" class, but more precise estimation would place it very near the mean.

A stature distribution provides a pleasing example of something in real life that closely resembles a Gaussian curve — pleasing to teachers of elementary statistics and pleasing to those who, in the history of statistics, applied the "Gaussian curve of error in physical measurements" to biologic variation. This is one reason why the habit of calculating the mean has spread to other bell-shaped distributions, for it is very important in a Gaussian curve.

The Mean in a Gaussian Curve.   It is not very difficult to visualize the enthronement of the mean in the field of physical measurements if we recall the problem that faced physical scientists in the 18th and 19th centuries. Improvement in the manufacture of instruments prompted astronomers and others to strive for very accurate measurements; but however good their instruments, they could never reach the "true" value because of observational error.

They wished to find the "best" estimates of the "true" values. The line of thought of the mathematicians who tried to help them can apparently be summarized by an imaginary soliloquy as follows:

"The variable errors of observation produce a Gaussian frequency distribution. The 'true' value of the measurement is at the center of the distribution, or is separated from it by a systematic error which can be determined. The central value in a Gaussian distribution is equally the mode, the median and the mean; but in estimating the central value from a sample of measurements the most 'efficient' of the three is the mean of the sample."

"Greater efficiency" in this context has the usual meaning of greater output for given input. In this instance it means closer approximation to the center of the Gaussian distribution from samples of a particular size (N). Let us suppose that we inscribed on disks the measurements from a truly Gaussian distribution (obtained from mathematical tables), then took random samples of size N, and found the mode, median and mean of each sample. By increasing N we could come as close as we wished to the center of the Gaussian distribution, whichever of the three estimates we used.

We would find, however, that for any particular value of N, the sample medians would vary more — would be more erratic — than the means from the same samples. That is, if we wished to come within a certain specified distance of the center of the distribution we would have to increase N much more if we used the medians than if we used the means. For example, if the mean of a sample of 1000 would bring us close enough to the center for our purposes, we would require a sample of more than 1500 to bring us as close to it by the use of the median. The sample mode is likewise an inefficient estimate, and in small samples it is of course difficult or impossible to determine it.

Returning now to the mathematician's imaginary soliloquy, we note that its basic assumption or belief, the Gaussian distribution of variable errors, does not really hold true, even in physical measurements. In biology and medicine intersubject variations do not form strictly Gaussian distributions; and therefore, except in some instances in which extensive data have been studied, we do not know how far apart the mode, median and mean may lie. We would like to form an estimate of the center (median) of the parent population of our sample, and perhaps of the mode as well. The sample mean may lead us very efficiently toward the population mean, but that is not where we want to go. Even if we knew the mean very exactly, it would not tell us the position of the median or mode. Whatever other uses the mean may have, clearly the most reliable guide to a population median is the sample median.

Limitations of Averages

However mentally satisfying averages, especially medians and modes, may be, they often fail to give us the information for which we collected the data, namely, the extent of variation between individuals. In fact, averages can mislead us greatly. I have seen a statement, made by a medical worker who was acquainted with statistical techniques, that the mean stature of a population was the "true" stature of that population. This was obviously a carry-over of the physical scientists' concept of a "true" value at the center of a crowd of erroneous readings. The mean of the students' statures in Table 5 was 5′8.82″, but it is extremely unlikely that a single one of the thousand students would have been found to possess that stature even if they could have been measured with that degree of precision. Even the modal class, 5′8″, contained only 17.1 per cent of the total students.

When we have a sample of measurements we may speak of the "true" mean measurement (or median, or mode) to indicate the mean (or median, or mode) in the parent population; but this does not imply that this value is in some way "true" of the members of the population. Nor does it imply that this value "ought to be true" of the individuals — that the average, or commonest, or typical, is in some way better than the extremes. We have already seen how a merely random interplay of plus and minus effects can produce a bell-shaped distribution.

Individual Variation

Cut-off points in the formation of clinical standards or "norms" have already been discussed in general. Here we look at a particular way of selecting these points. Later we will see that the same simple method can be used to express the differences among individuals in any series of measurements. Some workers still express the variation in a sample of measurements by stating only the observed maximum and minimum. This is obviously not satisfactory. If the sample is small we can nearly always be certain that a larger sample would contain measurements outside its range. If the observed sample is large, its extreme values will very likely be rare in its parent population. What we require is information regarding how often measurements lie, and can be expected to lie, beyond certain values.

The following example is from a table of measurements of boys and girls at half-yearly intervals, from age 5 to age 18 — weight, height, hip width, chest circumference and leg girth. The basic data were collected, during the years 1930–1945, from Iowa City children of northwest European ancestry, at the University of Iowa experimental schools (Stuart and Meredith):

	From 235 Boys Aged 5 Years				
Percentile	10	25	50	75	90
Weight (pounds)	36.6	39.6	42.8	46.5	49.7
Height (cm.)	105.3	108.3	111.3	114.2	116.7
	From 210 Girls Aged 5 Years				
Percentile	10	25	50	75	90
Weight (pounds)	36.1	38.6	41.4	44.2	48.2
Height (cm.)	105.0	107.2	109.7	112.9	115.4

Before we discuss the "percentile" method it is desirable to mention three points to be remembered by anyone who applies any such standards, whether they are expressed in percentiles or some other form:

1. Use exactly the same methods of measurement as were used in establishing the standard.

2. Expect regional and racial differences. Stuart and Meredith recommended users of their tables to look for systematic differences from the Iowa norms, and then establish their own.

3. Recall that estimates from small samples may differ considerably from the parent population values. We will later apply the methods of Chapter XI to some of the figures just given.

The report that contained the above table appeared somewhat apologetic for using percentiles instead of standard deviations. We will see later that no apology was necessary.

Percentiles

If a set of measurements of a variable (X) is arranged in ascending order of magnitude, the 10th percentile (10 per cent point) is defined as the value of X that separates the lowest 10 per cent of the measurements from the other 90 per cent. The other percentiles, such as the 25th and 90th (the upper 10th) percentiles, are defined in a similar fashion.

This percentage expression has nothing to do with a percentage of the variable X itself. For instance, with reference to human weights the percentile expression should not be confused with another method that is still in use, the "percentage of average weight." By that system, if the standard table showed a median of 40 pounds a child weighing 36 pounds would be called "10 per cent underweight." That is obviously an undesirable system. We ought to be concerned, not with how a child's weight compares, in pounds or percentages, with the median, but with the proportion of healthy children that are as far from the median as he is, or farther.

If the measurements number several hundreds, a point can be found that will divide the series almost exactly into a lower 10 per cent and an upper 90 per cent, but with smaller series some difficulties arise. If the number (N) is 20, a point between the second and third items cuts the series exactly; but if $N = 28$, say, a point between the second and third items would cut off less than 10 per cent below and leave more than 90 per cent above, while a point between the third and fourth items would throw the weight in the other direction. However, what we usually wish to find is not an exact cut-off point in a sample but an estimate of the cut-off point in the parent population. The rule for this estimation is simple.

Estimation of Population Percentiles

We have seen that to estimate the median (the 50th percentile) we write $(N + 1)/2$, or 50 per cent of $(N + 1)$. Similarly, to estimate the 10th percentile we write 10 per cent of $(N + 1)$ or $(N + 1)/10$; for the 25th percentile, we write $(N + 1)/4$.

Let us suppose that the lowest three of 20 readings (ranks 1, 2 and 3) of X are 2, 7 and 10 units. $(N + 1)/10 = 2.1$, i.e., the estimated 10th percentile has a rank of 2.1. It lies 0.1 of the distance from the second to the third readings, i.e., 7 units plus 0.1 of 3 units = 7.3 units.

We can reach the same point by numbering the readings from the other end, and estimating the 90th percentile from that end: 90 per cent of $(N + 1) = 18.9$. In the new numbering, the original third and second items are now the 18th and 19th items respectively. Therefore the cut-off point is at 0.9 of the interval (3 units) between 10 and 7 units, i.e., at $10 - 2.7 = 7.3$ units as before.

If the lowest three measurements in a series were the same as before (2, 7 and 10 units), but the set contained 28 measurements, the estimated 10th percentile would have rank $(28 + 1)/10 = 2.9$. That is, the cut-off point would be at 7 units + 0.9 of 3 units = 9.7 units.

The kind of thinking that underlies this simple rule is as follows:

1. Whatever may be the shape of the parent distribution (bell-shaped, multimodal, J-shaped, or other), and whether it is continuous or discrete, we can, except in peculiar circumstances, be certain that the population would contain measurements lying in the gaps that exist in our sample.

2. It is very likely, also, that measurements outside the sample range would be found in the population, except in special cases, e.g., when an instrument cannot register above the highest value found in the sample.

3. The relative position of the measurements in a sample is a guide to their relative positions in the population. In terms of the samples just shown (N = 20 and N = 28), the first contained only 18 measurements greater than 7 units, whereas the second contained 26 such measurements. Therefore it is likely that the true (population) 10th percentile in the second case would be farther along in the interval between 7 and 10 units than in the first case.

Applying these concepts, we visualize the 19 intervals between the measurements in a sample of 20, with measurements in the population that would be spread evenly in each interval. In addition, we visualize a rank of zero below rank 1, and a rank of 21 above rank 20. There are then 21 intervals, and we take the first 10 per cent of them to give us the estimate of the 10th percentile.

What we would like, of course, is a method that would give us an "unbiased" estimate of population percentiles. That is, we would like to be assured that if we could take more and more random samples from the population, and could estimate from each of them a particular percentile, say the 10th, the average of all our estimates would lead us closer and closer to the population 10th percentile as we continued. With many kinds of measurements the method described above meets this requirement, because the population frequency distribution is almost continuous and is smooth; i.e., the intervals between adjacent measurements are very small compared with the total range, and the differences in frequency among neighboring values of the variable are small compared with the total frequency. Many measurements in healthy subjects (e.g., statures, weights, blood pressures) have these characteristics.

Even with such populations, however, the smaller the sample the less confident we can be that our method of interpolation will give us an unbiased estimate, because in small samples the intervals between the observed measurements are often wide and we do not know how evenly the missing measurements would be spread in the intervals.

We are in still greater uncertainty when we have a small sample and know little about the irregularity of measurements in the parent population. For all we know, there might be gaps where no measurements would ever be found. In such cases there is no method that guarantees an unbiased estimate, but when we use our simple method we know that it will generally be more likely to give us an estimate that is near the desired population percentile than if we used any of the actual measurements in the sample, or if we arbitrarily took, say, the midpoint between two observed measurements that would enclose the desired percentile.

The Problem of Tied Ranks. In large samples, even if the measurements are made with high precision, many individuals often have the same value, and therefore should have the same rank. In estimating percentiles in such cases it is customary to proceed as we did in estimating the median stature from the data in Table 5 (p. 253). In estimating the 10th percentile from that table we note that up to and including the class 5'5" (5'4.5" to 5'5.5") are 87 students. Therefore, to make up 100 we require 13 from the next class, which contains 84 students. Since 13/84 = 0.15, we take this fraction of the distance (1 inch) above the lower boundary of the class, and give the 10th percentile as 5'5.65".

Tied ranks occur also in smaller samples. Let us suppose that 20 measurements are:

X (units)	2	7	10	12	13	14	15	16	18	Total
Frequency	1	2	1	2	4	1	3	4	2	20

The very fact that there are multiples in the outlying parts of the sample suggests irregularities in the parent population, and with such a small sample even elaborate methods would give only a crude estimate of population percentiles.

In reporting such data, and even data from much larger samples, the best thing is to present the figures themselves, and then point out the limitations of the percentile estimates that could be made from them.

Errors in Estimated Percentiles

We have seen that a percentile estimated from a small sample may contain an unknown degree of bias (systematic error); but even if the sample is fairly large (one hundred or more individuals) and even if the parent population is, for practical purposes, continuous and smooth, we must think about sampling errors. As always, in order to form any kind of estimate of the sampling error, we have to step into the world of random sampling. The 10th percentile for body weight, estimated from 235 boys aged 5 years was 36.6 pounds. We might ask: "If this were a random sample of an indefinitely large population of 'standard' boys aged 5 years, how far might 36.6 pounds lie above or below the population 10th percentile?" This, however, is not exactly the information that we would like to have in evaluating a boy's weight. Rather, we should ask: "If we always used 36.6 pounds as the 10th percentile, what proportion of boys in the standard population might we misclassify — that is, what proportion might we place on the wrong side of the population 10th percentile?"

We require estimates of population limits, and we can use a simple procedure based on the methods of Chapter XI. Let us imagine that the 235 boys constitute a random sample from a binomial population in which the X's are boys who weighed less than 36.6 pounds and the not-X's are boys who weighed more than 36.6 pounds. In a sample of this size almost exactly 10 per cent of the boys would therefore be X's. In Table II at X per cent = 10, we find the following figures for population percentages of X:

	Lower Limit	Upper Limit
N = 200	6.2	15
N = 300	6.8	14

For N = 235 we can say that the limits would be approximately 6.5 and 14.5 per cent X's. That is, by using 36.6 pounds as the cut-off value we might actually be using anything between the 6.5 percentile and the 14.5 percentile. Under random sampling conditions we would be "unlikely" (in the sense defined in Chapter XI) to be using percentiles below 6.5 or above 14.5.

Avoidance of Underestimation. In human weight assessment such a range of possible error is probably not serious; but in assessing other variables, for clinical or other purposes, we might wish to feel confident that we were not classifying too few individuals as below the 10th percentile. Even in assessing weights, we would remember that the samples which provided the standards were not strictly random — particularly that they might have included subjects who were not in optimum health. We might therefore wish to play safe, and set our standard higher than the sample indicated.

We could then ask a question of this type: "In the sample of 235 boys, where should we place a cut-off point to insure that, in a population randomly represented by the sample, we would be unlikely to exclude *fewer* than the lowest 10 per cent of weight measurements?" In Table II we look at N = 200 and N = 300, working up from X per cent = 10 until we come to X per cent = 15. We stop there because we find that the lower limit at N = 200 is 10 per cent X's. Hence, in a random sample of between 200 and 300 subjects, the sample 15th percentile would give us considerable assurance that by using it we would not exclude fewer than the lowest 10 per cent of subjects in the parent population.

Estimates from Small Samples. Samples of 200 to 300 are large compared with many of the samples from which clinical and laboratory norms are derived; and in most small-scale medical research in which we wish to measure and display individual variation, our samples are very small indeed. As an example, we can use the sample of 20 measurements which began as follows:

X (units)	2	7	10	12
Frequency	1	2	1	2

The estimated 5th percentile would lie between 2 units and 7 units. If we call any measurement that lies below that point "X" we have one X in a sample of 20. Table I shows that the population limits are 0.13 per cent and 25 per cent X's.

Regarding the 10th percentile, all that we can say, without making questionable assumptions, is that it appears to lie in the neighborhood of 7 units. If we call measurements of 7 units and less "X," we have 3 X's in a sample of 20 (15 per cent X's); but the population limits (Table I) are 3.2 per cent and 38 per cent X's.

For information on the reliability of sample percentiles from continuous distributions, and for a general discussion of the percentile method in determining clinical "norms," reference should be made to the paper by Herrera (1958).

To those who have developed the standard-deviation habit, the percentile method may appear inaccurate, unsophisticated and even retrogressive. Therefore, we must try to see how standard deviations came to supplant percentiles in the description and estimation of individual variation.

The Nature of Standard Deviations

Although the arithmetic mean has misled us considerably in medicine, the standard deviation has done much more damage. Its very name is misleading. I have seen medical speakers present human physiologic and biochemical measurements of various kinds in which they marked the interval from 1 SD below the mean to 1 SD above the mean as the "normal" range — as if this were a biologic standard, with implications of pathology outside it. More often it is ± 2 SD that receives this honor as a biomathematical discovery — obviously because this quantity is used as a criterion of "statistical significance."

It is well to remember that a "standard" is something "set up"; and, except in theological discussions, those who set up standards for human action are human beings. As we saw in Chapter XI, the standard deviation was set up as a yardstick for use with the Gaussian curve, and presently we will look at it there.

Calculation of Standard Deviations

We can calculate a standard deviation for any set of N measurements or other items expressed as numbers. They do not need to belong to any curve or to anything else in particular. If we let x represent each of the individual items, $\bar{x}$ their mean, and S "the sum of such quantities as," we can find the standard deviation by the formula:

$$SD = \sqrt{S(x - \bar{x})^2/N}$$

The answer comes out with the same units as the original x's. $S(x - x)^2$ is the sum of squares of deviations from the mean. If we are estimating a population SD from a sample, we replace N as divisor by $(N-1)$, because it has been found that division by N tends to underestimate the population SD.

Other Names for the Standard Deviation. The standard deviation has been called the "root-mean-square deviation from the mean," and it is a pity that this phrase is seldom used now by English-speaking workers.

It is almost self-explanatory, and it lacks the air of authority and permanence suggested by "standard" deviation. We can avoid a cumbersome phrase, and also the overtones of "deviation" (something erroneous or aberrant), by calling the mean of the sum of squares of differences simply the "variance." The standard deviation is then the square root of the variance. There is, however, much to be said for the use of "sigma" (σ) as a name for the standard deviation of a population of items, because it suggests what it is — part of a mathematical operation. (When "sigma" is used for the population SD, "s" (lower case) is often used to represent an estimate of sigma from a sample of the measurements.)

Gaussian Standard Deviations

We call the standard deviation an expression of the variation among measurements, but an expression is hardly of much use unless it expresses something more than the way in which it was manufactured — in this instance, the calculation of the root-mean-square deviation. It is all very well to say that the standard deviation gives us a single quantity, a kind of "average scatter," to save us the difficulty of trying to comprehend, and to handle, the scatter of individual measurements in a table or dot diagram. To be of any value in that connection, the expression must give to us, and to those with whom we are trying to communicate, a way of finding, or at least estimating, the actual individual scatter of the measurements.

In Chapter XI we saw that the standard deviation gives us exactly that ability in a Gaussian distribution. It enables us to find what proportions of items lie between, or beyond, any fractions or multiples of itself. The Gaussian curve is an artificial or abstract thing; but when the curve has been shown experimentally to be reliable with real data, the standard deviation functions usefully and safely. Chapter XI exemplifies this in relation to binomial data; and so does Chapter XII, though not explicitly, for the standard deviation (or more strictly the variance) is hidden in the chi-square test.

In its proper place, then, the standard deviation is valuable; but if we wish to find the average scatter (average deviation) of a series of measurements, why not merely find their deviations from the mean, drop the plus and minus signs, add them and divide by N? The result would be the "mean absolute deviation from the mean (MD)." This is very little used. Of course, most of us avoid it because we have been told to use SD; but the initial reasons for the preference were: (1) the greater "efficiency" and (2) the greater "tractability" of SD.

In an actual Gaussian curve, MD could be used as a yardstick, either directly or by conversion to SD, because the ratio SD/MD is 1.2533. But, just as in the case of median versus mean, the sample MD is an inefficient estimate of the population MD, as compared with the sample SD used as an estimate of the population SD. In samples, of course, the SD/MD ratio is seldom the same as in the population.

By the "tractability" of SD the mathematicians mean that it can be handled in various rather simple ways to produce short-cuts to useful information. Several examples of this are in Chapter XIV, but there are many other instances. Indeed, the standard deviation, or more exactly the variance, forms the basis of the most extensive developments of statistical techniques in biology during the last 40 years, called "the analysis of variance."

Standard Deviations in Medical Data

The efficiency and tractability of a mathematical device, used in an abstract relationship, are not in themselves sufficient to justify the use of the device in the real world. We have to test it by empirical methods. Let us suppose that we were working with some particular type of measurement, such as the concentration of blood sugar in persons under certain specified conditions, and that we wished to use the quantity, mean $\pm$ 1.2816 SD, to cut off 10 per cent of the measurements at each end of the frequency distribution, as it does in a Gaussian curve. We would have to try it on a large number of individuals (at least several hundred) under these conditions, in order to see whether the Gaussian approximation led us seriously astray, according to our standard of "seriousness."

Misuse of Standard Deviations

For each of the infinite variety of measurements that we meet in medicine, if we wished to use the Gaussian approximation, we would have to perform the test just outlined; and it has been performed for relatively few types of data. Nevertheless, the standard deviation is presented in reports as if it had a "Gaussian" meaning. It even appears, without comment, in cases in which Gaussian multiples are clearly not applicable. Thus, we may see: Mean duration of pus formation in an abscess = 13.8 days; SD of series = 12.0 days. Now, mean − 1 SD excludes about one sixth of the items at the lower end of a Gaussian distribution; so we begin to wonder whether in nearly one sixth of these patients the pus formation ceased *before* the abscess had formed!

Even in less extreme cases than this, when a bell-shaped distribution is positively skewed, a given multiple of SD will exclude a smaller percentage of items below the mean than above it. To compensate for this (to pull in the right-hand tail), the original measurements are often replaced by their logarithms, because log X does not increase as fast as X. The result is called a "log normal" (i.e., log Gaussian) distribution; but again only actual testing of large numbers can tell us whether it is sufficiently Gaussian to make the Gaussian SD a safe yardstick in estimating percentages of individuals at various distances from the mean.

Causes of Overconfidence in SD

The wholesale use of the standard deviation as a measure of individual variation, regardless of frequency distribution shape, seems to have arisen, at least partly, in the following way. The arithmetic means of samples of measurements are commonly compared by a method based on the Gaussian distribution. Although the justification for this practice is not as thorough as many research workers imagine, there is considerable evidence in its favor. In particular, it can be shown that, even if a frequency distribution of individual measurements is multimodal and skew, the frequency distribution of the arithmetic means of random samples from it is much more nearly Gaussian. Now in the process of comparing the means of two samples, we estimate the standard deviation of the individual measurements that compose the samples; but this is only a single step in the test. It does not imply that this estimate can be used with Gaussian multiples, as if the actual distribution of measurements were Gaussian; but it has apparently led people to believe that it does.

Another cause of faith in the standard deviation is probably the fact that it takes into account all the individual measurements in a sample, whereas a percentile subdivision merely counts the measurements above and below a certain value. This is an illusory gain unless we know the distribution shape of the sample's parent population.

Perhaps akin to this illusion is a belief that a standard deviation is much more accurate than the corresponding percentile estimate. We can compare the two only when we know the parent population. When we do so, the superiority of the standard deviation is often not very striking.

Let us suppose that we have a sample of 40 measurements and 4 of them (10 per cent) are below a certain value. If we wish to know the risk of using the sample 10th percentile, we can go to Table I and find the lower limit estimated for 4 X's with $N = 40$, namely 2.8 per cent. That is, the sample 10th percentile might lead us to exclude only about 3 per cent of the population. On the other hand, let us suppose that we knew that the sample came from a mathematically exact Gaussian distribution of measurements. We could use the mean minus 1.2816 SD as a cut-off point for the lowest 10 per cent; and then some calculation based on the Gaussian distribution would show that this sample estimate of the 10th percentile might well be about the population 6th percentile. This is better than the 2.8 percentile obtained by the percentile method without bringing in Gauss, but not extremely good.

Again, if we have a sample of 100 and use the sample 10th percentile, Table I shows that we may cut off anything from 5 per cent to nearly 18 per cent of the population. If we knew that the parent distribution was truly Gaussian and used 1.2816 as before, we might cut off anything from 7 to 13 per cent of the population. These figures are nearer to 10 per cent than those obtained by the other method, but hardly so close that we need lament our ignorance of the exact shapes of most of our frequency distributions of measurements.

Versatility of Percentile Method

The percentile method is a simple way of obtaining understandable information from any sample of measurements or counts; but even more important is the fact that, without making any assumptions regarding the shape of the parent population's frequency distribution, it is possible (e.g., by the use of Table I) to make allowance for sampling variation.

The diversity of application of the method can be illustrated by six types of data on which it has been used. In the first edition of this book two of these examples (Nos. 2 and 6) were used to illustrate the application of Gaussian-curve techniques, because the data form bell-shaped distributions that resemble the Gaussian distribution. This has been the customary method of treating such data, but I have come to feel that it depends too much on an individual investigator's interpretation of figures. We may say that a Gaussian-derived technique will not lead us "far astray," but how far is "far"? Although in certain instances we lose something in precision by refusing to accept a Gaussian assumption, we gain in confidence by being able to remove that assumption from our estimates.

1. Total and differential leukocyte counts. Percentile charts of these, similar to standard weight charts, can be used in assessment of individual patients.

Table 6. Numbers of Valves in Left Cephalic Veins of 59 Dalhousie University Cadavers, 1938 – 1947

(Students' records, checked by instructors.)

No. of Valves	No. of Cadavers	No. of Valves	No. of Cadavers	No. of Valves	No. of Cadavers
0	0	6	6	12	1
1	0	7	11	13	0
2	2	8	9	14	1
3	2	9	6	15	1
4	6	10	2	16	0
5	10	11	2		
				Total	59

2. Numbers of valves in the cephalic vein (Table 6). Here are data in which we cannot visualize the gaps between valve numbers being filled, however many subjects were examined; and we may refuse to accept the assumption that a vein in any subject might contain no valves at all. We can report, for instance, that 4 out of 59 cadavers (approximately 7 per cent) had 3 valves or less, and that the median number was 7 valves.

We might wish to know, however, what the median might be in a population randomly represented by this sample. This kind of question may arise with regard to any set of measurements or counts. We note that 20 of the 59 subjects had 5 valves or fewer, and that 26 had 6 valves or fewer. In Table I we can use $N = 60$ instead of 59, and we see that for 20 X's out of 60 the upper limit is 47 per cent X's; for 26 X's it is 57 per cent. Therefore this sample would be "rare" if 50 per cent of the population had 5 valves or fewer, but not if it had 6 valves or fewer. Next we note that 22 subjects had 8 valves or more, and the upper limit for 22 X's out of 60 is approximately 50 per cent. Therefore, adopting the 2.5 per cent error risk of Table I, we could say that the population median might be 6, 7 or 8 valves, but would be unlikely to be outside that range.

3. Duration of life after appearance of symptoms in tuberculous meningitis — data collected on 75 children during the period when this disease was fatal, i.e., before the discovery of an effective antibiotic. In a report on such data the complete frequency distribution should of course be given, but the salient features can be expressed by a statement such as the following: Days to death ranged from 1 (in one child) to 63 (in one child). The median was 17 days. Twenty-one children (28 per cent) were dead before the 12th day, and 58 (77 per cent) were dead by the 25th day. The median was much nearer the lower end than the upper end of the distribution, and this is a common feature in frequency distributions of the duration of disease, whether it ends in death or recovery. The distributions are positively skewed.

4. Clearance of diphtheria bacilli from the throats of carriers. Subjects were examined at 5-day intervals from the beginning of treatment and the data were presented in the following form:

Days	No. of Positives
5	457
10	297
15	229
. .	. . .
65+	27

As in many other collections of survey data, the purpose here was not merely to find out what happened under certain circumstances, but to compare this with what happened under other circumstances. In this instance the comparison was with another form of treatment designed to remove the bacteria. Such a past-and-present comparison may have some value if we remember that other things differ besides the things that we are looking at (here the treatments). The most suitable analytical technique is often a contingency table, but we must remember that no cell in such a table can contain individuals that are in any other cell. The present data would have to be rearranged in the form:

Days	No. Who Became Negative
5 – 10	160
10 – 15	68
etc.	etc.

5. Amount of change in symptoms and signs during a drug trial. Drug A may have been followed by improvement in a higher proportion of cases than drug B, and the difference may be "statistically significant." That information may be useful, but probably more useful is an answer

to the question: "How much improvement and in what proportion of patients on each drug?" To answer this question we first arrange the cases in order of change from the extreme negative change (greatest deterioration, e.g., greatest increase in erythrocyte sedimentation rate) to the extreme positive change (greatest improvement). Then we divide by selected percentiles, e.g., 5th, 10th, 25th and so on. In a summary report of a trial in rheumatoid arthritis (Mainland and Sutcliffe, 1962), the form adopted was the median and the 90 per cent range (5th to 95th percentile). These were shown for the following measures of change (posttreatment reading minus pretreatment reading): duration of morning stiffness, number of clinically active joints, grip strength, time required to walk 50 feet, and erythrocyte sedimentation rate.

6. The variable error in volumetric analysis. We usually estimate the variability of routine laboratory techniques by duplicate or triplicate analyses; but we should visualize each pair or trio as a tiny sample of a large population of such analyses conducted under the same conditions. To illustrate this concept and to discover the magnitude of the error in a particular case, urine that contained 2 to 3 gm. of glucose was diluted with distilled water (1 volume of urine to 9 volumes of water) and 5 liters of it, covered with toluol to prevent fermentation, were stored in a well corked bottle. On this solution a practiced observer made 100 determinations of glucose by Benedict's quantitative copper solution, 25 ml. for each determination. The readings showed no evidence of observer's fatigue or of changes in the urine from day to day. The frequency distribution of the estimates for the original undiluted urine were:

Gm. Glucose per 100 ml. Urine	Number of Estimations
2.300 – 2.319	2
2.320 – 2.339	6
2.340 – 2.359	17
2.360 – 2.379	23
2.380 – 2.399	21
2.400 – 2.419	12
2.420 – 2.439	10
2.440 – 2.459	3
2.460 – 2.479	2
2.480 – 2.499	2
2.500 – 2.519	1
2.520 – 2.539	0
2.540 – 2.559	1
	Total 100

The median is approximately 2.38 gm., and the mean from the ungrouped data was 2.387 gm. The standard deviation was 0.0422 gm. and therefore 2 SD, measured on each side of the mean, would exclude about 5 per cent of the values, but all of them would be at the upper end of the series. This is a reflection of the positive skewness of the distribution and a percentile expression would give a truer picture. (Incidentally, it should be noted that in routine work, unless we have at least three readings in each test we cannot tell whether the parent distribution is skew or symmetrical.)

These figures were obtained about 25 years ago in an effort to find out what really happened when a method commonly used in clinical chemistry was applied repeatedly to the same material. They seemed to provide a commentary on two statements that were made to me about that time. One was made by a physicist who informed me that the proper way to estimate laboratory error was by a mean-square method, which turned out to be based on the assumption of a Gaussian distribution. The other statement was obtained from a chemically oriented biochemist who said that in many analyses a maximum "allowable" error could be estimated — for example, by allowing for a mistake of one scale division in each buret reading and one drop in each titration. Contemplation of the glucose distribution will show that neither the physicist's nor the biochemist's theory was very realistic.

Error estimates from the above distribution could not, of course, be assumed reliable in routine work, even performed by the observer who made the hundred determinations. The distribution serves, however, to emphasize what we need to know, even if we have to depend on duplicate analyses. If we keep that picture in mind it may help when we are trying to elucidate statements that various laboratory workers make regarding their allowance for variable error.

For example, what, in terms of these data, might a laboratory worker mean if he said that he allowed for a 5 per cent (or a 2 per cent) error? Or if he took a series of readings (two or more replicates) and calculated a "mean error"? Or if he used, as a standard, the mean difference between duplicates? None of these standards or calculations will give him the information that he needs, unless it tells him how often differences of certain sizes between duplicates, or other replicates, can be expected to occur — the kind of information that the percentile method gives in a simple and direct fashion.

CHAPTER XIV

COMPARISONS BY MEASUREMENT

If we wish to compare the effects of treatments A and B by measurement rather than by enumeration, we can nevertheless assign the treatments in the same three ways. (1) We can apply each treatment to a different group of subjects without trying to match individuals. (2) We can use matched pairs of subjects. (3) In some types of experiments we can apply the two treatments at different times to the same individuals. The advantages and disadvantages of these methods have been discussed already. Here we look at the analysis of the resulting measurements. Designs (2) and (3) produce matched-pair data, and we will consider them first.

Data from Matched Pairs

An obstetrician wished to use a certain drug to strengthen uterine contractions in labor. Knowing that a drug that would cause contraction of nonstriated uterine muscle would probably affect arterial muscle also, he feared that it might be dangerous in women with cardiovascular weakness. He did not wish to subject to a possible risk any more women than were necessary. Therefore he injected the drug into 5 women and took diastolic blood pressure readings before and after injection.

	Blood Pressure (mm. mercury)		
Serial No. of Patient	Before Injection (B)	After Injection (A)	Difference (A-B)
1	98	102	+4
2	86	96	+10
3	88	100	+12
4	98	98	0
5	72	90	+18

This investigation was performed long ago, and would now be recognized as not being a proper experiment, in that there was no contrast (control) group of uninjected women. However, the figures are useful for demonstration purposes, because they are few in number and possess certain features of special interest. They could have been produced from an actual experiment on matched pairs, e.g., 5 pairs of litter mates in a comparison of treatments A and B, assigned within each pair by the toss of a coin or by odd and even random numbers. We could suppose that the readings (98, 102, and so on) were made from some baseline (perhaps zero), and the question would then be: "If in reality A and B did not differ in their effects, how often could we meet such an amount of evidence, pointing to an A-B difference, but produced solely by our randomization?"

The "amount of evidence" is the sum of the A-B differences: $4 + 10 + 12 + 0 + 18 = +44$. (Average $= +44/5 = +8.8$ mm. Hg.) The arithmetic average (mean) difference is inserted by reflex action, but it will soon be seen that it is quite unnecessary for an answer to our question.

The Direct Method of Analysis

We will continue to look at the data as if they came from an experiment in which A and B had been applied within pairs, such as litter mates, and as if the treatments did not really differ in their effects. Whichever treatment was applied, one member of the first pair would give a reading of 98 units and the other member a reading of 102 units. The randomization would have decided which of these two readings would be labeled "A" and which would be labeled "B" — that is, whether the A-B difference, 4 units, would be $+4$ or -4.

If we repeated the randomization many times, we would approach equal frequency of $+4$'s and -4's. The same would happen with the next difference, 10 units; and so, out of these two pairs the randomization would in the long run produce, in equal frequency, the following amounts of evidence regarding the A-B difference:

$$+4 +10 = +14$$
$$+4 -10 = -6$$
$$-4 +10 = +6$$
$$-4 -10 = -14$$

Incorporating the third difference, 12 units (equal numbers of $+12$'s and -12's), we obtain the following eight sums, in equal frequencies: $+26, +2, +6, -18, +18, -6, -2, -26$. Leaving the zero difference aside temporarily, we can incorporate the fifth difference, 18 units; and then we find the following sums in equal frequencies, except that zero has twice the frequency of the other values:

$$-44 \ -36 \ -24 \ -20 \ -16 \ -12 \ \ -8 \ \ \ \ 0$$
$$\ \ 0 \ \ +8 \ +12 \ +16 \ +20 \ +24 \ +36 \ +44$$

It will be noted that if there are N items in a sample the total number of possible sums is 2^N. Here, $2^4 = 16$.

Returning now to the zero difference (No. 4), we might dismiss it by saying that it adds nothing to our information regarding the difference between A and B; but it is probably better to visualize what would actually happen in the randomizations. In half of them, one of the 98's would be assigned treatment A and in half of them the other 98 would be assigned that treatment. There would then be two —44's, two —36's, and so on. The result would be 32 possible arrangements, with double the number in each class. Then $+44$ would comprise $2/32 = 1/16$ of the total, just as when the zero difference was disregarded.

We can now answer the question: "How rare would be the observed amount of evidence (a sum of 44) in favor of a difference between A and B?" We would meet sums of 44 (half of them plus and half of them minus) in 2 out of the 16 possible arrangements, i.e., 1/8 or 0.125 or 12.5 per cent. This is far greater than the usual 5 per cent maximum "rarity" (P not greater than 0.05).

Indeed, it would be impossible to reach the 5 per cent standard with a sample of 5 pairs. There are only $2^5 = 32$ possible arrangements; and the most extreme values, in which all the differences are of the same sign, comprise $2/32 = 1/16$ of the total.

With $N = 6$, the possible arrangements are 64. Therefore, when all 6 differences have the same sign their sum comprises $2/64 = 1/32$ of the total frequencies. That is, a sample of 6 pairs enables us to detect rarity on our 5 per cent standard. It does not, however, enable us to apply our 1 per cent standard (P less than 0.01). Nor does a sample of 7, because 2^7 shows that there are 128 possible arrangements, and the largest sum (one sample at each end of the distribution) comprises 1/64 of the total frequency. With 8 pairs, however, $2^8 = 256$, and therefore we can cut off at each end a tail containing one sample in which all differences have the same sign, and these samples together comprise $2/256 = 0.0078$ of the total frequency.

Matched Pairs in Surveys

In an experiment, in which we actually randomize treatments within pairs, the analysis springs directly from the randomization. In the production of the blood pressure data with which we started, however, there was no randomization, i.e., the data were equivalent to survey data.

In order to see what the matched-pair analysis can tell us after a survey, we have to visualize a somewhat different picture from that of an experiment. We visualize an indefinitely large population of women of the type that provides the sample of five, and subjected to the same conditions, including the injections. We imagine that on each woman an earlier and a later blood pressure reading was made, and that some showed differences of 4 mm., others of 10, 12, zero and 18 mm. We know nothing about the sizes of other differences and make no assumptions about them. Our "null hypothesis" is that nothing (e.g., the course of labor or injection of the drug) affected the population in such a way as to make the blood pressure rise rather than fall during the interval between the readings. Then if the reading differences were always expressed as A minus B, in half the women with a difference of

18 mm. it would be +18 and in half of them it would be —18. The same would be true regarding the other differences (12 mm., 10 mm. and 4 mm.). Therefore, if we obtained strictly random samples of 4 women containing these differences (or 5 women containing in addition one zero difference), we would obtain the same frequency distribution of possible arrangements as was described above — or, to be exact, we would approach that distribution by continued sampling.

The question to be answered regarding the obstetrician's sample of 5 women was: "Would this be a rare type of random sample from such a population?" We have seen that the sample was too small to answer that question according to the usual (5 per cent) standard of rarity. If it had been larger, and had qualified as "rare," questions regarding the interpretation of "significance" verdicts on survey data would have arisen — for example: "Was the injection or the process of labor responsible?" "Was the selection biased?" Such questions have been sufficiently discussed in earlier chapters.

A Shortcut — Signed-ranks Analysis

Without an army of clerks, or perhaps an electronic computer, we could not display all possible arrangements of positive and negative differences, except in very tiny samples. In a similar predicament during the analysis of fourfold contingency tables in Chapter XII, we turned to Fisher's "exact" test, which gives the frequencies of all possible random arrangements in two binomial samples. There is, however, no one formula that would fit the infinite variety of possible measurement data and we turn to a method which at first sight appears crude, but which, as will be seen, is remarkably accurate. It is the "signed-ranks" test devised by Wilcoxon, but employed here in a slightly different form from the one shown by its originator. Using the blood pressure differences, we proceed as follows:

1. Drop the zero difference because, just as in the analysis of the actual measurements, its inclusion has no effect on the result.

2. Arrange the measurements, regardless of sign, in ascending order of magnitude: +4, +10, +12, +18. If there were, say, a —5, it would lie between +4 and +10.

3. Number the measurements in order of rank:

Measurement	+4	+10	+12	+18
Rank	1	2	3	4

4. Give to each rank the plus or minus of the corresponding measurement; then add the ranks: +1 +2 +3 +4 = +10. (This is the "algebraic" sum, because minus signs, if present, would have a negative effect.)

For sample sizes up to N = 40 this completes the arithmetic, because we can find in Table VI whether our sum of ranks is "significant" or not (see Appendix). For samples larger than 40, a simple formula is available. However, before using Table VI or the formula we must show what "significance" in this connection means numerically, by a step-by-step exact test, which shows the frequencies of occurrence of sums of ranks as in a randomization experiment.

Exact (Randomization) Test of Sums of Signed Ranks
This test is exactly the same as for the measurements themselves — a display of all possible arrangements. For our sample of 4, we proceed as follows:

$$
\begin{aligned}
+1 \quad +2 \quad +3 \quad +4 &= +10 \\
+1 \quad +2 \quad +3 \quad -4 &= +\ 2 \\
+1 \quad +2 \quad -3 \quad +4 &= +\ 4 \\
+1 \quad +2 \quad -3 \quad -4 &= -\ 4 \\
\end{aligned}
$$

$$
-1 \quad -2 \quad -3 \quad -4 = -10
$$

We have then the following 16 arrangements:

Sum of ranks	−10	−8	−6	−4	−2	0	+2	+4	+6	+8	+10
Frequency	1	1	1	2	2	2	2	2	1	1	1

The sum of ranks in the observed (blood pressure) sample was $+10$, and is at the extreme end of the distribution. There is a corresponding sample (-10) at the other end, and together these comprise $1/8$ of the total samples, as was found when the measurements themselves were analyzed. Such exact equivalence does not always occur, but this does not seriously impair the usefulness of analysis by ranks.

Since the most extreme sums of ranks occur in more than 10 per cent of the samples produced by randomization, no figures for $N=4$ are shown in Table VI. Therefore we examine a larger, and more complex, example.

A More Complex Example of Signed Ranks
In a search for age differences in the knee joint interspace by body-section roentgenography of healthy men aged from 20 to 84 years, the vertical distance between the tibia and the lateral condyle of the femur was measured in both knees of 33 men, and corrected for magnification due to x-ray dispersion by reference to a special scale exposed alongside each knee. The following sample of right-left differences in 8 men was selected for the present demonstration in order to include both positive and negative signs and also two readings that are numerically identical. The R-minus-L differences (in mm.) were:

$$+1.8, \quad -0.4, \quad -0.7, \quad +0.2, \quad -1.1, \quad -1.7, \quad -0.2, \quad +0.1$$

Clearly there was no suggestion of a predominance of right or left side, but we can use the sample to illustrate the signed-ranks technique.

The easiest way to arrange the measurements in order of magnitude is to write each of them (with its sign) on an index card and then sort the cards without reference to signs. Having allotted rank 1 to the 0.1 mm. reading, we meet the two 0.2 mm. values — the problem of tied ranks. If another decimal figure were available we would probably find that one pair should receive rank 2 and the other rank 3. Not having this information, we give to each the average rank, 2.5. If there had been three 0.2 mm. readings, occupying ranks 2, 3 and 4, we would again have assigned to each the average rank, 3.

Except with the smallest samples, it is best to postpone the averaging of tied ranks until all ranks have been assigned, and we have checked to see that the highest rank is the same as the number in the sample (excluding zero differences, which do not contribute to N). (If the tied ranks have the same sign, plus or minus, the averaging is obviously unnecessary.)

In the summation of ranks it is useful to add the negatives and positives separately, because then we can check the arithmetic from our knowledge of what the total of all ranks, without signs, should be, namely: $1 + 2 + 3 + \ldots + 8 = 36$. This total is easily found for any number (N) of ranks by two steps:

1. Add the first and last rank and divide by 2 to find the average rank.
2. Multiply the average rank by the number of ranks.

$$\text{Thus, } N(1 + N)/2 = (8 \times 9)/2 = 36$$

In the present example the sums of ranks are as follows:

Negative sum $= -24.5$
Positive sum $= +11.5$
Total with sign $= -13$
Total without sign $=\ \ \ 36$

We could now take the signed-ranks sum to Table VI and find its "significance," but before doing so we will again show the results of an exact (randomization) test and thereby learn what the figures in Table VI really mean.

Exact (Randomization) Test of Eight Signed Ranks

The frequency distribution obtained by creating all possible sums of ranks 1 to 8, with equal numbers of plus and minus signs allotted to each rank was as follows (SR = Sum of ranks, F = Frequency):

SR	−36	−34	−32	−30	−28	−26	−24	−22	−20	−18	−16	−14	−12
F	1	1	1	2	2	3	4	5	6	7	8	9	10

SR	−10	−8	−6	−4	−2	0	+2	+4 . . .	+36	Total
F	11	12	13	13	13	14	13	13 . . .	1	256

The distribution was perfectly symmetrical; therefore in marking the cut-off points for either tail we can disregard signs.

The cumulative sum from the extreme end, up to and including SR = 30 is 5/256 = 1/51.2, which is less than 1/40 (2.5 per cent); but if we include SR = 28 we have 7/256 = 1/36.7, which is greater than 2.5 per cent. Therefore we mark the 2.5 per cent point in each tail between SR = 28 and SR = 30.

The 0.5 per cent point in each tail (to exclude not more than 1 per cent of the total distribution) must be placed so as to cut off only the single rarest sample, SR = 36, in which all signs are minus or all signs are plus.

The sum of signed ranks in our sample was −13; and such samples are far more central than the cut-off points. Our verdict on the sample would therefore be "Far from significant at the 5 per cent level." If, however, the sum of ranks in our sample had been −32 (or +32), the verdict would have been "Significant at the 5 per cent level." Translating this, we could say: "If, in an indefinitely large population of R-L differences, there were, for every positive difference (R greater than L), a negative difference of the same size, and if random algebraic sums of 8 differences were taken, it would be found that sums as large as in the observed sample were rather rare. If the differences were expressed as signed ranks, less than 5 per cent of the sums of ranks would be as large as in the observed sample — half of them positive and half of them negative."

Table VI — Sums of Signed Ranks

This table contains the salient information obtained from distributions of sums of ranks such as the one shown above. At N = 8, under P (both tails) = 0.05−, the sum of ranks is 30. This is the value next beyond the 2.5 per cent cut-off point in each tail (−30 in one tail, +30 in the other). Under P = 0.01−, the value 36 is the sum of ranks next beyond the 0.5 per cent cut-off point in each tail.

Preparation of Table VI. If we increase sample sizes by one individual (and therefore by one terminal rank) at a time, we can build up, step by step, the frequencies of all the various sums of signed ranks. Table VI was prepared in this way by M. I. Sutcliffe, in accordance with the patterns of the tabulated data in Tukey's Memorandum issued in 1949.*

For samples of N greater than 40, we obtain essentially the same information as in Table VI by using a method that will now be shown.

Gaussian Approximation in Signed-ranks Test

For N = 8 the random frequency distribution of sums of signed ranks looks like the beginning of a Gaussian distribution, and this prompts us to think that, as with many other distributions of samples produced by random processes, we might, for samples beyond a certain size, substitute Gaussian distributions for exact distributions and use a standard deviation to determine the cut-off points for "rare" samples in the tails.

The SD of the N = 8 distribution is fairly easily found by the formula

* I am indebted to my former colleague, Lee Herrera, for assistance with the mathematical methods used in these computations and in the construction of Table VIII.

shown in Chapter XI. For instance, −36 is not only the value of the most extreme sum of ranks but also its deviation from the mean of the distribution, which is zero; and since the distribution is symmetrical we need to find the sum of squares of the deviations for only one half, and then double it. We must, of course, take into account the frequencies, e.g., $(-30)^2 = 900$, but this must be multiplied by 2, because that is the number of items in that class.

The sum of squares of deviations = 52,224. As divisor we use the total number of samples, 256, not 256 − 1, because it is the complete population that we are studying, not a sample of it. Therefore SD = $\sqrt{52,224/256}$ = $\sqrt{204}$ = 14.28.

In a Gaussian distribution, mean ± 2 SD gives approximately the 2.5 per cent cut-off points. In this distribution of rank sums it is $0 \pm 2 \times 14.28$, i.e., −28.56 and +28.56. The cut-off points therefore lie between SR = 28 and SR = 30, just as was found by examining the distribution itself. Even when N is as low as 6, this relationship holds true.

As N increases we have to use 1.96 SD instead of 2 SD, but if we do so the Gaussian substitution gives a very satisfactory 5 per cent cut-off point. Thus, at N = 40 the value of 1.96 SD is 291.6; and Table VI shows that the minimal sum on the 5 per cent standard is 292.

As a cut-off point at the 1 per cent level (0.5 per cent in each tail) 2.576 SD is not entirely satisfactory. It usually demands a rank sum greater by 2 to 4 units than the actual distribution shows to be necessary. Thus at N = 40, the value 2.576 SD is 383.3, whereas Table VI shows that rank sums of 380 and greater constitute less than 1 per cent of the randomization distribution. However, this is not a serious fault. Although we are using nominally the 1 per cent standard, we are applying a slightly higher standard − we are slightly overestimating the randomization frequency of samples like those that we are testing.

For P = 0.10 (not more than 5 per cent in each tail) the Gaussian-curve cut-off point is found by ± 1.645 SD. It often does not take us quite far enough out from the center (zero) in the exact distributions represented in Table VI, but if we add 2 units to 1.65 SD we come very close to the 10 per cent cut-off points shown in the table.

Formula for SD of Sums of Signed Ranks

The similarity of the Gaussian curve to the exact distribution of rank sums would of course not be of practical value if we had to display an exact distribution before we could calculate its standard deviation. Fortunately, owing to the regularity of the series of ranks, 1, 2, 3, and so on, mathematicians have been able to produce a simple and exact formula for the standard deviation. Where N is the number of ranks the formula is:

$$SD = \sqrt{N(N + 1)(2N + 1)/6} \quad \text{(The figure 6 is a constant.)}$$

For example, if

$$N = 8, SD = \sqrt{(8 \times 9 \times 17)/6} = \sqrt{204} = 14.28,$$

exactly the same value as we already found by the step-by-step procedure.

This is the formula which, along with the Gaussian-curve multipliers (1.65, 2 and 2.58) enables us to go beyond Table VI. Even within the table, it enables us to show roughly how far from the 5 per cent standard our evidence lies. Our sample of 8 R-L knee joint interspace measurements gave a sum of ranks $= -13$. With $N = 8$, $SD = 14.28$. Then $13/14.28 = 0.91$, and the table of excerpts from the Gaussian distribution (Table VII) shows that P (both tails) lies between 0.3 and 0.4. That is, between 15 and 20 per cent of random allocations of signs to ranks 1 to 8 would produce negative rank sums as great as the observed sum (-13) and greater. The actual frequency distribution showed 19 per cent.

An Example for Practice. The sample of 8 knee joint interspace differences already used for illustration were selected from the following series of 33 such measurements (R–L in mm.):

+1.8	0.0	−1.7	+2.0
+1.6	+0.1	+0.5	−0.3
−0.4	−0.8	−0.9	+1.1
−0.7	0.0	−3.2	+0.3
+0.2	−3.9	+0.6	−1.2
−1.1	−0.8	+1.5	−2.6
−1.7	+0.8	−0.7	
+1.2	−0.3	−1.3	
+1.5	−1.3	−0.2	

Omitting the two zeros, we have a sample of 31 measurements, and in order to apply the exact (randomization) test we would have to display 2^{31} possible arrangements, i.e., over 2000 millions. Show that the sum of signed ranks is -101, which is far smaller than the minimal value (202) required by Table VI for a randomization frequency of less than 5 per cent. Show also that the SD of sums of ranks is 102.1, and that therefore Sum of ranks$/SD = 1$ approximately, which corresponds in Table VII to a P value, in both tails combined, of about 0.3. Finally, express the verdict with less jargon.

Measurement Analyses versus Frequency Analyses

Having shown at considerable length how to analyze a sample of differences as measurements (or as equivalent ranks) we now ask why we should do so at all — why not simply use the sign test as in Chapter XI? Such a question has been previously met in more general terms. Here we ask it with reference to a particular type of data: measurements of matched pairs.

With reference to the sample of knee joint differences, we might ask a still more fundamental question: "Why do we perform a 'significance test' at all?" When rather precise direct measurements of right and left organs or segments of the body can be made, it is apparently common to find a tendency for one or other side to predominate in size. The question in this study was therefore: "Does body-section radiography reveal (or produce) a tendency for the right or left knee interspace in x-ray films to predominate in size?"

For the purpose of the study the distinction between "reveal" and "produce" (by an artifact, such as the positioning of the limb) was unimportant. In setting up a standard series of interspace dimensions against which to test subjects suspected to have abnormal narrowing (by reduction of thickness of cartilage), it would be desirable to know whether separate standards should be set for the right and left knees. If there were no suggestion of a predominance, detectable by x-rays, only half the labor, and exposure to radiation, would be required, in comparison with what would be needed if a separate right and left series were to be set up.

The 33 measurements contained 13 positive and 18 negative signs, and Table I shows that 13 positives would be quite compatible with a population value of about 60 per cent positives. Differences of 13 versus 18 would often occur in random samples from a population containing 50 per cent of each sign. Although we cannot exclude the possibility that a large survey would show negatives (L greater than R) in the majority, the sample gave no suggestion that this would be so.

We may therefore ask: "What more have we shown through analysis of the measurements (by ranks) than the sign test would have told us?" In this instance, perhaps nothing of consequence; but in general we have to remember that the two tests do not tell us quite the same thing. The sign test tells about frequencies; the signed-ranks test tells us about magnitudes. For instance, let us suppose that in a sample of 24 measurements 12 were negative and 12 were positive. There would be no suggestion of a difference in frequency of signs. But let us further suppose that all 12 negative differences were of smaller magnitude than the positive differences. The sum of signed ranks would be +144, which Table VI shows is "significant" at the 5 per cent level. In a bell-shaped distribution centering about zero, great disagreements of verdicts from frequencies and from measurements are very uncommon, but this kind of discrepancy can occur in some experiments in which two treatments are applied to the same subject — if, for example, some subjects are very susceptible to the effect of treatment A and others are not, while treatment B does little or nothing. Therefore, although we speak of measurement tests as more sensitive (more able to detect a real difference) than frequency tests, we should not argue automatically from measurement differences to frequency differences or vice versa.

Comparison of Two Groups of Subjects

Fourteen patients with rheumatoid arthritis were randomly divided into two groups of 7, the A-group to receive a placebo, the B-group to receive a certain drug. (All patients continued to take aspirin.) The grip strength of the right hand was measured by the squeezing of a rubber bag attached to a mercury manometer. In each patient the pretreatment reading was subtracted from the reading after one week of treatment, and the following measurements of change (in mm. of mercury) were found:

> Group A: +32, +20, −10, +90, − 9,   0, −60
> Group B: +40, +52, +20, +52, +95, +54, +84
> Totals (and arithmetic means): A + 63 (+ 9.0 mm.)
>   B + 397 (+56.7 mm.)

Again the arithmetic means are inserted although we do not need them, and again we postpone discussion of the way in which they can be used in such comparisons.

The "null hypothesis" was that nothing except the randomization was responsible for the intergroup difference in the totals. Therefore the question is: How often would random division of these 14 measurements into two groups of 7 produce differences of such magnitude? However, before going to the trouble of analyzing the measurements we ought not to overlook simpler evidence, obtainable from frequencies.

Frequency Tests

When some measurements are negative and others positive we can perform a kind of "sign test" by arranging data in a fourfold contingency table (A versus B; positive versus negative). In this instance we could say that there were 4 failures to increase grip strength in the A-group and none in the B-group; but Table III shows that this difference could often be produced by the randomization alone.

Such a test is, of course, very insensitive, but there is another more sensitive frequency test that can be applied even if all the measurements have the same sign. We arrange all the measurements in order of magnitude and find the median as closely as we can, in this instance +36 mm. mercury. Then we arrange the two groups in a contingency table thus:

Treatment	Below Median	Above Median	Total
A	6	1	7
B	1	6	7
Total	7	7	14

We can then calculate chi-square (with Yates' correction) = 4.6; or we can consult Table III, which shows that fewer than 5 per cent of randomizations would produce differences of this magnitude. If we adopt the 5 per cent standard of rarity we will conclude that something in addition to the randomization was responsible. This test can be called the "median test," and it can be applied to unequal as well as to equal samples.

Randomization Experiments

This procedure was applied on a small scale to the 14 measurements shown above. Each measurement was written on a card and then on each card 100 two-digit random numbers were copied from Fisher and

Yates' *Statistical Tables*. The cards were then sorted in the ascending order of the first random numbers on each card. The first seven cards were called "A," the last seven were called "B," and the totals of the measurements in each group were recorded. The process was repeated with the second random numbers on each card, then with the third random numbers and so on, until 100 experiments had been performed. The tails of the distribution showed the following values:

Sum in A	Sum in B	B —A	Diff. of Means (mm. Hg)	Frequency
+413	+ 47	—366	—52.3	1
+406	+ 54	—352	—50.3	1
+384	+ 76	—308	—44.0	1
+383	+ 77	—306	—43.7	2
+381	+ 79	—302	—43.1	1
. . .	. . .	. . .	. . .	. . .
+ 88	+372	+284	+40.6	1
+ 87	+373	+286	+40.9	1
+ 65	+395	+330	+47.1	1
+ 63	+397	+334	+47.7	1
+ 54	+406	+352	+50.3	1
+ 35	+425	+390	+55.7	1

It will be noted that A = +383, B = +77 occurred twice, but the components of the samples were different in the two cases. This kind of duplication occurred 12 times in the series, and one pair of sums occurred 3 times. The sample under test had the values A = +63, B = +397. In the tail of the distribution where these values lie there are two more extreme A-B differences. Therefore the 2.5 per cent cut-off point would not place it in the "rare" class; P (one tail) in this set of 100 experiments was 0.03. We will return to these results later.

Display of All Possible Arrangements

The number of possible divisions of 14 measurements into two groups of seven is $14!/(7! \times 7!)$, where 14! stands for "factorial 14." This gives a total of 3432 possible divisions. This method, called Pitman's "exact" test (Kendall, 1952) is obviously practicable with only tiny samples, but it should be examined, because it is the basis for the two-sample rank analysis, which is a simple and practical substitute.

The following 8 of the above hand-grip measurements were chosen for the demonstration — with unequal samples because they present slightly greater difficulties than do equal samples:

5 A's: +32 +20 —10 +90 —9   Total = +123   Mean = +24.6
3 B's: +40 +52 +95   Total = +187   Mean = +62.3
Grand total = +310

The total possible divisions of the 8 measurements into groups of 3 and 5 are $8!/(5! \times 3!) = 56$.

For convenience we work with the smaller sample, labeled N_1, because the total for the larger sample (N_2) will always be $+310$ minus the total for N_1. We begin with N_1 as it occurred, and then substitute for its last measurement, $+95$, each of the remaining measurements in turn:

$$
\begin{aligned}
+40 \quad +52 \quad +95 &= +187 \\
+32 &= +124 \\
+20 &= +112 \\
-10 &= +\ 82 \\
+90 &= +182 \\
-\ 9 &= +\ 83
\end{aligned}
$$

Then we substitute for the second measurement, namely, $+52$:

$$
\begin{aligned}
+40 \quad +95 \quad +32 &= +167 \\
+20 &= +155 \\
&\text{etc.}
\end{aligned}
$$

The 56 different arrangements produced the same sum twice in only five instances. The tails of the distribution were as follows:

Sample B (N_1)		Sample A (N_2)		Frequency
Sum	Mean	Sum	Mean	
$+\ 1$	$+\ 0.3$	$+309$	$+61.8$	1
$+\ 13$	$+\ 4.3$	$+297$	$+59.4$	1
$+\ 21$	$+\ 7.0$	$+289$	$+57.8$	1
$+\ 33$	$+11.0$	$+277$	$+55.4$	1
$+\ 42$	$+14.0$	$+268$	$+53.6$	1
$\dots$	$\dots$	$\dots$	$\dots$	$\dots$
$+187$	$+62.3$	$+123$	$+24.6$	1
$+205$	$+68.3$	$+105$	$+21.0$	1
$+217$	$+72.3$	$+\ 93$	$+18.6$	1
$+225$	$+75.0$	$+\ 85$	$+17.0$	1
$+237$	$+79.0$	$+\ 73$	$+14.6$	1

The distribution is, of course, nonsymmetrical and the differences that are of equal rarity in the two tails are not equal in size; e.g., at the one end, Mean A minus Mean B $= 61.5$ mm., at the other end it is -64.4 mm. Since $1/56 = 0.018$, the 2.5 per cent cut-off point excludes only the terminal value in each tail. The value in the original sample ($+187$ in B) is far from the cut-off point. Samples containing that value and larger values in the same direction comprise $5/56$ (8.9 per cent) of the total samples; i.e., P (one tail) is 0.089, or nearly 0.10.

Two-sample Ranks Tests

Although we cannot apply an exact test to the actual measurements in most of our samples, we can come close to the same results by converting measurements into ranks. The test described here is based on the one that was devised by Wilcoxon for equal samples and by White for unequal samples. We will exemplify it first by the samples of 5 and 3 hand-grip measurements, for comparison with the Pitman test already applied to these measurements. We proceed as follows:

1. Arrange the measurements in order from the extreme negative to the extreme positive.
2. Assign ranks to the measurements in that order (1, 2, 3, ..., 8). (If two or more measurements were the same, and had the same sign, i.e., if two or more ranks were tied, we would assign to each measurement the mean of the tied ranks.)

Measurement	−10	−9	+20	+32	+40	+52	+90	+95
Rank	1	2	3	4	5	6	7	8
Treatment	A	A	A	A	B	B	A	B

We do not affix signs to the ranks because the relationships and differences would remain the same if the whole series were moved to the right by some fixed amount, so that all items would be positive.

3. Find the sum of ranks of the smaller sample (N_1) and also of the larger sample (N_2), because they act as a check on each other by reference to the sum of ranks 1 to 8, found by the formula already shown.

Sum of ranks for smaller sample (B) $= 5 + 6 + 8 = 19$
Sum of ranks for larger   sample (A) $= 1 + 2 + 3 + 4 + 7 = 17$
Sum of all ranks $= 8\,(8 + 1)/2 = 36$

The test is completed by taking the sum of ranks of the smaller sample to Table VIII (see Appendix), but before doing so we ought to find out what that table tells us. We do so by looking at the randomization of ranks in the present example.

Randomization of Ranks. If we repeatedly assigned ranks 1 to 8 by random numbers to two samples, one containing 5 items and the other 3 items, we would ultimately display all possible such arrangements; but with such small numbers it is possible to do this on paper without much labor. We proceed exactly as with the measurements themselves, and we need use only the smaller sample because the sum of ranks in the larger sample will be the total (36) minus the sum in the smaller sample.

$$1 + 2 + 3 = 6 \qquad\qquad 7 = 10$$
$$4 = 7 \qquad\qquad 8 = 11$$
$$5 = 8 \qquad\qquad 1 + 3 + 4 = 8$$
$$6 = 9 \qquad\qquad 5 = 9 \text{ etc.}$$

The total 56 divisions produced the following frequencies (F) of the sums of ranks (SR) in the smaller sample (B):

SR	6 7 8 9 10 11 12 13 14 15 16 17 18 19 20 21
F	1 1 2 3 4 5 6 6 6 6 5 4 3 2 1 1

The smallest possible sum of ranks (6) in the B-sample indicated the largest possible difference in favor of A. It was formed by the summation of ranks 1, 2 and 3. The corresponding sum of the actual measurements was $-10 -9 +20 = +1$, the smallest possible sum of measurements in the B-sample. Whether we tested such a sample by summating the measurements or by summating the ranks, we would classify it as beyond the 2.5 per cent cut-off point at the one end of the distribution.

The same verdict would apply to the extreme sample at the other end (rank sum = 21; sum of measurements = $+237$). No other sample in the total 56 could qualify as rare on this standard. It is this verdict of rarity that we find when we enter Table VIII at $N_1 = 3$ and $N_2 = 5$ and find the sums of ranks 6;21 under P less than 0.05. It is impossible in 56 items to find one that is rare enough to qualify for the column P less than 0.01.

The sum of ranks does not always occupy the same position in the frequency distribution as does the corresponding sum of measurements. For instance, the B-sample of 3 measurements with which we started had a rank sum of $+187$, which is fifth from the upper end of the randomization distribution, i.e., its P value (one tail) = 5/56 (8.9 per cent). This combination of measurements produced a rank sum of 19 and two such values occupy the third and fourth positions from the end of the distribution; P = 4/56 (0.071 = 7.1 per cent). The difference is slight and, what is more important, the same verdict regarding rarity (relationship to the 2.5 per cent cut-off point) would be obtained by either test.

Application of the Two-sample Ranks Test

We can now return to the actual pair of samples containing the readings of hand-grip changes in 7 patients on treatment A and 7 patients on treatment B. When we arrange the measurements in order from the extreme negative to the extreme positive value, assign ranks and indicate treatments, we have the following series:

Measurement (mm. Hg)	Rank	Treatment	Measurement (mm. Hg)	Rank	Treatment
-60	1	A	$+40$	8	B
-10	2	A	$+52$	9 or 10	B
-9	3	A	$+52$	9 or 10	B
0	4	A	$+54$	11	B
$+20$	5 or 6	A	$+84$	12	B
$+20$	5 or 6	B	$+90$	13	A
$+32$	7	A	$+95$	14	B

Of the two 20's, one is in A and one is in B; therefore we assign to each of them the average of ranks 5 and 6, i.e., 5.5. The two 52's are both in B, and it is immaterial which receives rank 9 and which receives rank 10.

$$\begin{array}{lll} \text{Sums of ranks:} & A = & 35.5 \\ & B = & 69.5 \\ \text{Total} & = & \overline{105.0} \end{array}$$

As a check, we find that the total of 14 ranks is $14(14 + 1)/2 = 105$.

In Table VIII at $N_1 = 7$ and $N_2 = 7$, under P less than 0.05, we find 36;69. This means that if all possible groups of 7 were selected from ranks 1 to 14 inclusive, the 2.5 per cent cut-off points would lie between 37 and 36 in the one tail and between 68 and 69 in the other tail. The observed sums of ranks were 35.5 and 69.5. Therefore for brevity we can say that the A-B difference was significant at the 5 per cent level; but the following statement is more explanatory. When the two-sample ranks test was applied, it was found that the difference in sums of ranks, 35.5 and 69.5, and greater differences, would occur in less than 5 per cent of random divisions of ranks 1 to 14 into two samples of seven.

Obviously, the true P (one tail) for this sample would not be much less than 0.025; and it is interesting to compare this result with the results of two other tests applied to the same data. The series of 100 randomizations of the actual measurements (p. 281) gave $P = 0.03$. The median test (p. 280) gave a chi-square value of 4.6; therefore, P (one tail) would be beyond the 2.5 cut-off point, and the exact fourfold-table test (Chapter XII) showed that it was 0.015.

Preparation of Table VIII. Miss Sutcliffe built up part of Table VIII as in Table VI by increasing the sample sizes by one individual (one terminal rank) at a time. Beyond that area she derived the cut-off points from Auble's tables, and checked them where possible by the methods and tables of Fix and Hodges.

When N_1 or N_2 is greater than 20, we use the Gaussian curve instead of Table VIII.

The Gaussian Curve and Sums of Ranks

The distribution of the sums of ranks in the sample of 3 (p. 284) looks like the beginning of a Gaussian distribution. It is symmetrical, with a center (median and mean) at 13.5. This value can be easily found without having to display the distribution. The total of ranks $1 + 2 + 3 + \cdots + 8$ is 36. If there were no difference in the effect of A and B, we would expect the samples to share this total in proportion to their size, 3:5. More explicitly, in a long series of random assignments, each rank (1, 2, 3, and so on) would be shared by the samples in the 3:5 ratio. Therefore the average of all the randomizations would show the sample of 3 with 3/8 of $36 = 13.5$.

As always, if we intend to try using the Gaussian curve instead of an exact distribution, we must find the standard deviation. The step-by-step method applied to this frequency distribution gave the value $\sqrt{11.25}$ = 3.3541. As with signed ranks, however, there is a formula that obviates the need for displaying the actual frequency distribution. If N_1 and N_2 are sample sizes the standard deviation of sums of ranks for either of the two samples is given by the following formula:

$$SD = \sqrt{N_1 N_2 (N_1 + N_2 + 1)/12}. \text{ (The divisor 12 is a constant.)}$$

In the present example,

$$SD = \sqrt{3 \times 5(8 + 1)/12} = \sqrt{11.25} = 3.3541,$$

which is exactly the same as was found by the step-by-step method.

We have now to see where, as sample sizes are increased, the Gaussian curve can safely be substituted for the exact distributions of sums of ranks in a two-sample test. We begin with the sample-pair in which $N_1 = 3$ and $N_2 = 5$. The SD of the sums of ranks is 3.3541. If we take twice 3.3541 = 6.71, and measure it below and above the mean, 13.5, we mark the points which in the Gaussian curve would cut off at each end slightly less than 2.5 per cent of the total distribution. In the distribution of rank sums it cuts off the most extreme value at each end, and thus correctly classifies those items as "rare" on the 5 per cent standard. The Gaussian approximation is not always so reliable with such small samples, but with slightly larger samples it becomes safe for most purposes, as in the following examples.

Examples of Gaussian-curve Approximations. Three examples with small N's permit us to make comparisons with the exact values in Table VIII (in parentheses here). (SR = sum of ranks.)

Av. SR in N_1	$N_1 = 7, N_2 = 7$	$N_1 = 5, N_2 = 20$	$N_1 = 20, N_2 = 20$
± 1.65 SD	39.6;65.4(39;66)	40.7;89.3(40;90)	349.02;470.98(348:472)
± 2 SD	36.8;68.2(36;69)	35.6;94.4(35;95)	336.1;483.9(337;483)
± 2.58 SD	32.3;72.7(32;73)	27.02;102.98(28;102)	314.6;505.4(315;505)

Clearly there is no reason to doubt the reliability of the Gaussian curve with samples larger than those in Table VIII, except, perhaps, where one sample is very much larger than the other; but such cases are exceptional, and when they occur a frequency test is often sufficient to provide an adequate verdict.

The question that we have not yet fully faced in these descriptions of rank-order tests is their justification as substitutes for certain popular methods of analyzing measurement data as such. We will now look at those methods.

Gaussian-curve Analysis of Measurements

In the first edition of this book and in its predecessor (Mainland, 1938) measurement data in matched pairs and in two-sample comparisons were analyzed by the very orthodox and widely used "t-test." This is a test derived from the Gaussian curve and applied directly to the measurements. It is not a Gaussian-curve technique substituted for an exact test after being investigated for its reliability, as with the ranks tests.

The reasons for emphasizing rank sum tests in this edition will emerge after we have looked at the t-test. Look at it we must, if we are to have any rational grounds for using it or for refusing it, or for passing judgment on conclusions that are drawn from it in almost every kind of medical journal. The purpose here is not to teach techniques of t-tests. Those can be found, with arithmetical shortcuts, in many statistical textbooks. What we need to know chiefly is what t tells us, what it does not tell us, what assumptions it is based on, and why we go through certain procedures in calculating it.

Basic Structure and Function of t

When we examine the essential structure of the quantity t, it appears almost surprisingly rational — the kind of thing that an experimenter might invent if he desired some kind of "index of confidence" in his results. As an example, let us use again the five blood pressure differences (mm. Hg) shown at the beginning of this chapter: $+4$, $+10$, $+12$, 0, $+18$.

Almost automatically an experimenter would find the arithmetic mean, $+8.8$ mm. Hg. If asked why, he might say that because samples differed in size it was always desirable to express the sum of a set of measurements on a per-unit basis. Or he might say that this sample was for him a representative of a large group (a population) of similar units, women treated in the same way, and the per-unit expression was necessary so that the sample could give an estimate applicable to the indefinitely large group.

The experimenter would wish to know how far he could trust the sample mean as a guide to the population mean — the mean that he would approach if he took a larger and larger sample of the same kind of subject. He would like an index that would be larger if he could have more confidence in his sample mean, and smaller if he could have less confidence. A ratio is a suitable form of expression because it can vary all the way from zero to almost infinity, depending on what we use as numerator and denominator.

The most obvious choice for the numerator would be the sample mean difference, because the larger the mean difference the greater would be the experimenter's confidence that he would not find a zero mean difference in the population. But mere size of the mean would not satisfy him. If the individual measurements in the sample agreed closely with each other (and therefore with the mean) he would have more confidence in the mean than if the individual measurements differed greatly. The denominator of the ratio would therefore appropriately contain some kind of expression of the variation within the sample.

Finally, the larger the sample the more confidence it would induce in the experimenter. Therefore sample size, or some quantity derived from it, would be appropriate in the numerator, or as a factor to reduce the denominator, which comes to the same thing.

The threefold ratio thus developed would be almost identical with the t-ratio that is used for testing the mean of a set of matched-pair differences. Other t's have a corresponding structure — for example, the t for testing the difference between the means of two samples and the t for testing the slope of the straight-line relationship between X and Y variables.

In all forms of t the measure of variation that goes into the denominator is a standard deviation, and for each kind of thing that we test we must use the appropriate standard deviation. In testing a mean of a sample of N measurements we need not only the SD of the individual measurements but the SD of means of samples of N measurements. In testing a difference between means of samples we need an SD of differences. These SD's are often called "standard errors," but this causes confusion, and if we meet the term "standard error" we should always translate it as "standard deviation." Before we reach t, we must look at some of these standard deviations.

Standard Deviation of Means

Often this is called the SD (or SE) of *the* mean, as if it belonged to the particular mean that we are testing. This is misleading. We ought to picture a population of measurements (or of any other numbers) and a large number of random samples of size N from that population. When we take such samples we find, of course, that their arithmetic means differ from each other. We can express this variation as a standard deviation, which we can find in exactly the same way as if the means were individual measurements. In actual research, however, a problem arises. We commonly have only one sample representing a particular population. Therefore, how are we going to find (or estimate) the SD of means of such samples?

If we actually knew the SD of the parent population of individual measurements the answer would be simple, as was illustrated by an experiment on the 1000 students' statures shown in Table 5 (p. 247). This series was large enough to be used as an "indefinitely large" or "infinite" population in a sampling demonstration when the samples are small. Each stature was marked on a disk and 1000 random samples of 5 disks were taken. The frequency distribution of the means of these samples is in Table 7.

Table 7. Frequency Distribution of Mean Statures in 1000 Random Samples of 5 from the Statures in Table 5

Mean of Sample (inches)	Frequency (No. of Samples)	Mean of Sample (inches)	Frequency (No. of Samples)
64.0 — 64.9	0	69.0 — 69.9	335
65.0 — 65.9	3	70.0 — 70.9	128
66.0 — 66.9	36	71.0 — 71.9	21
67.0 — 67.9	167	72.0 — 72.9	2
68.0 — 68.9	308	73.0 — 73.9	0
		Total	1000

Comparison with Table 5 shows that the means varied less than did the individual statures; and this is not difficult to understand. If one member of a sample is far out from the center of the distribution of individual measurements it will be more often accompanied by more central values than by values from its own region. This is the familiar averaging process that occurs with samples taken from any set of numbers, not only from bell-shaped distributions.

The mean of the thousand arithmetic means was 5′8.82″, the same as the original population mean. The SD of the means was 1.08″, whereas the SD of the individual statures was 2.45″. If, however, we divide 2.45″, the population SD, by the square root of 5, the number in each sample, we find that $2.45/\sqrt{5} = 2.45/2.24 = 1.09''$. Except for the last digit, this is the same value (1.08″) as was found directly from the thousand sample-means.

This illustrates a relationship which can be demonstrated mathematically and expressed in general terms. If SD is the standard deviation of an indefinitely large population of measurements or other numbers, and if random samples of size N are taken from it, the standard deviation of the means of those samples can be found by the formula:

$$\text{SD of means} = \text{Population SD}/\sqrt{N}$$

The more samples we take, the closer do we approach to this relationship.

If instead of the SD of the population we use the variance (mean square deviation), we can say that just as we divide the sum of a set of numbers by N to obtain the mean, so we divide the population variance by N to obtain the variance of means. (Note that the divisor is N, not N—1.) The relationship holds true regardless of the shape of the frequency distribution of the original population, and is equally true, however small N may be. (For small *finite* populations, an extra term, based on the size of the population, has to be introduced into the formula, but that need not concern us here.)

The impediment to our use of the formula is of course that in most research we do not know the population SD. The larger our sample (if random) the more closely does its SD of individual variation approach that of the population; but many of our samples give poor estimates. For instance, with samples of 25 from a known (Gaussian) population it is not uncommon to find that the sample SD must be increased by nearly 30 per cent, or decreased by nearly 13 per cent, to give the population SD.

Presently we will see how the t-test removes this impediment; but first we must look at the SD of differences, because it is used in the comparison of means.

Standard Deviation of Differences

If we have two populations (A and B) of measurements or other numbers, we can take a series of random samples, one individual from each population, and obtain a series of A-minus-B differences. These vary from each other, and we can express this variation by a standard deviation. If, however, we know the SD's of the original populations we can calculate the SD of the differences without even finding a single one of the actual differences. If SD_A and SD_B are the population SD's, the formula is:

$$\text{SD of (A-B) differences} = \sqrt{SD_A^2 + SD_B^2}$$

This relationship can be shown mathematically and illustrated experimentally to be true for populations with any shape of frequency distribution. The formula has to be changed somewhat if A- and B-readings are correlated with each other. For example, it would not hold exactly if we were studying the differences between right and left hand-length, or right hand-length and right foot-length, in a series of subjects. However, this does not concern us here.

The populations A and B can be composed of the arithmetic means of samples; and the samples can be of the same or different sizes in the two populations, but in any one of the populations they must all be of the same size. The relationship holds also if we take random samples from the same population, and find the difference between the first and second sample in each pair.

Out of all this emerges a well known rule for estimating the standard deviation of differences between the means of pairs of random samples (A-minus-B). (1) Estimate the variance of means of A-samples and the variance of means of B-samples. (2) Add the variances and (3) take the square root. In applying the rule, however, we meet the same impediment that we met earlier. To make a reliable estimate of the variance of means, we need the variance of the original population of measurements; and we commonly know little or nothing about that, except what our sample tells us. We will now see how the t-test can help us in this problem.

Testing a Mean Difference by t

Let us suppose that we have a sample of five differences, such as the women's blood pressure differences (in mm. Hg) already discussed: +4, +10, +12, 0, +18. If we decide to apply the t-test, we proceed as follows:

Mean difference = +8.80

Deviations from mean (without sign) = 4.8, 1.2, 3.2, 8.8, 9.2. (We do not discard the zero difference in this test.)

Sum of squares of deviations from mean = 23.04 + 1.44 + 10.24 + 77.44 + 84.64 = 196.80.

To estimate the variance (mean square deviation) of measurements in a population randomly represented by this sample, we divide the sum of squares by one less than the number of items in the sample, i.e., by $N - 1 = 4$. The estimated variance is therefore 49.20, and the estimated SD is $\sqrt{49.20}$.

To estimate the SD of means of samples randomly represented by the sample of five, we use the full sample size, not N — 1. SD of means $= \sqrt{49.20} \div \sqrt{5} = \sqrt{9.84} = 3.1369$ mm. Hg.

Of course we do not trust this estimate, because we do not trust $\sqrt{49.20}$ as an estimate of the population SD. What we trust, in the sense described below, is the ratio t.

t = mean/estimated SD of means = 8.80/3.1369 = 2.805. (The sign of the mean, plus or minus, is dropped at this stage.)

The Meaning of the t-Test

We now take 2.805 to Fisher's table of the distribution of t, which is in his *Statistical Methods*, also in Fisher and Yates' *Tables*, and has been reproduced in many books, including Arkin and Colton's *Tables for Statisticians*. We look for n = 4, i.e., N — 1, the same as the divisor used in estimating the population variance, and we find:

P	0.1	0.05	0.02
t	2.132	2.776	3.747

These t values are cut-off points in the random sampling distribution of t, and P is the probability (in both tails combined) of finding values beyond the various cut-off points. To state what the figures tell us we must begin with three "if" clauses:

If (a) we have a Gaussian distribution of measurements, if (b) its center (mean = median) is at zero, and if (c) we take an indefinitely large number of random samples of 5 measurements and calculate t as shown above, we will find 5 per cent of the t values greater than 2.776. In half of this 5 per cent, the sample means will be below zero, and in half of them it will be above zero; or, if we leave the plus and minus signs attached to the t, half of these rare t's will be negative and half will be positive.

We can picture a series of symmetrical bell-shaped curves of t values with their centers at zero — a slightly different curve for each value of n. In both tails of each curve would be marked cut-off points, such as the 2.5 per cent points in the curve for n = 4, at t = —2.776 and at t = +2.776. The curves are not Gaussian, but are derived from the Gaussian curve, and they become more and more Gaussian as n becomes larger. That is indicated by the last line of the table; at n = "infinity" the cut-off points are those of the Gaussian curve, e.g., 1.96 for P = 0.05 (P = 0.025 in each tail) and 2.576 for P = 0.01 (P = 0.005 in each tail).

We could produce the table of t experimentally by writing on disks the measurements from a table of the Gaussian distribution, then taking random samples and calculating t for each sample.

The t from the sample of 5 women's blood pressure changes, 2.805, lies just beyond the 5 per cent cut-off point, 2.776. Therefore we can say: "The t value was significant at the 5 per cent level, though barely so." Would this tell the investigator what he wanted to know? An investigator who uses a t-test wants it to tell him how much confidence he can have in what he is testing, e.g., a mean change in a certain measurement, or the difference between two sample means, or the slope of a line — confidence that the value of this thing in his sample's parent population would not be zero.

To see what the t-test actually tells him, we must refer to the three "if" clauses in the statement made above:

a. If the frequency distribution of the parent population is Gaussian. Of course we know that it is not truly a Gaussian distribution, which is an abstraction like a "perfect circle"; so we have to say "sufficiently like a Gaussian distribution that the t-test will not mislead us."

b. If the center of the distribution is at zero.

c. If the samples are strictly random.

Unfortunately, we have developed the habit of looking only at clause (b). The t from the five women was beyond the 5 per cent cut-off point, but we translate this as "the mean change in blood pressure was significant, i.e., differed significantly from zero." We take this as indicating the likelihood that, if we could build up a population of women of the same kind and treat them in the same way, the population would, on the average, show a rise in blood pressure. What we ought to say is: "The observed t was beyond the cut-off point. Therefore, either the conditions (a), (b) and (c) were true and something happened that occurs in less than 5 per cent of random samples, or one or more of the three conditions did not hold true."

This picture of multiple conditions or multiple "null hypotheses" becomes confusing, and we may look back with longing to the simple concept of the exact test (display of all possible arrangements) or its substitute, the signed-ranks test. We recall that these tests showed that, if there were a 50:50 chance for the five readings (or for the four readings other than zero) to have plus or minus signs, the most extreme cases (all plus signs or all minus signs) would comprise one eighth of the total possible arrangements, i.e., P from both tails = 0.125. This is very different from the t-test result, P less than 0.05. Looking at conditions (a) and (c) we ask two questions:

1. What is the evidence for a belief that blood pressure changes in such women would form a distribution near enough to the Gaussian curve to make a t-test safe?

2. Do the verdicts disagree because the tests ask different questions? The t-test visualizes a population comprising a great and unknown variety of blood pressure changes, and asks about the differences between random samples from that population. The exact test and the signed-ranks test confine themselves to the blood pressure changes that were actually observed and they ask about the effect of random allocation of plus and minus signs in all possible combinations.

We will return to these questions after seeing how t is used in the comparison of two means, because similar questions arise there also.

Comparison of Two Means by t

As an illustration we take again the two samples of hand-grip changes (in mm. Hg) already analyzed by the exact test and by the two-sample ranks test.

    5 A's: +32, +20, −10, +90, −9   Mean = +24.6
    3 B's: +40, +52, +95   Mean = +62.3

Difference between means (B − A) = +37.7.

Underlying Principles. In applying the t-test we should visualize an indefinitely large population of measurements (hand-grip changes) with a Gaussian frequency distribution. The position of the center (mean change) is quite immaterial. We picture ourselves taking a random sample of 5 measurements and labeling it "A," then (or simultaneously) taking a random sample of 3 measurements and labeling it "B." We find the mean for each sample and the difference between the means, B − A. If we repeated this procedure many times we would create a frequency distribution of differences. Since A and B are merely labels representing treatments that do not differ in their effects on hand grip, we would find an equal number of (B − A) positive and negative differences of the same size. That is, the distribution would be symmetrical, and its mean would approach zero as we continued to build it up. Indeed, it can be shown experimentally and mathematically that it would be of Gaussian shape, with its center at zero.

The variation of the distribution would be expressible as a standard deviation of differences and, as we have seen, if we knew the SD of the original population of blood pressure changes we would not need to perform the sampling experiment at all. In applying the t-test we start by making an estimate of the SD of the original population. Each sample gives us a bit of information about it, and since the hypothesis that we are testing is that the samples originated from the same population, we pool the information from the two samples.

Performance of the Test. In sample A we subtract the mean (+24.6) from each reading to obtain the following deviations: +7.4, −4.6, −34.6, +65.4, −33.6. The sum of squares of deviations for A = 6679.20. In sample B the deviations from the mean (+62.3) are: −22.3, −10.3, +32.7. The sum of the squares of deviations for B = 1672.66. (We are breaking the rule, previously mentioned, about carrying two more decimal figures than we require in the final answer, but essentially the same t value was obtained when the rule was obeyed.)

Pooled sums of squares = 6679.20 + 1672.66 = 8351.86.

At this point, some students have asked: "Since we are by hypothesis treating the two samples as if they belonged to the same population, why do we not find the grand mean of all 8 measurements and the sum of squares of deviations from that mean?" After a little thought, the questioners have seen that we would thereby include in the denominator of t the difference between the samples, and this is what we wish to test by putting it in the numerator of t. In essence, we divide the total variation into two parts: (a) between the A and B samples, and (b) between individuals treated alike. The aim of the t-test is to show whether the difference between these two variations is too great to be adequately accounted for by random assignment of "A" and "B" to the two groups.

To find the variance, we divide the sum of squares by $(5-1) + (3-1) = 6$, i.e., we use $N-1$ from each sample. The estimate of the SD of the parent population of measurements is therefore $\sqrt{8351.86/6}$ mm. Hg. We now use this to estimate the SD of means for each sample size, dividing the population variance by the appropriate N.

$$\text{Sample A: } \sqrt{8351.86/(6 \times 5)}$$
$$\text{Sample B: } \sqrt{8351.86/(6 \times 3)}$$

The estimate of the SD of differences between the means is therefore:

$$\sqrt{8351.86/(6 \times 5) + 8351.86/(6 \times 3)} = \sqrt{742.39} = 27.25 \text{ mm. Hg}$$

Finally, $t = 37.7/27.25 = 1.38$.

The Result of the Test. Turning to Fisher's table of the t distribution we look for $n = 6$, because that was the divisor used in estimating the variance of the original (hypothetical) population of measurements. We find:

P	0.3	0.2	0.1	0.05
t	1.134	1.440	1.943	2.447

The t from our sample-pair (1.38) is far from significant at the 5 per cent level. It lies between 1.134 and 1.440. Therefore it would be exceeded in more than 20 per cent of randomly obtained sample-pairs from the same Gaussian population. In half of these sample-pairs (more than 10 per cent of the total) the t would be positive as in our own sample-pair. That is, there would be a greater mean change in hand grip in the sample of three, labeled "B."

We can now compare the t-test verdict with the verdicts of the randomization tests applied to the same data — the display of all possible divisions of the 8 items into groups 5 and 3. These tests were applied to the measurements themselves (p. 282) and to the ranks substituted for the measurements (p. 283).

Test	P (One Tail)
Randomization of measurements	0.089 (8.9%)
Randomization of ranks	0.071 (7.1%)
t-test	greater than 0.1 (greater than 10%)

The ranks test agrees more closely with the measurements test than does the t-test, but with reference to the 5 per cent standard (2.5 per cent in one tail) the verdicts of the three are equivalent.

Comparison of Three Tests

The same eight hand-grip measurements can be used for further comparisons of the three tests. On p. 282 are shown the tail regions of the frequency distribution which displayed all 56 possible divisions of the 8 measurements into groups of 5 and 3. One of the tails (with some additional entries) is reproduced here, along with the corresponding frequencies obtained by display of all 56 possible divisions of sums of ranks and also the results of the t-test applied to the differences between means.

	Means (mm. Hg)		P (One Tail) Expressed as Percentage Actual Frequencies		
A	B	A — B	Measurement Sums	Rank Sums	t-Test of Diff. between Means
26.2	59.7	+33.5	12.5	12.5	10 to 15
25.6	60.7	+35.1	10.7	12.5	10 to 15
24.6	62.3	+37.7	8.9	7.1	10 to 15
21.0	68.3	+47.3	7.1	12.5	5 to 10
18.6	72.3	+53.7	5.4	7.1	2.5 to 5
17.0	75.0	+58.0	3.6	3.6	1 to 2.5
14.6	79.0	+64.4	1.8	1.8	0.05 to 0.5

Two noteworthy features of this display are:

1. In the extreme tail regions, where decisions are most crucial, the t-test gave the impression of greater rarity than was actually found.

2. Although the rank-sum frequencies are not quite parallel to the measurement-sum frequencies, they are much closer to them than are those inferred from the t-test.

Still another comparison of the three tests can be obtained from the 100 randomization experiments in which 14 hand-grip changes were divided into two groups of 7 (p. 281). To each of the sample-pairs in the tail regions of the distribution the two-sample ranks test and t-test were applied. We show here the results in one tail; those in the other tail were similar. (The P values for rank sums were obtained by the same method as in Table VIII, but with narrower intervals.)

Difference of Means (B — A, mm. Hg)	P (One Tail) Expressed as Percentage		
	Measurement Sums	Ranks Test	t-Test of Diff. between Means
+29.1	10	gr. than 10	10 to 15
+31.4	9	sl. gr. than 10	5 to 10
+31.7	8	" " " 10	5 to 10
+38.6	7	5 to 10	2.5 to 5
+40.6	6	4 to 5	2.5 to 5
+40.9	5	5 to 10	2.5 to 5
+47.1	4	1 to 2.5	1 to 2.5
+47.7	3	2.5 to 4	1 to 2.5
+50.3	2	1 to 2	1 to 2.5
+55.7	1	1 to 2	0.5 to 0.1

The t-test again exaggerates the rarity of the rarest sample-pairs, and we are reminded of the two questions that arose when there was discrepancy between the t-test of matched-pair differences and the randomization tests (measurement sums and rank sums) of the women's blood pressure data:

1. Did the Gaussian-curve origin of the t-test render it unsuitable for the data?

2. Was the discrepancy due to the difference in the questions asked by the t-test and the randomization tests? In terms of hand grip, the randomization tests (on measurements and ranks) take into account only the observed measurements of change, along with the randomization that was performed in assigning the A and B treatments. The t-test, conceiving the A and B sets of measurements as random samples, implies the potential existence of a population containing many other values of the same variable.

To approach the answer to these two questions we would require a large collection of the same kind of data, and if we obtained the answer it would be of little value beyond this particular investigation. Therefore we take another approach to the comparison of tests — a consideration of what we wish the tests to do for us.

General Requirements in "Significance" Tests

In any such test we desire assurance regarding two features: (1) its Type I error, and (2) its Type II error, or, conversely, its "power." By the randomization test of measurements (direct or by ranks) we can fix our Type I error at any desired level, e.g., we can be sure that we will not classify as "rare" more than the extreme 2.5 per cent of the sample-pairs in frequency distributions produced solely by randomization.

If we actually knew that our measurements came from a Gaussian distribution, we could determine the Type II error (and power) of a test that was derived from the Gaussian curve, but to do so with a randomization test we would require an endless series of large experiments. We would have to set up "treatment groups" between which we had introduced differences of various magnitudes, and then perform sampling experiments and find out how often the test enabled us to detect the difference.

Having done one such experiment, we could not feel confident that the results would apply to other data of the same general type. For example, in an experiment to test the effect of injecting ragweed pollen extract as a possible preventive of hay fever in children who were allergic to that pollen, one measure of effect was the number of antihistamine tablets taken by children to relieve hay fever symptoms during the ragweed season. Having satisfied ourselves about the power or sensitivity of a test on such data, we could not assume that it would be the same in data obtained in a study of rheumatoid arthritis, in which one measure of the effect of a drug is the number of aspirin tablets taken by the patients.

Perhaps sometime it will be possible for most research workers to put their data (from matched pairs, two-sample and other comparisons) into an electronic computer and obtain in a few seconds the results of a randomization test of the actual measurements. In the meantime we have to choose between t-tests and ranks tests, bearing in mind the two criteria — the Type I error and the power or sensitivity.

Choice between t-Tests and Ranks Tests

During recent years considerable attention has been paid to ranks tests. They are no longer thought to be second-class methods, suitable only for observations that cannot be made by scale measurement, or quick but crude substitutes for t-tests. It is therefore not necessary or desirable to try to map out, as in the first edition of this book, the kinds of data with which t-tests could be considered safe, or to discuss "transformations" (logarithmic, square-root and others) that have been devised to make non-Gaussian data more suitable for analysis by methods derived from the Gaussian curve (see Chapter XIII).

This does not imply a wholesale condemnation of t-tests, or of transformations when they have been fully explored on large bodies of real data; but it certainly seems desirable to ask ourselves what we gain by continuing to practice an old habit, instead of adopting a newer method which is not only simpler to use but easier to understand.

If we were living in a truly Gaussian world of measurements we would do better by using tests of Gaussian origin than even an "exact" (randomization) test, because in such a world we would know more about a sample and its population than the sample itself could tell us. Our tests would be more "powerful" — our experiments would be more "efficient," i.e., able to detect a particular size of difference with smaller samples than is possible in the real world.

The world of medical research is, however, far from Gaussian. An instrument scale may be linear, but often the systematic error and the variable error differ at different parts of it. Our measures take many forms — pH's; antibody titers; percentage measurements; percentage frequencies to be analyzed as measurements; numbers of days during the ragweed pollen season on which an allergic child has a running nose; and a host of other measures, which more than justify the remark made by White in presenting his ranks test for unequal samples: "Biologists at times measure bizarre variates, such that one can have little intuitive feeling as to what form the frequency distribution of the measurements in the population is likely to take; and any attempt to investigate the distribution may involve much more work than the experiment in hand."

In clinical research, moreover, our samples are heterogeneous. A group of patients with a certain disease may have been chosen by very strict criteria, but may very well contain two or more subgroups or variants, which may become distinguishable years after this particular group of patients has been studied. In the meantime it is probably safest to visualize our sample's unknown parent frequency distribution of any variable as being irregular, with two or more peaks.

Another feature of medical measurements can be illustrated by reference to hand-grip readings. In the series of 14 grip changes already discussed, the greatest gain was 95 mm. Hg and the greatest loss was 60 mm., and there appears to be no reason why in such a series the loss in some patients should not be 95 mm. or more. Actually, however, patients for clinical trials are selected by certain criteria — not specifically hand grip or potential for gain or loss of grip strength, but by criteria of severity of disease, and this is partly reflected in, or correlated with, hand grip. For all we know, the selection method in a particular trial might exclude patients who could lose (or gain) more than a certain amount in hand grip. In many experiments on animals and human beings we are ignorant of the upper and lower limits of possible change in our subjects. Our frequency distribution might be sharply lopped off at one or both ends.

All the foregoing considerations lead us to feel safer if we confine ourselves to testing the measurements that were actually made, instead of basing our test and its conclusions on the assumption that other measurements (as in a Gaussian distribution) could have been made. Ranks tests enable us to avoid that assumption; and the question is: "How reliable are they?"

Reliability of Ranks Tests

We have seen that ranks tests, being essentially randomization tests, permit us to set with assurance our Type I error — the frequency with which we will classify as "rare" extreme events that are due solely to randomization. Moreover, experiments with small samples have shown that this classification — "rare" versus "not rare" — agrees closely with the classification of the same samples by the randomization test of the actual measurements.

Although it would require endless experimentation to determine the power or sensitivity of ranks tests in all our various kinds of data, there is one situation in which their power can be detected, namely, when samples from a mathematically exact Gaussian distribution are tested by ranks tests and by t-tests.

When that was done it was found that, except in very small samples, the signed-ranks tests and the two-sample ranks test have about 95 per cent of the power of the corresponding t-test. In other words, to obtain from the ranks tests a power equal to that of the t-tests we need to increase the sample sizes by only about 5 or 6 per cent. It has been shown further that, in some non-Gaussian distributions, ranks tests are even more powerful than t-tests.

Therefore, apart from the other advantages of the ranks tests, we can be confident that we are losing little in efficiency, and perhaps gaining some, when we employ those tests instead of t-tests.

Nonparametric Methods

At this point it may be useful to introduce a term to distinguish t-tests and related but more elaborate analyses mentioned later (analysis of variance), from ranks tests, measurement-randomization tests, sign tests, median tests and others. In the t-test and related tests, estimates are made of population measures (means and standard deviations). These measures are called "parameters" and the tests that use them are called "parametric methods." The others, which do not involve estimation of population parameters are called "nonparametric methods."

Ranks versus Measurements

In spite of the foregoing evidence in favor of ranks tests, those of us who have been brought up in the worship of actual measurements may still feel qualms about converting them into ranks — the kind of assessment that has been used, for example, in beauty contests. We may fear that by arranging the actual measurements at unit (inter-rank) intervals we are distorting the data. That fear should prompt us to consider the kind of information that we obtain when we apply a scale to anything, in order to obtain a "real" measurement.

One arthritic patient's hand grip increases in a week by 90 mm. Hg, while another patient's hand grip increases by 54 mm., a difference of 36 mm. This is a convenient but arbitrary measure. We do not believe that the 36 mm. properly represents the physico-chemical or pathologic differences between the two patients in the tissues responsible for the respective readings, or that it is a linear measure of the difference in drug effect if the patients are on different drugs. Nor does the 36 mm. necessarily measure the difference in effectiveness of the hands in everyday activities.

We do not know what functions of the 90 mm. and 54 mm. would be appropriate for such purposes, but whatever they were, the measurement differences between these patients and between other patients in the same series would almost certainly be altered. It seems very likely, however, that their relative positions (rank order) would show little or no change.

In the laboratory we measure the contraction time of an isolated muscle in milliseconds, but the differences between the measures of time, under different conditions in the same muscle or in different muscles under the same conditions, are not necessarily related linearly to the differences in the tissues that are responsible for the differences in the contraction times.

Between the complex and crude hand-grip strength and the rather simple and precise muscle-contraction time, lies a great variety of types of measurements — clinical measurements such as duration of pus formation in days, and numbers of medicinal tablets consumed in a particular period, and also a host of laboratory determinations made on body fluids and tissues. With regard to all of them the question arises: "How valid are the actual differences, in the units that we use, as measures of differences in the relationships and processes that we are trying to assess?" Usually we do not know the answer. With this in mind, we can have fewer qualms when we translate measurements into ranks in the testing of differences.

The Meaning of the Mean

Even if we have disregarded the arithmetic means of our samples in order to perform a ranks test, we may still feel that the means, being derived from all the actual measurements, must tell us something more about the samples and their populations than we can learn from ranks or from the medians of the samples.

In Chapter XIII we saw that the arithmetic mean of an individual sample is not as informative as we might imagine in view of its widespread use. In the comparison of two or more samples we have got into the habit of speaking about "comparing their means." In such a comparison we try to answer a question of this kind: "Would the total measurements in these two samples, A and B, often (or rarely) differ as much as this, if the measurements had been divided between A and B solely by random shuffling?" If the samples are unequal we have to add a qualifying clause: " . . . when allowance is made for difference in sample size."

The easiest way to make allowance for sample size is to express the measurements in each sample on a per-unit basis, i.e., to take the arithmetic average; but this is not necessary. Even in the t-test there is a method, very useful in machine computation, whereby sample means are not calculated. Instead, the samples are given weight in proportion to their N values, and the results are exactly the same as when we start out by calculating the means.

It would probably clarify our thinking if we used the term "arithmetic average" instead of "arithmetic mean" in this connection, because "average" leads us back to the early days of marine insurance. When some part of a cargo had to be thrown overboard to save the ship, all merchants whose goods were on the ship shared the loss, averaging it among them in proportion to the value of their portion of the cargo. (The word "average" is said to have come from "havaria," which meant at first damage to cargo in transit and then the compensation to be paid by each individual [Moloney].)

The word "mean," on the other hand, indicates "middle," and that is appropriate in a Gaussian or other symmetrical distribution, but may be uninformative or even misleading with reference to the parent populations of many kinds of data.

The Reputation of t and Variance-ratio Tests

Although a strong case can be made for the supplanting of t and variance-ratio tests by nonparametric tests, it may appear strange that doubt should be cast on the reliability of a test that has been so widely used as t. The t-test first became easily available to the scientific public in 1925, in the first edition of Fisher's *Statistical Methods for Research Workers,* and it might be thought that the myriads of t-tests performed since then must have established its reliability — that otherwise it would have been discarded. On the surface this is a sensible argument, but deeper thought makes it questionable, to at least one former t-test devotee.

How would we, during those 35 years, have discovered that t-tests were unreliable? Presumably by finding that our conclusions from those tests, and our actions based on those conclusions, were wrong — that the tests had led us astray. We might find this after we had acted directly as a result of a test, or we might explore our material more abundantly and find that an action based on the t-test verdict would have been wrong.

Now there are many occasions on which other tests would lead us to the same conclusion, and the same action, as a t-test. The same verdict — "very significant" or "far from significant" — would be obtained from a frequency test (a sign test, a median test or the like — even an "eye" test). In these instances we could say that t was at least no less reliable than the other test; but then t would be superfluous.

It appears, therefore, that in studying the reliability of t we would have to look at those instances in which our actions based on it would be different from our actions based on one of the other tests. But how could we find out the frequency with which t had led us astray in such cases? An action of some sort is based on the verdict obtained from a certain investigation, but the setting of the action is not as a rule the same as the setting of the original investigation. Other variables are introduced, and also the results of other investigations. Then, as a result of this particular action another step is taken, and then another. After a while we or someone else may discover that we have taken a wrong turning; but there are so many causes of wrong turnings in a research path that it would seldom be possible to pin the blame on a t-test that should not have been trusted.

The same line of thought can be pursued with reference to the more elaborate forms of analysis of variance (variance-ratio tests), mentioned later. Here, however, we meet a greater temptation to smother our doubts. There is often no simple substitute for an ingenious system, which is adaptable to a great variety of experiment designs, and is practiced without apparent qualms by authorities in the field — a system, more-over, which any of us, by carefully following arithmetical instructions, can apply successfully, and emerge with a sense of accomplishment as we look at our set of apparently definitive verdicts.

If indeed a complex experiment design is desirable, and if there is not available a test that does not rest on unprovable assumptions, we should not assume that the only choice is the orthodox arithmetic. My present thoughts on this matter run along the following lines.

Let us suppose that an investigator had performed an experiment in which a certain factor was present, and that he had observed a certain event, e.g., an intergroup difference in a certain measurement. If he could perform a hundred such experiments from which the factor was absent, and could see how often the event occurred, he would probably feel that he could make up his mind whether the factor had been responsible for the event in his original experiment. It is true that if he looked at our Table I he would find that an event that occurred 3 times in 100 experiments might occur in 9 per cent of a much longer series of experiments. He would have to set up his standard of judgment before he started his 100 experiments, and he might decide that 200 would be preferable.

The 100 (or 200) experiments are, of course, randomization trials. Each individual is represented by a card or sheet of paper on which are recorded the observations made on him, and also 100 (or 200) random numbers. The writing of numbers can be avoided by making photocopies of sections of a random numbers table on thick paper, and using these sheets to represent the individuals. After each sorting, the numbers already used can be marked off before the next sorting starts.

It is important in the sorting to imitate exactly the procedure of randomization used in the original experiment; and the separation of the individuals into groups and subgroups should follow the skeleton of the appropriate analysis of variance, for it is not the scheme of analysis that is in question, but the "significance" testing that is applied to it.

These experiments take time, but if the original experiment has taken some months to perform there seems no reason to begrudge a few days or a week on additional experiments which can be performed by a meticulous and monotony-tolerant technician or clerk.

Estimates of Population Differences

We have repeatedly emphasized the need to go beyond significance testing to estimation of limits of population values. In relation to two-sample comparisons, the question arises: "What population value are we to estimate, and how?" If we assume Gaussian distributions of measurements, with SD's very accurately known, we can estimate upper and lower limits of the difference between the mean in population A and the mean in population B, the usual formula being: Difference between sample means ± 2 SD of differences.

In view of former discussions, however, the assumptions are not very appealing, and we seem to have no basis for our estimate. But how useful would any estimate of the range of possible differences between population *means* really be, even if we could depend on it? Let us suppose that hand-grip changes in rheumatoid arthritis formed Gaussian frequency distributions, and that we had a thoroughly reliable estimate that the superiority of drug B over drug A, as measured by difference in group-mean increase in hand grip (mean B minus mean A), lay between the limits +20 and +50 mm. Hg. When we remember that the mean of a Gaussian distribution is its center — that 50 per cent of the measurements lie above it and 50 per cent lie below it — we begin to wonder what of value we learn from the estimated limits.

It appears that much more meaningful information about limits of differences could be obtained from samples of measurements without questionable assumptions. For illustration we refer to the 14 patients' changes in hand grip (mm. Hg) already studied:

Group A: +32, +20, −10, +90, −9,   0, −60
Group B: +40, +52, +20, +52, +95, +54, +84

The difference has already been shown to exceed what we ordinarily attribute to randomization; but we note now that of the 7 A-treated patients only 3 showed an increase, whereas all 7 B-treated patients did so. It might be of interest to ask whether this difference was compatible with the following population figures:

Treatment	Decrease or No Change (X)	Increase (Not-X)
A	50%	50%
B	30%	70%

This is a matter of estimation of differences between binomial populations, discussed in Chapter XVI, sect. 2. The dividing line could be set at any point that was considered to have practical importance. For example, one of the A's and five of the B's showed an increase of more than 50 mm. Hg. One might ask whether this was compatible with the occurrence of 50 per cent of this class in the A-population and 60 per cent in the B-population.

Required Sample Sizes

The principles of sample size estimation discussed in Chapter VIII, and illustrated by frequency data, hold true also for measurement data, but are difficult to apply to them. Even if we had accurate information about the variation of measurements in a very large sample of A-treated subjects, and even if we knew that their distribution was almost Gaussian, we would seldom know what the B treatment would do to the variation or to the shape of the distribution, and pilot-study samples are as a rule too small to give us that kind of information. Therefore we seldom have a reliable basis for saying that samples of some particular size N would insure that 95 per cent of our experiments would be "successful" in the comparison of the average measurements of A-treated and B-treated groups. If we disregard distribution shapes and use rank-sum methods we are still in difficulty, because we still do not know what difference in variation would be produced by the use of B instead of A.

However, if we follow the line of thought suggested in the discussion of population limit estimates we may see a solution of the problem. Is it so very valuable to know how many individuals would be necessary to establish a difference between the *averages* of the A- and B-treated subjects? In application of results it is often frequencies, above and below a certain value, that we wish to know, rather than averages. Let us suppose, then, that we postulate the population median for A-treated subjects as +20 units of some kind, and call measurements below +20 units "X's." Then we could say: "If a B-treated population would contain only 25 per cent X's, what size of sample would we require to establish the superiority of that treatment?" Table V would provide the answer. If we intended after the experiment to test the difference by average measurements (or rank sums) and not by frequencies, our estimate of N would be needlessly high. We do not know exactly by how much; but we could probably safely reduce it by a fifth.

Comparison of More than Two Samples of Measurements

The two-sample t-test puts into the numerator the difference (variation) between the samples and puts into the denominator the variation within the samples; i.e., it is a form of analysis of variation (commonly called analysis of variance). After it was developed, the same principle was applied to the invention of tests for the comparison of more than two samples, including data from various experiment designs already mentioned, such as randomized blocks, factorial experiments and cross-over experiments. This more elaborate analysis of variance is based on Gaussian distributions as is the t-test and is therefore open to the same doubt when applied to the bizarre data that we create in medicine; but nonparametric methods have not been very extensively developed. However, even somewhat complicated designs produce data of the two-sample form, and therefore are suitable for the simple ranks tests. An example is the two-treatment cross-over experiment.

Analysis of Measurements in a Cross-over Experiment

The data* in this example (Table 8) were used in Chapter XII to show how frequency data (numbers improved, unchanged or deteriorated) in a cross-over experiment can be analyzed, and that section should be reread at this point, because the general principles are the same as in the following analysis. The data were selected from an A-versus-B trial in which the extent of a skin rash was estimated as a percentage of the total skin area by a scheme called the "rule of nines" (head 9 per cent, each arm 9 per cent, anterior trunk 18 per cent, posterior trunk 18 per cent, each leg 18 per cent, groin 1 per cent); the severity of the lesions was graded on a scale of 0 to 4.

We rank the twelve differences – change during period (1) minus change during period (2) – from the extreme negative to the extreme positive, and then we compare the sequences thus:

Sequence	Sum of Ranks
AB	53
BA	25
Total	78

* I am indebted to Dr. R. L. Black, National Institutes of Health, U.S. Public Health Service, for permission to use these data.

Table 8. Extent of Skin Involvement (Per Cent of Total Skin Area) in a Cross-over Trial of Treatments A and B

(Dr. Roger L. Black's data)

Init. = initial value (at beginning of treatment period).
Rank orders are in parentheses after actual values.

Patient	Period(1)			Period(2)			Total $(I - F)$ P(1) + P(2)	Diff. $(I - F)$ P(1) − P(2)
	Init. (I)	Final (F)	Diff. (I−F)	Init. (I)	Final (F)	Diff. (I−F)		
Sequence AB								
Rob.	42	37	+5	37	3	+34	+39 (9)	−29 (3)
Rh.	92	30	+62	30	11	+19	+81 (11)	+43 (12)
Ros.	29	11	+18	11	9	+2	+20 (8)	+16 (9)
Ni.	78	58	+20	58	67	−9	+11 (4)	+29 (11)
Pe.	26	9	+17	9	9	0	+17 (6)	+17 (10)
Ke.	12	10	+2	10	15	−5	−3 (1)	+7 (8)
Sequence BA								
El.	27	31	−4	31	9	+22	+18 (7)	−26 (4)
La.	70	94	−24	94	7	+87	+63 (10)	−111 (1)
Wr.	6	6	0	6	0	+6	+6 (3)	−6 (6)
Ol.	100	87	+13	87	0	+87	+100 (12)	−74 (2)
Ir.	8	7	+1	7	5	+2	+3 (2)	−1 (7)
Sh.	17	19	−2	19	1	+18	+16 (5)	−20 (5)

In Table VIII (see Appendix) under $N_1 = 6$ and $N_2 = 6$, we see that, if we adopt the 5 per cent standard of rarity, a rank sum of 26 in N_1 (or in N_2 since the N's are equal) is small enough to make us conclude that something more than randomization was responsible for the difference (and a rank sum of 52 is large enough to do the same). Since this trial was conducted in such a way that the randomization was responsible for the bias, the "something more" would be the difference in treatment— the fact that the period (1) treatment was A in the AB sequence and B in the BA sequence.

In order to find out whether the sequence *per se* had any influence on the outcome, we use from each patient the sum of his changes, period (1) + period (2). If, for instance, in the BA sequence a benefit from B were continued into the second (A) period, but if A's effect were not carried over in the AB sequence, the total (or average) improvement in the BA group would tend to be larger than in the AB group. In this instance the sums of ranks were identical (39) in both sequences; therefore there was no suggestion of a sequence effect.

Measured Changes versus Qualitative Changes. In Chapter XII the observations in this experiment were recorded, for each period in each patient, as simple direction of change: improvement, no change, deterioration. No convincing difference in the effects of the two treatments could be discovered; and this shows what can be lost in a cross-over experiment when this is the only form of assessment possible. If the same verdict is given for a patient in both periods he cannot contribute information regarding the treatment difference. On the other hand, if we can in some way measure a preference between the outcome in the two periods, a frequency analysis may be sufficient to answer our question regarding the difference in treatment effects. In this experiment the results were as follows:

Sequence	Period of Greater Improvement		Total
	(1)	(2)	
AB	5	1	6
BA	0	6	6
Total	5	7	12

Chi-square (with Yates' correction) $= 5.5$; P (both tails) less than 0.05.

Variation between Individuals
Sometimes it is desirable to know whether the variation among the individual measurements in one sample exceeds the variation in another sample to a greater extent than we can readily attribute to random processes. It is then customary to compare the standard deviations, but the significance test is actually applied to the variances. The larger variance is divided by the smaller, and then a table of variance ratios is consulted, in order to see how rarely the observed ratio is found in sampling from the same Gaussian distribution. With much medical data this is probably even more risky than the t-test. A nonparametric test can be employed instead. For instance, we can, in each sample, find the absolute distance of each measurement from the sample median, and compare these two sets of differences by the rank-sum method.

Individual Variation Relative to Absolute Size
Mice could not possibly vary as much as men in absolute units of length. If we wished to compare them we would ask: "Do they vary as much in proportion to their scale of size?" However, in less extreme comparisons this qualifying clause may be forgotten. An anatomist compared the intersubject variation of (1) lengths of adult human vertebral columns and (2) adult human statures. The intersubject standard deviation was 2.45 cm. for vertebral columns, whereas the usual SD for statures is about 2.5 in. (6.35 cm.) He interpreted the difference as indicating some special stability or growth regulation in the vertebral column; but he overlooked the difference in average length of the column (59.6 cm.) and stature (say, 69.0 in. $= 175.3$ cm.).

The common way of adjusting for differences in size scale is to express each SD as a percentage of the corresponding mean, and call the result the "coefficient of variation." Here are three examples from large series of adult human subjects:

	Mean	SD	CV
Vertebral column	59.6 cm.	2.45 cm.	4.1%
Stature	69.0 in.	2.5 in.	3.6%
Right male femur	46.33 cm.	2.25 cm.	4.8%

There is little difference between the three coefficients, and the ground for the anatomist's inference has disappeared.

The coefficient of variation is used also in the comparison of inter-subject (and intermeasurement) variation when the units of measurement in the two groups differ, e.g., statures and weights. We should, of course, be clear about the rationale of such comparisons. For example, it would perhaps be more sensible to compare the variation in statures with the variation in the cube roots of weights.

In the comparison of the coefficients of variation for vertebral column lengths, statures and femur lengths, there was no need to perform a "significance" test, because the coefficients were so much alike. When two coefficients differ by an amount that would be important if due to more than sampling variation, we are in difficulty regarding tests of significance. Long ago a formula was invented for a standard deviation of the CV, to represent the variation among coefficients of variation calculated for different random samples from the same Gaussian distribution of measurements; but we do not know how far to trust it with samples from non-Gaussian distributions, or even with small or moderate-sized samples from approximately Gaussian distributions. A two-sample ranks test would seem to be appropriate here. It would be applied in the same way as was mentioned for the absolute differences in measurements, except that each difference from the median could be expressed as a percentage of the median.

CHAPTER XV

CONCOMITANT VARIATION
AND TRENDS

The topics encompassed by this chapter heading are multitudinous, and some of them have been the subjects of individual monographs and books. The discussion here is confined to what appears most essential to medical workers — what we need to grasp first and most firmly in this mysterious area. These needs are the same for those who do research as for those who merely try to be rational in the midst of numerical statements produced by increasingly complex mathematical concepts and machines. A few of the simple techniques are essential in much of our small-scale medical research. They are discussed here, but detailed instructions are not given, because the danger of using these techniques without the personal help of a suitable guide is even greater than in the techniques described in the preceding chapters. The discussion is concerned with what we ought to know before we seek guidance. It may also help us to determine whether we have obtained a suitable guide.

Examples of Concomitant Variation

(1) A spring balance becomes progressively longer with increase in the weight attached to it. (2) The longer a child lives, the taller he grows, until he reaches adulthood. (3) As the partial pressure of oxygen in blood plasma increases, the degree of saturation of hemoglobin with oxygen increases also. (4) As the concentration of carbohydrate in a contracting muscle diminishes, the concentration of lactic acid increases. (5) After a single dose of penicillin, as time passes the blood level of that drug rises and then falls. (6) The taller men are, the greater is their average weight. (7) When 60 mice are randomly assigned to 6 dose levels of procaine varying from very low to very high (10 mice at each level), the higher the dose the higher, on the average, is the mortality. (8) During the past few decades the main trend in the reported incidence of diphtheria has been downward. (9) In a study of rheumatic fever in a certain city that contained 23 districts, it was found that the greater the average number of persons per room in apartments

and houses in the various districts, the higher was the incidence of the disease during a 3-year period.

These various relationships are most clearly represented by graphs, with the independent variable along the horizontal (X) axis and the dependent variable along the vertical (Y) axis. We must remember, however, that the term "dependent variable" does not imply an effect of the independent variable (Q II – 1). In each of the nine examples the first-mentioned variable would generally be chosen as X, but not necessarily. If we wished to find the relationship of average stature to weight, we would choose weight as the independent variable.

Before drawing any conclusions from a graph, we must, of course, recall its potential dangers (Q IX – 23).

Cumulative Effects versus Independent Evidence

All the nine examples resemble each other in their general XY form, and we can fit lines, straight or curved, in all of them by similar arithmetical techniques; but actually the first five examples differ in their structure from the remaining four. We attach an ounce weight to a spring balance and measure the distance of the pointer from zero. When we add another ounce and again measure from zero we are measuring the combined effect of the first and second ounces. In measuring penicillin level in the blood we are on each occasion including the effects of accretions and removals that have occurred since the dose was given.

By contrast, in showing the relationship between stature and weight in a group of men, or between mortality and procaine dose level in mice, we obtain independent pieces of information regarding Y at each value of X. Diphtheria incidence presents an interesting feature. Numerically the incidence in any year is free to be higher or lower than in the preceding year, because we do not include in it the previous incidence. Biologically, however, it may not be quite free. For example, even apart from preventive measures, in one year the disease may have caught the most susceptible subjects, or a relatively high incidence may have resulted in the spread of immunization effects among the community. Whenever X represents time we should think of the possibility of cumulative effects.

In this chapter we are concerned with data that give independent evidence of Y for each value of X. In analyzing phenomena in which cumulative effects are present, we must try to see whether they are merely arithmetical. To do so, we can make X represent successive equal intervals, and Y the *change* in the dependent variable during each X-interval; e.g., the growth of a child in each successive 6-month period, or the change in length of a spring with each additional ounce. To see whether the new Y is related to X, we can use the methods discussed here.

The Approach to Analysis

First, we must ask ourselves what we wish to find out. Do we wish to find out whether there is an XY relationship? Do we already know that a relationship exists but wish to define it more precisely? If so, for what purpose? For illustration of detail we can take one of the most familiar of the nine examples, the stature-weight relationship, pretending that we do not know that it exists and that we are making a preliminary study.

Such a simple example can illustrate basic principles common to many kinds of data, but we must not let it mislead us. There are many different purposes that prompt people to analyze concomitant variation, and special techniques are necessary for some of those purposes. None of these are discussed in detail here; but two examples may be mentioned.

The procaine-mortality example was based on an actual experiment which was designed to give an estimate of the dose that would kill 50 per cent of mice. This takes us into an area in which a rather elaborate statistical technique has been developed in connection with dose-response relationships, particularly for use in bioassay of drugs that cannot be isolated as individual chemical compounds.

The diphtheria-incidence example calls to mind infectious-disease studies with various purposes, such as attempts to predict future incidence by reference to observed rhythms, and the testing of theories regarding the spread of diseases.

The Stature-Weight Relationship

Except that many data on statures and weights are crude and unreliable, they illustrate the safest way to find out whether relationships between variables exist, and to measure them — by collecting large masses of data, displaying them in tabular form and doing some simple arithmetic, such as medians and other percentiles. The eye is then often a sufficient test of "significance." In many studies, however, this vast accumulation of data would be a waste of time, at least in the preliminary stages; and in very many cases it would be impossible to obtain large enough samples, because even a sample of several hundred measurements is small when it has to be divided into a number of subgroups, representing a number of different variables or different values of the same variable. Therefore we have to use more complicated methods.

Table 9. Statures and Weights in a Random Sample of 20 Male University Students

Stature (X) (inches)	Weight (Y) (pounds)	Stature (X) (inches)	Weight (Y) (pounds)
64	132	69	153
66	159	69	130
67	137	69	149
67	130	70	215
68	168	71	166
68	136	71	145
68	142	72	150
68	169	72	169
68	133	73	182
69	135	73	138

Table 9 shows the statures and weights of 20 men taken at random from the records of the thousand male students utilized for illustration of stature frequencies in Chapter XIII. With the pretense that there was no prior information regarding the relationship of stature and weight, a scatter diagram (dot diagram) was drawn, with X as stature and Y as weight, each student represented by a dot. If a reader wishes to repeat this graph he will probably not be convinced that a stature-weight relationship existed, unless he lets himself be influenced by his prior knowledge. In an actual study, however, he would wish to know whether there was evidence of anything beyond a random scatter of the Y's in relation to the X's.

Frequency Tests

With some types of data a frequency test will tell us all that we wish to know about XY relationships. If so, we can divide the data into quadrants by taking a point at or near the median of X and the median of Y. Here we can take 69 inches and 147 pounds, and construct a fourfold contingency table:

	Below 147 Pounds	Above 147 Pounds
Below 69″	6	3
69″ and over	4	7

Chi-square (with Yates' correction) $= 0.8$ approximately, and does not suggest anything but a random relationship. The stature-weight relationship that existed in the thousand students was not strong enough to be demonstrated in this sample by this method.

Rank-order Relationships

More sensitive than a frequency test is one that makes use of the relationships of the individual X and Y measurements to each other. It is possible to do this by assigning ranks to X and Y and expressing the relationship of the ranks by an index. This method will be outlined later. It is a simple method, useful if we are seeking only for evidence of a slope, upward or downward, of one variable as we pass from lower to higher values of the other variable. However, it does not tell us about the gradient of the slope, or its position in relation to the X and Y axes. Moreover, it does not open the door to the study of more complex associations, such as curvilinear relationships of X and Y, or multiple relationships, e.g., between weight, stature and pelvic width.

The method that gives us information about gradients and positions of lines, and can also be used for the study of complex relationships, is called "regression analysis."

Straight-line Regression

The basic meaning of "regression," i.e., "going back," does not help us to understand its present technical meaning. The method gives us an average trend or slope of the dots in a scatter diagram; and as a first approximation we usually represent this average by a straight line.

If we had to find this straight line on our own, without knowing anything about "regression," it would seem reasonable to start at the center of the series of dots, i.e., at the median of X and the median of Y. Through this center we could draw a horizontal line and then rotate it, trying to fit it as closely as possible to the dots. To find the closeness of fit we could measure from it vertically, up and down, to each dot, i.e., we could find the "deviation" of each Y value from the line. We could add the deviations together, without signs, and decide to accept as the "best-fitting" line the one that produced a smaller sum of deviations than any other line. We would, however, have no guarantee that only one position and slope of the line would meet this criterion, and in any case we would soon become frustrated by this trial-and-error method.

We might then adopt another approach — to find an average slope first and then draw a straight line with that slope through the center of the series of dots (medians of X and Y). To calculate the average slope we could find for each dot its deviation from the median X and from the median Y, and write: Slope = Y-deviation/X-deviation. For example, if the medians were 69″ and 147 pounds, a stature of 72″ and a weight of 169 pounds would produce the ratio $+22/+3 = +7.3$. The average of all twenty ratios could be taken as the average slope of the line. We would, however, have no assurance that the line would fit the dots closer than, or even as close as, many other lines.

We can get ourselves out of these difficulties if we are willing to accept:

1. The arithmetic means of X and Y, instead of the medians, as the center-point through which the line must be drawn.

2. The minimum sum of squares of Y-deviations from the line as the criterion of "best fit."

For any set of dots in a plane there is only one straight line that meets these conditions, and it can be found by a rather simple calculation.

We will see later something of the origin of this method, but at present we may note that the minimum sum of squares does not appear so arbitrary if we recall that in any set of measurements (or other numbers) the sum of squares of deviations from the mean is less than the sum of squares of deviations from any other quantity. That is, if we were forbidden to find the mean directly, we could find it by trial and error, taking first one figure and then another, and finding each time the sum of squares of deviations from it, until we arrived at the figure that produced the least sum of squares. When using the regression method we are seeking an average line instead of an average point, but we adopt the same criterion, the minimum sum of squares of deviations.

Linear Regression Equations

In order to see the structure and function of the equation that enables us to draw a straight regression line, let us suppose that we choose x, any value of the X variable, and wish to find the value of Y on the regression line vertically above x. If $\bar{x}$ is the mean of the observed X's, $\bar{y}$ is the mean of the observed Y's, and b is the slope of the line, the rectilinear (or linear) regression equation is:

$$Y = \bar{y} + b(x - \bar{x})$$

Since $\bar{y}$ and $b\bar{x}$ are numerical constants we can add them and write: $Y = bx + k$.

For the data from the 20 students (Table 9), with statures in inches and weight in pounds, the equation becomes:

$$Y = 151.90 + 3.32(x - 69.10) \text{ pounds; or } Y = 3.32x - 77.51 \text{ pounds.}$$

This equation shows, for those students, the linear regression of weight on stature (W/S). Obviously, if we choose the mean stature as our x value we have Y = mean weight. Therefore if we wished to insert this line in the dot diagram we could use the mean values as one point and take one other point calculated from the equation, but it is better to use three points as a check on our arithmetic.

Linear Regression Coefficients

The coefficient b, with its plus or minus sign, indicates the slope of the line — both its direction and gradient, or rate of change of Y per unit change of X, in this example 3.32 pounds per inch.

The structure of b looks rather puzzling. Letting $(x - \bar{x})$ stand for any X-deviation, $(y - \bar{y})$ for any Y-deviation, and S for "sum of all such quantities," we have:

$$b = \frac{S\{(x - \bar{x})(y - \bar{y})\}}{S(x - \bar{x})^2}$$

The mean of the sum of products of deviations is called the "covariance" of X and Y, i.e., the concomitant variation of the two variables. The mean sum of squares for X is the variance of X. Since the divisor (sample size) is the same for the covariance and variance, we disregard it; but actually the regression coefficient is the covariance divided by the variance of the independent variable.

A few lines of elementary calculus show how the coefficient b acquires its structure when we start with the requirement that the sum of squares of Y-deviations shall be as small as possible; but the details of this need not concern us. What we would like to know is why we should use the least-squares method at all.

The Least-squares Method

It is pleasant to have a simple automatic device for inventing a straight line to fit our data; but we should ask such questions as: "Is the device anything more than a convention?" "If we select an X value and then find the corresponding Y value from the equation, what does it tell us about the real X's and Y's in our sample, or about the X's and Y's in a population randomly represented by our sample?"

In order to have some basis for answering such questions, we must glance at the origin of the least-squares method. To its originators early in the 19th century it was more than a convenient device for inventing a line. It arose as part of the effort to find a "best" estimate to be derived from physical measurements that differed from each other because of experimental error — the effort that led to the development of the "Gaussian curve of error." Recalling the remarks in Chapter XIII about arithmetic means, we can say that the arithmetic mean of a random sample from a Gaussian distribution is the "best" estimate of the center of that distribution because:

1. It is unbiased; that is, as we take larger and larger random samples we are led toward the true center (mean, median and mode) of the parent distribution.

2. Sample means vary less from each other than do other estimates of the center of the distribution, such as the median. Therefore they are more "efficient" than the other types of estimates — they require smaller samples to give us the same proximity to the true center.

We can, with a modification, extend this statement to any kind of measurements. Without restriction to any distribution-shape, we can say that, in the sense just defined, sample means provide the "best" estimates of population means; but they are not, of course, estimates of the centers of the parent distributions unless those distributions are symmetrical.

With these ideas in mind we can try to picture in an elementary fashion the concepts of those who developed the least-squares method. Let us visualize, at each X-value in the graph, a very large number of Y's arranged in frequency distributions. The bases of these distributions would lie along the vertical lines (ordinates) of the graph, and their tops (frequencies) would stick up into the air at right angles to the graph paper. At first, of course, Gaussian distributions were visualized, representing the supposed "law of error"; but it was subsequently shown that the shape need not be Gaussian. The essential feature is that the mean Y-values of these distributions shall form a straight line, which would be the "true" or population regression line of Y on X in the graph.

Let us now suppose that we took random samples from the Y-distributions (one or more items from each) and found for each sample a straight line by the least-squares method, just as was done for the statures and weights of the twenty students. The lines would be very unlikely to coincide with the population regression line. Some would be above it in the graph, others below it, and their slopes would vary. However, they would have the same desirable qualities as do the means of samples from single distributions of measurements:

1. They would be unbiased — as we increased our sample size we would come closer and closer to the population regression line.

2. The variation between the lines would be less than if we invented lines by some other method than the least-squares technique.

It is these mathematically demonstrated facts that justify the use of the least-squares technique in the artificial world that we have visualized. The important question is: "How is the method justified in the real world?"

Discrepancies in the Real World.   A straight line is an abstraction. Even in the most familiar everyday example of a straight-line relationship, a spring balance, we know that by more and more precise measurement we would find irregularities as we added weights by small increments from zero to the maximum capacity. For each balance we could find an irregular curve of weight-length relationship; but in the manufacturing and standardizing of a balance all that is necessary is to attach in succession a series of standard weights, mark the position of the pointer at each weight, and then divide the intervals between these marks into equal segments. The approximate straight-line relationship is safe within these intervals, the width of which will depend on the purpose for which the balance is to be used.

Biologic material is even more irregular than physical material. If we have a sample of adult statures and weights it may show no evidence that a curve would represent the true stature-weight relationship better than does a straight line; but we can easily imagine the existence of a curved relationship in the population. For example, let us suppose that among tall men those who had the same height-weight relationship as did the medium-sized or short men had a lower survival rate than those who were not so heavy in proportion to their height. There would then be a tendency for the population regression line to reduce its upward slope in the higher stature classes. In this instance we could look for evidence of the relationship by examining more subjects; but in most research we wish in the first place to find out whether Y has an overall relationship to X that can, to a large extent, be represented by a straight line. The question then is: "What are the advantages in the least-squares method of inventing a straight line by which to test that hypothesis?"

Some Advantages of the Least-squares Method

Three points may be mentioned in support of the least-squares method:

1. In some respects this technique resembles many other techniques that we use in medicine. A blood pressure reading, made by arm cuff and sphygmomanometer, does not give us a patient's intra-arterial pressure, nor do we know the correction terms that would enable us to calculate that pressure in each particular patient. Nevertheless, external blood pressure readings are found useful when made by a simple and uniform procedure. Similarly, neither the least-squares method nor any other technique will enable us to find from a sample the true (population)

values of the mean Y's corresponding to the X's, and we seldom know what correction to make for the discrepancy; but the least-squares method is easy to learn and it is, of course, so uniform that anyone who does the arithmetic properly will obtain the same answer from the same set of observations.

2. We might, of course, adopt some other simple and equally objective method such as the one mentioned earlier, whereby an estimate of the slope was made, from each pair of X and Y measurements, in the form of a ratio, and then the ratios were averaged. It is interesting to note one difference in the effects of the two techniques. Let us suppose that there are dots on the graph at some distance apart and that we use them in estimating the slope of the line.

Dot No.	Deviation $(x - \bar{x})$	Deviation $(y - \bar{y})$	Ratio $(y - \bar{y})/(x - \bar{x})$	Product $(x - \bar{x})(y - \bar{y})$
(1)	+2	+4	+2	+8
(2)	+8	+16	+2	+128

In the ratio method the contributions of (1) and (2) to the average slope would be the same($+2$), whereas in the regression equation dot(2) would contribute much more than dot(1) to the numerator of the regression coefficient. When we observe that dot(2) has carried the same slope much farther from the center than dot(1) it seems appropriate that dot(2) should carry more weight in the regression coefficient.

3. A strong argument in favor of the least-squares method is that it can be taken far beyond the fitting of a straight line — to curve fitting and to the simultaneous analysis of the interrelationships of more than two variables.

In a more orthodox presentation a fourth argument in favor of the least-squares method would be adduced — that it leads directly to significance testing and to estimation of population values. For reasons that will emerge later, that argument is not used here; but we must look into these problems of inferences from regressions that have been found in samples.

Inferences from Sample Regressions

Having found a straight regression line from our data, if we follow the orthodox procedure we can obtain an impressive array of figures:

1. We can test the "significance" of the regression coefficient by a t-test which will answer, or purport to answer, the very important question: If the slope of the regression line in the population were zero, and we took random samples of the same size as our observed sample, would we rarely find as large a value of b as in our sample?" The t ratio in this test is built up very sensibly, as are the t's mentioned in Chapter XIV. The coefficient b is the numerator. The denominator contains a standard deviation which is derived from the scatter of the observed dots (their

deviations from the regression line), because obviously our confidence in an apparent slope should be greater if the dots are close to the line than if they are more widely scattered. We can find the P value corresponding to t by using the same (Fisher) table as was mentioned in Chapter XIV.

2. We can estimate limits for the population value of b.

3. We can estimate limits for the population value of any Y that we calculate from the regression equation.

4. We can estimate the range of variation of individual measurements in terms of a standard deviation derived from the scatter of the dots, and then we can draw lines on each side of the regression line at multiples of SD; e.g., ± 2 SD purports to include 95 per cent of all the dots in the population, excluding 2.5 per cent above the regression line and 2.5 per cent below it.

The catch in all this procedure lies in the picture that we must visualize and accept as real, in order to have faith in the values that emerge from our arithmetic. In visualizing the distributions of Y-values at each X-value, we must now picture not only the mean Y's lying along a straight line as described above. We must visualize all these distributions as Gaussian, and all their standard deviations must be the same. We have to stretch our imaginations even more than when dealing with Gaussian-derived tests and estimates in Chapter XIV. If we had so many hundreds of observations that we could feel confident that the various conditions were sufficiently well met, we would hardly need to go through the regression calculation in the first place.

If, however, we decline to make such assumptions about the parent population of our sample, we do not need to forfeit the least-squares method of fitting a regression line, nor do we need to forego testing the data to see how often random processes alone might have created the apparent XY relationship. The following remarks are merely suggestions, but they indicate how the "nonparametric" methods discussed in Chapter XIV might be extended.

A Nonparametric Test of Slope.   Having drawn through the mean X and mean Y, on graph paper or in our imagination, a straight line found by least-squares or any other method, we can insert a horizontal line that also passes through the means. Then we can pose the following question: "If the observed Y-values were assigned to the observed X-values by a strictly random method such as card shuffling, and if the assignment were repeated many times, how often would we find as much evidence in favor of a sloping line as we did in the actual experiment?" In trying to answer that question, we need not perform the randomization. For each of the observed Y-values we can find its deviation (vertical distance) from the sloping line and from the superimposed horizontal line. Omitting the signs of the deviations, we can find for each Y-value the difference between its deviations from the two lines, and then we can affix plus signs to those cases in which the deviation from the horizontal line is the greater, and minus signs where the reverse is true. The signed-ranks test (Chapter XIV) can then be applied. (It might be argued that, in accordance with the least-squares principle of fitting, the squares of the deviations should be used in this test rather than the absolute deviations; but the purpose here is to suggest a principle rather than prescribe a specific technique.)

Scatter of Individuals

Having decided that we will not accept random processes as a sufficient explanation of the slope of a line, we often behave in the same way as we do after comparing two samples of measurements. There we act as if the difference between the two averages was the most important feature; here we often attach the same importance to the average trend, i.e., the regression line.

Even when we measure the scatter of individuals in relation to the regression line we often confuse a small scatter, measured in absolute units, with high precision. Some cadaver bones were x-rayed and their shadow densities were determined by a photoelectric method. Then the bones were analyzed chemically and their mineral content (Y) was plotted against their shadow densities (X). A regression line was calculated and the scatter of points about the line, in absolute units of mineral matter, was impressively small. This was taken as evidence that x-ray densitometry could be substituted for chemical analysis, which is not only time-consuming but destroys the material under study.

Apparently no attention was paid to the size of the possible error in relation to the total mineral matter of a bone; but examination of the published figures showed that the densitometric method would not uncommonly over- or underestimate the mineral content by more than 10 per cent. For estimation of the average mineral content of a group of bones, densitometry might well be satisfactory, because the variable error (the plus and minus deviations from the regression line) would tend to average out; but the method hardly seemed adequate for individual bones.

Reduction of Intersubject Variation by Regression Analysis

In tables of standard adult human weights, statures are given in order that we can assess individuals more precisely, because the weight variation within each stature class is smaller than the weight variation when stature is disregarded. If we joined the mean weights of the various stature classes we would produce an empirical weight-on-stature regression line; and this illustrates the effect of the regression analysis, which we must use when, as is commonly the case, samples are too small to provide reliable mean Y-values for each value of X.

We can express the effect in general terms thus: Variation of Y represented by Y/X regression + Variation from regression line = Total variation of Y. Indeed, if we express variation as sums of squares of deviations (from means and from regression lines) this is an exact arithmetical statement regarding any set of paired (X and Y) measurements. It does not depend on any assumptions of population values or distribution shapes.

Let us suppose, now, that we did not know the relationship of weight to stature, that stature measuring was a difficult or expensive procedure and that we wished to find out whether it would provide a profitable adjustment or correction term in assessment of the weights of individuals. We might take 100 subjects, probably fewer in the first instance, and find the weight/stature regression line. If we planned to use the upper and lower 10th percentiles (or any other values) as cut-off points in weight assessment, it would be impossible to mark these points reliably for each individual stature value. Therefore we would act as if the weight variation from regression were equal at all statures. We would then arrange all the deviations from regression in order, from the largest negative to the largest positive deviation, and insert the cut-off points that we had decided upon. We would thus avoid the assumption that the individuals were scattered around the regression line in a Gaussian distribution.

In order to see what benefit might accrue from the use of the weight/stature regression, we would have to realize that, whether we took stature into account or not, we could always classify the same *proportion* of subjects (e.g., 20 per cent) as lying outside our chosen range. Having used the weight/stature regression, we could take each subject and find out how we would classify him (e.g., on the 10th percentile standard) by the two methods: (a) without taking account of stature, (b) by use of the deviations from weight/stature regression. Any subject that was classified differently by the two methods would be considered a "misclassification" because the more sensitive method (b) would be taken as the standard. The percentage of misclassifications would afford a measure of the advantage of correcting for stature.

Regression in Intergroup Comparisons

The foregoing imaginary weight/stature example illustrates one of the chief uses of regression in research — to increase precision or sensitivity. This function is particularly useful in the comparison of groups. A classical example is an animal-feeding experiment. Two or more different diets are randomly assigned, usually each diet to the same number of animals. After a certain period the changes in weight of the groups are compared with each other.

It is known that animals that have different initial weights may show different amounts of weight gain, even on the same diet. With small laboratory animals the effect may be avoided by choosing a very narrow range of initial weight, but with larger animals this may materially restrict the number of suitable individuals. In any case a wider generalization is possible if experimental subjects are more varied than if they are highly selected — provided that the variation can be prevented from seriously lowering the sensitivity of the experiment.

In this connection we should note that if we paid no attention at all to initial weight, either by selection of animals or by adjustment of the data, the randomization would nevertheless provide a valid inference. If we found, at the end of the experiment, a treatment-group difference in weight gain that was, say, "significant at the 1 per cent level," we could say: "This may be the result of a bias due to many factors, including differences in initial weight; but the randomization would cause that amount of bias less than once in a hundred trials." Our concern about variation in initial weight is, therefore, not fear of a spuriously significant difference, but fear that a real effect will be masked.

Percentage gains may be used as a means of correcting for initial weight differences, but that involves an assumption, or demonstration, that this is an appropriate method. It seems more sensible to let the data themselves produce a correction term, and that is what is done by regression analysis. Using only two dietary groups for simplicity, we can picture the procedure, in essence, as follows. We find the regression of weight gain (Y) on initial weight (X) among animals that are on the same diet (each dietary group provides a contribution to this estimate). We draw the regression line through the mean X and mean Y of all the animals, and then we insert a dot for each group to show its mean gain plotted against its mean initial weight.

The mean gains of the two groups may not differ very much, i.e., the two dots may be about the same height on the Y-axis — say, +60 gm. Let us suppose, however, that they differ considerably in mean initial weight, and that the regression line slopes upward — the greater the initial weight, the greater, on the average, is the gain in weight of animals on the same diet. Then the two dots will have different relationships to the regression line. Let us suppose that the group (A) with lower initial weight is 10 gm. (in weight gain) above the line and that the other group (B) is 10 gm. below the line. Group A has gained more than would be expected simply from the relationship of gain to initial weight, and group B has gained less than would be expected. To adjust for difference in initial weight, we take the sum of the distances from the regression line, i.e., $10 + 10 = 20$ gm. Such differences are usually tested for "significance" by t (or by the variance-ratio test, mentioned in Chapter XIV, if there are more than two groups), but this is a secondary matter, because ranks tests or other nonparametric tests could be used.

When we employ the regression method in this way after a properly conducted experiment it is reassuring to remember that we do not thereby commit ourselves to assumptions about linearity of means in the parent populations (or even in the samples), or Gaussian distributions, or equality of variation of Y at all the X-values. It may well be that the XY relationship is not the same at certain values of X as at other values; i.e., the correction may not be equally good among all animals or subgroups. Perhaps, therefore, our regression line ought to be higher at one part and lower at another part, and perhaps curved; and our final verdict about the difference in dietary effects may be due to this. Our protection, as usual, is the random assignment of subjects to treatments. This assures that the various sources of bias, including possible defects in the adjustment by regression, will not lead to false verdicts of "significance" any more often than we decide when we set our Type I error.

The correction or adjustment by straight-line regression is called "covariance adjustment"; but we can do the same kind of thing by curved regression lines.

Correction by regression analysis is useful also in surveys, but there we must remember as usual that because we cannot randomize the variables that are under examination, when we come to test for "significance" we are at the mercy of uncontrolled and unknown biases, and in this case these include biases due to defective correction methods.

More Complex Regressions

There are two kinds of regression that are more complex than the two-variable (XY) linear reression: curvilinear regression and multiple regression.

The discussion under Q IX – 23 to Q IX – 26 emphasizes the importance of applying good sense before and after the fitting of curves and expressing complex relationships mathematically. Here we give a little more detail.

Curvilinear Regression. There are many types of curves that can show concomitant variation of X and Y, but for only a few of them are systematic methods of least-squares fitting readily available. Sometimes the problem can be removed by transforming one or both variables, so that the relationship becomes approximately linear, e.g., X or Y or both of them may be replaced by their logarithms.

If we wish merely to find whether a simple curve fits the data better than a straight line, a parabola, represented by a quadratic equation, $Y = b_1x + b_2x^2 + k$, is useful; and the fitting by least-squares has been developed into a simple routine procedure. Higher orders of the same (polynomial) series contain also x^3, x^4, and so on.

Multiple Regression. The idea of making allowance for more than one variable at a time is familiar in medicine. If we use pelvic widths as well as statures in assessing men's weights, our estimates will have less error than if we use either statures or pelvic widths alone, and this relationship is applied in some of the weight tables used for clinical assessment. We can express the relationship by saying that even among men of the same stature the weight varies according to breadth, which is measured by pelvic width. This could be represented by an equation:

$$\text{Weight} = b_1(\text{stature}) + b_2(\text{pelvic width}) + k$$

We call this a *multiple regression* equation because it shows more than one relationship. It is called also a *partial regression* equation because it shows the weight-stature relationship and the weight-width relationship separate from each other. The particular equation shown here represents straight-line relationships, but multiple regression equations can represent curved relationships also, e.g., x^2 can be introduced.

The numerical values of the b's and of the constant k are calculated by the least-squares method. Ordinarily the b's are tested for "significance" by the t-test, and population estimates are also made by methods derived from Gaussian distributions. That is, the tests and estimates depend for validity on the same conditions as in the two-variable linear regression. However, this does not in itself deprive multiple regression of usefulness, because nonparametric methods could be used in testing. Of greater importance are certain features inherent in the equation itself. In the weight-stature-width equation, for example, when changes are made in the two X's their effects on Y are additive; and the effect of a particular change in X_2 is the same for all values of X_1. For instance, if a difference of 1 inch in pelvic width in men 66" tall was accompanied by an average weight difference of p pounds, the equation implies that a 1-inch pelvic width difference in men 72" tall would also be accompanied by an average weight difference of p pounds.

The computation required for an equation containing more than three independent variables is somewhat heavy for a desk calculator, because many digits have to be retained from one step to the next. Electronic computers have, of course, made it possible to work with enormous numbers (even hundreds) of independent variables, and have thereby introduced a problem that ought to be looked at, even by those medical workers who will themselves never produce even a simple two-variable regression line.

The Problem of Many Variables

In a proposed study of the factors that affected the utilization of hospitals in a certain state the following plan was drawn up. Two hundred randomly selected administrative areas out of the total 307 such units in the state were to be studied. In each unit the dependent variable (hospitalization rate) and fourteen independent variables were to be recorded. The hospitalization rate for a particular year was defined as the number of persons discharged from hospitals in that year per thousand population. (For technical reasons which need not detain us, discharge rate was chosen in preference to admission rate.) The independent variables were in three groups:

1. Patient variables, such as the rural-urban population ratio, percentage of persons over age 65, index of educational level, and percentage coverage by medical care insurance.

2. Hospital variables, such as the number of hospital beds per thousand population.

3. Physician variables, such as the number of physicians per thousand population, percentage in general practice, and average length of time since graduation.

This example has not been chosen in order to stigmatize the methods of sociologists or other behavioral scientists, but for three reasons:

1. Social scientists make more systematic efforts to study multiple variables than is commonly done in medicine, and therefore they provide more complex examples.

2. Social scientists are now exploring problems of patient care, and we should be able to appreciate their difficulties and evaluate their results.

3. Now that MD's and electronic engineers are getting together, it will probably not be long before many-termed multiple regression equations will appear in medical literature that will purport to tell us what factors determine the occurrence, frequency and severity of various diseases, and to predict their outcome. It should not be difficult to translate the remarks that will be made about the present example into terms applicable to etiology and prognosis. Indeed, some of the sociologic variables might well be transferred directly.

A Complex Equation. In the plan of the hospitalization study a regression equation was visualized, constructed from the 200 pieces of information that would be obtained (one from each unit) on each of the 15 variables. Y would be the hospitalization rate and each of the 14 independent variables would be an X, with its appropriate coefficient b, and there would, of course, be a numerical constant k.

The first thing to notice about this equation (and about the complete list of 15 variables) is that a certain independent variable is missing — the number or percentage of sick persons (or of persons suitable for hospitalization) in each unit. This information would be difficult to obtain, but some investigators would probably decline to study the other variables unless they could characterize each unit area by some measure of the amount of sickness present. Even if medical and hospital care were covered entirely by insurance, it would be risky to assume that the ratio of hospitalized persons to the number of persons suitable for hospitalization was constant throughout the 200 areas. However, our concern should be chiefly with what the investigators thought that their equation would show them.

Inferences from the Equation. It was stated that the equation would show the order of importance of the independent variables and would provide clues to action, such as the development of medical care plans, building of new hospitals, and the training of physicians. If, as these statements seemed to imply, there were to be direct steps from the equation to action, those who took the steps might find, after enormous expense, that their feet were in fourteen *post hoc* fallacies. An equation is perhaps the most thorough disguise for the distinction between association and cause. By changing the value of X we change the value of Y — in the equation, but not necessarily in the real world, or to the same degree, or even in the same direction, as the equation indicates.

The equation might show that an increase in the proportion of city dwellers would increase the hospitalization rate, if all the other X's remained the same, but actually they would be very unlikely to remain the same. For example, the increase in city dwellers might well be due to an increase of younger people (in proportions not represented by the age-variable in the equation) and they would need less hospitalization per person than the city dwellers in the equation. Or the equation might show that an increase in medical insurance coverage would increase the hospitalization rate; whereas in fact increased coverage might prompt people to go to doctors earlier in illness and so prevent the need for hospitalization, and also, perhaps, prevent the spread of disease to others.

A regression equation, derived from a cross-sectional survey, thus presents a static picture of a number of abstract relationships. It is based on a "mathematical model," and we have to ask: "How do we know that the mathematical model represents the real phenomena completely enough for the investigators' purposes?" Before looking at the model, however, we should note a difficulty that would arise, even if the model were adequate, and even if the equation portrayed causal relationships. This is the problem of the relative importance of the various independent variables.

Relative Importance of Variables. One way of judging relative importance is to assume that if a particular regression coefficient is not "significantly" different from zero, the variable to which it is attached has in fact no effect, or very little effect. This is unsatisfactory because the decision depends on an arbitrary level of "significance," often a convention adopted without much thought. Obviously, one ought to ask: "How big may the effect of this variable be, if it actually has an effect?"

Even when regression coefficients are clearly "significant," their relative sizes do not show their relative importance. Let us suppose that the size of the regression coefficient attached to the number of hospital beds per thousand population were five times the size of the coefficient attached to the physicians' average length of time since graduation. That would mean that a difference of one unit in the hospital bed variable would have five times the effect on Y (hospitalization rate) that would be produced by a difference of one unit in the physicians' graduation variable; but clearly the ratio depends on the units used in measuring the variables.

Here we meet with a problem that is common to all studies of the relative weights of different kinds of factors, whether regression analysis or any other method is employed. When action is proposed, some common unit is necessary. Here it might be dollars required on the one hand for hospital building and on the other hand for the postgraduate education of doctors. Leaving that question to administrators, we return to the investigators' proposed mathematics.

The "Mathematical Model." In trying to find out whether the hospitalization rate equation is based on a model that would be safe in application to the real world, we are not concerned with the fact that the investigators planned to survey a random sample of administrative units instead of all the units in the state, or with the doubts that must arise when anyone applies to such data the methods of significance testing, and of estimating population values, that are derived from the Gaussian curve.

Perhaps the best way to grasp the problem is to imagine that the investigators had an indefinitely large "population" of administrative units, and of persons within each unit, subjected to the same factors that acted on the material that they planned to examine in the actual survey. That is, if some categories of persons, or some levels of the variables, had few or no representatives in the population, or if there were different relationships between the fifteen variables within the different subgroups, these features would not be due to scarcity of persons. They would be due to factors of various kinds — physical, pathologic, psychologic, sociologic, economic or other factors — that would prevent certain subclasses from containing individuals, and would create real differences in the relationships among the fifteen variables in different categories of the total population.

We are imagining a population so large that, without any regression calculation, the investigators could actually observe and record all the relationships among the fifteen variables. Let us suppose that, having done so, they pretended that they did not possess the information and performed a regression analysis on the total population, just as they planned to do on their sample of 200 units. The difference between the equation, thereby produced, and the relationships that they had actually seen in the population could be called the "systematic error" of the regression analysis, arising from the fact that the population did not fit the mathematical model on which the least-squares technique is based.

Even from our scanty knowledge of such data we can see that in some parts the fit would be very bad, much worse than with many physical and biologic measurements. For example, one of the variables was the ratio of rural to urban dwellers in each area; another was the percentage of the population engaged in farming. In areas where there was a very high proportion of city dwellers we could not visualize a wide range of percentages of farmers, against which to plot hospitalization rates; but the mathematical model pretends that we can do so, and that we will find the same relationship (a particular straight line or curve) as the one that we find in the areas where most persons live in the country.

And so we have to admit that, even as a static picture, we do not know how far the regression equation may be from the truth. Moreover, we cannot be reassured by finding that the measurements agree closely with the equation that has been derived from them. If we had one Y-value for each X-value in a graph and if we worked long enough we could find an equation for a line that would pass through every dot. Then the "prediction" of Y from X would be "perfect"; but it would not tell us how true a picture we had of the relationships in the population.

We can, of course, make moving pictures, as well as static pictures, by multiple regression — by longitudinal instead of cross-sectional surveys. Then the X's and the Y represent changes instead of absolute values; but the mathematical model and its ability to create fiction remain essentially the same as in a cross-sectional study.

The Attitude of Experimenters. Most sociologists and other students of populations recognize, at least verbally, the imperfections of the regression model; but few of them reject it as a tool. In justifying the use of it they say that there must be, as one of them expressed, "a constant checking of results obtained, by comparison with results obtained by other methods." This appears to be a sound principle, but I am not qualified to say how successful it is in sociology, or how often it receives mere lip-service, while inferences from multivariate analysis, unverified by other methods, win academic kudos for their perpetrators and impress other people, including administrators, because electronic computers have been used in producing the results. In medicine, certainly, this kind of thing can happen unless we are aware of the danger.

The method that has led to the advancement of scientific knowledge, in the search for causes or merely for association of variables, has been the formation of carefully considered hypotheses and the testing of them by methods that have eliminated or controlled variables other than those under study. More than one hypothesis can be tested at a time, as in factorial experiments, but always the design is systematic.

This kind of approach to survey data, the experimenter's approach, was mentioned under Q IV – 4. It is a method that requires much thought in the selection of relevant data, in order to test hypotheses with as little "contamination" as possible. It is a slow, awkward, often hesitant and frustrating process, in comparison with the automatic, streamlined and "sophisticated" multiple regression method. Also, it seems to tell us much less than does multiple regression, which will give us verdicts simultaneously on as many hypotheses as we desire, if we put that number of independent variables into the equation. In applying the experimenter's method to the same data we might not find enough diverse information about many of the variables to test the hypotheses regarding them.

But what is the use of fourteen verdicts, or forty, or four hundred, if we do not know how far we can trust any of them? The experimenter's approach would give us isolated pieces of information, but it would be much more likely to be information about associations that existed in the material under study. Out of it would come questions and suggestions for further investigation. Some of these suggestions could actually be in the form of equations, but specifically designed equations, to be tested on other data. It should be mentioned that this attitude to the use of multiple regression and other mass analyses of survey data (including "factor analysis," which is not the same as the factorial experiment design) is not confined to biologic or medical experimenters. It is the attitude of an increasing number of experimentally minded behavioral scientists.

Complex Mathematics in Medicine

The foregoing remarks should not be construed as skepticism regarding the value of higher mathematics and of electronic computers in the advancement of medical knowledge. Even as mere time-savers, computers are making possible more complicated and more thorough studies of phenomena than were previously possible. For instance, a physiologic instrument such as an electrocardiograph can feed its observations directly into a computer which, by previous "instruction," can store measurements and perform analyses that would otherwise require an impossibly large amount of time and labor. This is basically the same kind of help that a desk calculator provides; but computers have also opened a new kind of opportunity in research.

For example, when studying a complex system such as a neural mechanism or a metabolic process an investigator can imitate it in the machine — the technical term is "simulation." That is, he can introduce into the machine all that he knows about the system, and also factors that he thinks may account for certain features in the behavior of the system. When he sets the machine system in motion he is able not only to compare its results with that of the real system, but also to study the internal working of the machine system. For instance, if the production of a certain chemical substance in the real system is imitated in the machine system by the accumulation of a certain electric charge, the investigator can arrange that the level of the charge will affect the processes that lead to its accumulation, and thus he can study the effects of this "feed-back" mechanism. Then he can return to the real system and devise an experiment to see whether the same mechanism is acting there.

The words that should be capitalized in the last sentence are "return to the real system and devise an experiment." This is the motto that can prevent this newly opening path of research from leading to pseudo-science. It is also a yardstick by which those of us who are ignorant of the techniques can evaluate the reported results of computer work and other advanced mathematics in medicine.

Operations Research

The study of complex systems is entering medicine also in what is called "operations research" (in England, "operational" research). This has been defined as "the application of scientific methods to the sort of problems that confront executive authorities" (Bailey, in *Medical Surveys and Clinical Trials*, edited by Witts). It was developed during World War II as a means of solving such problems as the determination of the optimal size of a convoy of ships for protection against enemy attack. The method has since been applied to many types of activity, such as manufacturing processes and a bus transportation system; and now it is starting to be used in analysis of the operation of hospitals.

First, a definition of "optimal" efficiency of the system must be decided upon, which is not an easy task. Then records are made of variables in the system, and the relationships are analyzed mathematically, often with the aid of electronic computers, and sometimes "simulation" is used. Finally, recommendations are made for the improvement of the system. All this is usually done by engineers who have specialized in operations research. The rest of us, in evaluating proposals for, or results of, such a study, have to look at the behavior of the specialists with regard to those aspects of the problem upon which we are qualified to pass judgment. We can do so by questions such as the following set of nine:

1. Is the plan too global in scope? A hospital is a very complex universe containing many subuniverses or subsystems — the activities of doctors, nurses, patients, administrators, housekeeping staff, laboratory workers and others. Although the general objective is supposed to be "patient care," the specific objectives of these various groups can differ considerably and can even be in conflict to some extent. Moreover, to describe the whole hospital universe one must include its setting — the community that provides the patients, the financial support and the hospital employees.

The human body is also an extremely complex system composed of interacting subsystems; but physiologists would have made little headway if they had tried from the first to comprehend the total system and all the outside influences upon it. Their success has come from the study of subsystems, often very limited subsystems at first, followed by search for interrelationships between subsystems. The same approach is leading to understanding and practical success in the application of operations research methods to hospital systems. For example, the Operations Research Division of the Johns Hopkins Hospital turned its attention first to those areas that were most obviously in need of treatment. It has produced a method of reducing patients' waiting time in the outpatient clinic, a system for the distribution of bed linen, and a method whereby the members of the nursing staff are deployed more efficiently, because more flexibly in accordance with patients' needs (Flagle, 1962, and unpublished reports).

By taking problems that, though complex, are small enough to be handled, the specialists learn the methods necessary for work in the hospital environment, and by producing local successes they obtain opportunities to pass on to the study of still more complex interrelationships.

2. Does the operations research engineer appreciate the differences between the hospital system-complex and other systems that he may have analyzed with practical success?

3. Does he make real contact with all kinds of people involved in, or related to, the system that he is studying, not only with administrators?

4. How does he take into account the most important single factor in any human system — the psychology of human beings?

5. What is the definition of "optimal"? What are the various desiderata in the running of the system? Were some of them overlooked? How would the plan balance these desiderata? Here a medical person may be able to bring some of his own knowledge to bear. As a simple example, a scheme to reduce the waiting time of clinic patients would be of little use if it gave too little time for doctors, nurses or others to handle each patient properly, or if it left these personnel themselves with long periods of inactivity.

6. What allowance is to be made for variation in the load on the system?

7. Is the operations research engineer sufficiently aware of the peculiar features of medical data, or does he insure that he will work with someone who knows about these dangers? The hidden defects of routine clinical records and the mysteries of official vital statistics provide traps for clever mathematicians, even if they are astute in the handling of data from other applied sciences.

8. How, and how thoroughly, will the recommendations arising from the study be tested? The success of operations research in medicine — not only in hospital systems but in other problems of community health care, and in the study of diagnostic procedures — will rest with those specialists who realize that a systems analysis, however thorough its simulation in a computer may have been, merely generates hypotheses which have to be thoroughly tested in the real system.

9. How wide is the proposed generalization from the particular study? Some proposals for analysis of a hospital system state that, after the study of one, or perhaps two, hospitals, formulae will be issued which will enable other hospitals to be run more efficiently. This is carrying the principle of the "uniformity of Nature" far beyond the limits of our present knowledge of hospital systems.

For further study of this topic, one of the most useful discussions suitable for the general medical reader is that of Bailey, whose definition of operations research was quoted at the beginning of this section.

Mathematics in Medical Diagnosis

When an anthropologist makes certain measurements on a bone and as a result of those measurements decides whether the bone is more likely to have belonged to a male or to a female, he is making a diagnosis. In the 1938 edition of his *Statistical Methods,* Fisher presented an automatic method of assigning relative weights to the individual measurements to produce a compound expression which reduces the frequency of incorrect diagnoses — or, more generally, misclassifications — in a wide variety of material or phenomena. It is called the "discriminant function." The method is obviously applicable to certain problems of medical diagnosis. In the simple case of discrimination between two possible diagnoses, the necessary information would be a series of measurements (or even of semiquantitative assessments, such as 0, +, ++, +++, which can be converted into figures) on a number of different criteria in a group of patients, some of whom were known to have one of the diseases while the others had the other disease. Calculation on these data would then produce the necessary formula, which would then be used in classifying future patients whose diagnosis with respect to these diseases was in doubt.

The discriminant function is related to the multiple regression method and the coefficients (weights) are estimated by the least-squares technique; but its justification does not depend on assumptions about parent populations, because we can test its usefulness empirically. First, we find the proportion of misclassifications in the series from which we have created the formula, and then we ought to test it further on other groups in which the classification is already known.

The discriminant function could, therefore, be used in an attempt to make diagnosis more objective and more automatic. However, it is not a universally applicable method — for two reasons. First, many diagnoses depend on information about signs and symptoms of the "present or absent" type. Secondly, there enters into many diagnoses some information, however vague, about the relative frequency of various diseases at a particular time in a particular region and in particular kinds of persons. Consequently these two kinds of information form the basis of many current attempts to make diagnosis more systematic, more objective and more automatic, even "automated" ("machine diagnosis").

In outline this problem appears rather simple. One can collect a large number of records containing a variety of diseases, e.g., all records for several years in the hospital where the automatic technique is to be used. One can classify these diseases by the presence or absence of a wide range of symptoms and signs, and by various measurements determined clinically or in the laboratory. Then for each combination of symptoms, signs and measurements one can find the relative frequencies of various diseases. Actually, the procedure is visualized as a series of steps, beginning with coarse screening; but even at that stage the complexity of manifestations of disease presents big problems which have not yet been solved.

Undoubtedly it is very desirable to establish more extensive and more reliable information in order to permit inferences from frequencies of signs and symptoms to specific diseases or groups of diseases, even if only to assist clinicians in forming their judgments. There is also little doubt that some kind of mechanical weighting of complex frequency data, and of complex concatenations of symptoms, will be found useful in certain categories of diseases or at certain parts of diagnostic procedure. Therefore it is desirable to encourage those who are exploring "machine diagnosis," especially those who pay attention to the collection of sound basic data, and who explore the techniques thoroughly in certain well defined areas.

Correlation Coefficients

In a chapter headed "Concomitant Variation" it might have been expected that the term "coefficient of correlation" would have appeared in the first sentence of the first paragraph. It has been deferred until near the end of the chapter for good reasons. Of all the statistical expressions commonly used in medicine, perhaps the most mysterious, misunderstood and misleading is *Pearson's coefficient of correlation*, usually symbolized by "r." If it were abolished in medicine we would lose very little, because the valuable information that it contains can be found by straight-line regression analysis. However, it is not likely to be abolished; therefore in self-protection we must learn something about it.

We can see how closely regression and Pearsonian correlation are related when we compare the two coefficients. In the notation already shown for the regression coefficient b, we have:

$$b = \frac{S\{(x - \bar{x})\ (y - \bar{y})\}}{S(x - \bar{x})^2}$$

$$r = \frac{S\{(x - \bar{x})\ (y - \bar{y})\}}{\sqrt{S(x - \bar{x})^2\ S(y - \bar{y})^2}}$$

The only differences are that the correlation formula contains the sum of squares of Y-deviations and that a square-root sign is introduced. These differences do not change the plus or minus sign of b. We will not probe further into the formula, except to associate the numerator with the name commonly applied to Pearson's r — the "product-moment correlation coefficient." The moment of a force applied to a lever is defined as the product of the force and its distance from the fulcrum. If X is considered as distance and Y as force (or vice versa) the numerator of r (and also of b) is the sum of such products. Biologists and medical workers do not appear to benefit from this analogy with mechanics.

Information from r. Unlike the regression coefficient, the correlation coefficient does not indicate the gradient of the line representing the XY relationship. It is not a probability or a measurement expressing so many units of anything, or a percentage, although it is sometimes multiplied by 100 and called a percentage — a misleading practice. It is an index — a figure that indicates the *closeness* or *strength* of the XY relationship, which is just another way of saying that it indicates the closeness of the dots to the straight regression line. The larger the value of r, the closer are the dots to the line; but owing to its structure r cannot exceed unity. r = +1 (perfect positive correlation) indicates that all the dots are on an upward-sloping straight regression line; r = −1 (perfect negative correlation) indicates that they are all on a downward-sloping straight line.

In actual investigations perfect correlations are not to be expected if the measurements are fine enough. Absolute zero correlations (r = 0) are likewise not to be expected, even if we scatter dots randomly in a graph without any reference to X or Y.

Having estimated r from a sample, we must find how much allowance to make for differences between r values in random samples from a population in which there is no XY correlation. The "significance test" is a form of t-test, and is based on the same assumptions, regarding Gaussian distributions and equality of SD's in the parent population, as underlie the t-test for linear regression coefficients. In fact the t-tests for b and for r from the data are really the same test. However, it is possible to take a correlation direct to a table (Table VI in Fisher and Yates' *Tables*) and, after making a proper allowance for sample size, to determine its "significance" without further calculation. Since the answer about

"P" is the same as for the corresponding regression coefficient, if we wish to test the significance of b in the orthodox way (i.e., by t) we do not need to perform the actual t-test on the regression data. We can do the little extra arithmetic necessary to convert b into r, and then take r to the table.

Examples of r. It is helpful to remember a few typical correlation coefficients:

1. Correlation of the length of the proximal segment of the right index finger and the length of the same segment of the left index finger in 551 women: $r = +0.92$ — a high correlation (Whiteley and Pearson).
2. Correlation between stature and weight in adults of the same sex: $r = +0.5$ approximately — a moderate correlation.
3. Correlations of stature of uncles and stature of adult nephews: r between $+0.2$ and $+0.3$ — a low correlation. A similar correlation was found between intelligence quotients and head circumferences of boys (Boynton and Herbert).

The last example illustrates how r gives some indication of the practical value (or lack of value) of a relationship. We know that uncles' statures are a poor guide to their nephews' statures. Since the head-intelligence correlation coefficient is of similar magnitude, we see that the head size can be of very little value as a guide to intelligence; and this would still be true if the relationship were very real. How this comes about can be seen when we recall that a regression relationship can be used to divide the total variation of Y into two parts.

Partition of Total Variation. We have noted that the total variation (scatter of the Y-values around the mean of Y) is composed of the variation represented by the regression relationship plus the deviations from regression (scatter of Y-values around the regression line). From the regression equation we can find, for any X-value, the corresponding Y-value on the regression line; but when the scatter of dots around the line is not much less than the total scatter, the Y-value on the line tells us hardly any more about the actual individual Y-values than we knew before we found the regression line.

When we express the variation of Y-values as sums of squares of deviations, we can use r to show the actual numerical partition of the total variation which is $S(y - y)^2$. If we multiply this by r^2 we have $r^2 S(y - y)^2$, which represents the variation accounted for by the regression. Then clearly the residual variation, i.e., the sum of squares of deviations from the regression line, is:

$$S(y - \overline{y})^2 - r^2 S(y - \overline{y})^2 = (1 - r^2) S(y - \overline{y})^2$$

This result (except for slight effects of arithmetical rounding) is identical with what we find by the more laborious process of taking the vertical distance between each observed Y-value and the regression line, squaring it and summing the squares. Therefore r has some value as an arithmetical shortcut.

Even if we do not go as far as actually partitioning the variation, the trick with r^2 is useful, for it often shows that an XY relationship is not as important as it looks. If r is $+0.5$ (or -0.5) the regression accounts for $r^2 = 0.25$ of the total sum of squares, i.e., 25 per cent; and thus it leaves 75 per cent as residual variation. With a moderate degree of correlation, therefore, most of the variation cannot be accounted for by the linear regression relationship. Letting SS represent the total sum of squares of deviations from the mean Y, we have the following figures:

Coefficient of Correlation	Variation Accounted for by Regression (%SS)	Residual Variation (%SS)
0.95	90.25	9.75
0.9	81	19
0.7	49	51
0.5	25	75
0.3	9	91
0.1	1	99

Coefficients of Partial Correlation. These are r's that correspond to the coefficients of partial regression discussed previously. For example, in the weight-stature-width relationship we could calculate an r to represent the correlation between weight and pelvic width when stature was held constant, and another r to represent the correlation between weight and stature when pelvic width was held constant, and still another r for the correlation between stature and pelvic width when weight was held constant. Sometimes it is useful to calculate these coefficients before going to the greater trouble of calculating the corresponding b's. If a partial r is low we may decide that the relationship that it represents will have such a small effect in reducing the Y-variation that it is not worth putting it into a multiple regression equation.

Confusion from Correlations

A correlation coefficient is a measure of association and therefore the danger of fallacious causal interpretation should be heeded; but too often it is not. In fields like economics, psychology, sociology and education, in which opportunities for experimentation are, or are thought to be, limited, correlation has been extensively used in the search for causes; but the interpretations of the resulting coefficients have frequently been little more than untested speculations masquerading as inferences.

If in such speculations the possibility of time as an associated agent is overlooked, the conclusions can be entirely erroneous, because the passage of time can produce high correlations between otherwise unrelated variables. An investigator is reported to have found a correlation coefficient of about $+0.9$ between professors' salaries and the price of alcoholic beverages, and that might well be true because for many years there has been an upward trend both in commodity prices and in salaries. Although the figure seems to suggest a close relationship between professors and alcohol, it could equally well have been obtained if no professors had ever touched a drop of liquor.

Even when the correlation coefficient is used only as a measure of association, it tells investigators much less than many of them think it does. In order to see if estimation of free hydrochloric acid in gastric juice would provide a sufficiently close indication of the amount of pepsin in the same specimen of juice, certain physiologists found coefficients of correlation between these two variables in subjects with and without duodenal ulcer. The highest value was obtained from the fasting juice of 40 ulcer patients, $r = +0.85$. The investigators wrote as follows: "The fact that these coefficients are far from unity shows that often the acid titer and the amount of pepsin do not vary in the same way or to the same degree."

Actually, the observed coefficients could have been produced if acid and pepsin values had always varied in the same way (in the same direction) but with different relationships in different subjects. The important point, however, is that the correlation coefficient did not really tell the investigators what they wished to find out. Even if they had squared 0.85 and found that 18 per cent of the total variation in pepsin levels could not be accounted for by the regression of pepsin on hydrochloric acid, they would have been no nearer to an answer. The appropriate questions would have been: "How far from the observed pepsin value in each patient was the pepsin value estimated from the hydrochloric acid value?" "In what proportion of patients would the error be important in practice?" Only the individual patients' deviations from the pepsin/acid regression line could answer these questions.

Akin to this misuse of r is the habit of employing it to express the reliability of a technique when an observer has made duplicate measurements or when two observers have measured the same things. Even if the coefficient is $+0.95$ or higher, it does not tell us whether, for the purpose in hand, the differences between the duplicate readings are trivial or serious. The way to find this out is to look at the actual differences, note how frequently they exceed a certain value, and then estimate how often this frequency, or a larger one, might occur in a large sample (a population) of such pairs.

In the quotation from the pepsin study discussed above, it was interesting to meet a correlation coefficient of 0.85 that was not considered high, because often those of 0.8 (or even 0.7) are so designated. The designation seems to depend partly on whether the investigator wishes to find a strong or a weak relationship. Often, too, it appears that people are misled by the numerical form of the coefficient. When its value is 0.9 it is "90 per cent of what it could be, i.e., unity"; but this is an extremely uninformative statement.

Rank-order Correlations

Anyone who issues strong warnings against the hazards of correlation coefficients and then immediately recommends the use of one of them

lays himself open to the charge of inconsistency. The following remarks
may enable readers to evaluate the charge.

Let us suppose that we have a number of individuals of any kind, with
an X and a Y reading on each of them, that we arrange them in ascending order of X, and wish to find out whether the Y's tend to increase (or
decrease) as we pass from lower to higher values of X. We are not concerned with the question of straight or curved slopes, or with numerical
gradients, and we do not wish to make the assumptions that underlie the
orthodox significance tests of regression coefficients. All that we wish to
know is whether there is more evidence of an upward (or downward)
slope than could be easily accounted for by the random scattering of the
Y's in relation to the X's. "Tend to increase" and "evidence of an upward
slope" are, however, vague phrases. Do we mean, for instance, more
rises than falls of Y between each X-value and its neighbor above?
Do we mean that the total magnitude of the increases in Y from one X
to the next is greater than the total magnitude of the decreases?

We have to adopt a definition of the term "amount of evidence," but
having done so we could see how the question of random scatter could
be answered. We could enter each Y-value on an index card and,
with very small samples, we could arrange the cards in all possible
sequences in relation to the fixed X's. With larger samples we could
randomize the order of the Y's many times, and find out how often this
produced more evidence of slope, as we had defined the phrase, than had
occurred in our actual experiment or survey. This would, however, be
more laborious than a regression analysis followed by a nonparametric
test of significance of the b-coefficient, as suggested earlier in this chapter.
Instead, we seek for a rank-order method, such as is used in some
psychologic, educational and other researches in which values of the
variables can be arranged by relative magnitude but not measured on an
absolute scale.

Requirements in the Formula.   Let us suppose that we have 5 individuals, each with an X- and a Y-measurement. We replace the X-meas-
urements by ranks 1 through 5 and, quite separately, the Y-measurements
by ranks 1 through 5. Then we see how X and Y agree or disagree in
their ranks. There is as much agreement as there possibly could be —
"perfect agreement" — if we find:

$$\begin{array}{cccccc} X & 1 & 2 & 3 & 4 & 5 \\ Y & 1 & 2 & 3 & 4 & 5 \end{array}$$

There is the most complete possible reversal of order — "perfect disagreement," which is not at all the same as no relationship — if we find:

$$\begin{array}{cccccc} X & 1 & 2 & 3 & 4 & 5 \\ Y & 5 & 4 & 3 & 2 & 1 \end{array}$$

In terms of Pearson's product-moment correlation, perfect agreement
would be perfect positive correlation, and perfect disagreement would
be perfect negative correlation. It would seem desirable, therefore, that

a coefficient of rank-order correlation should reach its highest possible value at these two extremes, the same numerical value in each, but with a plus sign for agreement and a minus sign for disagreement. It would also be convenient if these extreme values were identical, whether there were 5 individuals in the sample, or 50 or 500.

Let us now consider two other possible arrangements of five pairs of ranks:

(1)	X	1	2	3	4	5
	Y	1	3	2	4	5

(2)	X	1	2	3	4	5
	Y	1	2	4	3	5

In both (1) and (2), two neighboring Y-ranks have been interchanged — minimal departure from perfect agreement. We would expect the formula to produce a coefficient with a plus sign, but the value should be less than the value for perfect agreement. Moreover, it would seem desirable that the value should be the same for (1) and (2) because in a random scattering all neighboring-rank interchanges would occur with equal frequency. Similarly, if we started with perfect disagreement and made a neighboring-rank interchange, it would be desirable that the numerical value of the coefficient be the same as when we start from perfect agreement, but it should have a negative sign. We can apply similar reasoning to interchanges between ranks that are farther apart; e.g., interchanges of ranks 1 and 3, or 2 and 4, or 3 and 5, should produce lower numerical values of the coefficient than a neighboring-rank interchange, but the values should be equal in all three cases. Of the formulae that have been proposed for expressing rank-order relationships, Spearman's coefficient of rank-order correlation is one that meets the specifications that we have outlined.

Spearman's Rank-order Correlation. When a formula to express the XY rank-order relationship was being sought, the most obvious first step was to try the simple X-Y differences in rank. In order to avoid too many zero sums of differences, the plus and minus signs have to be dropped, but even the absolute sums are found unsatisfactory. If, on the other hand, we square the difference between the X-rank and the Y-rank of each individual and utilize knowledge of the relationships that exist in arithmetic progressions (1, 2, 3, . . .), a formula can be developed that meets the requirements mentioned above, and has the advantage of numerical values of the same order as those of Pearson's coefficient. If N = number of individuals in sample, S = "sum of," and D = difference between X-rank and Y-rank of the same individual, the formula is:

$$\text{Spearman's } r = 1 - \frac{6S(D^2)}{N^3 - N} \text{ (The multiplier 6 is a constant.)}$$

This appears very mysterious, but the mystery here is not disturbing, because the formula is not based on imaginary straight-line relationships of measurements, Gaussian distributions and the like. It is a tool developed by mathematical maneuvers and then tested on the actual material for which it is developed, i.e., series of X-ranks and Y-ranks.

To see how the formula works, the reader can start with the series of five ranks in perfect agreement. Since there is no difference between any of the X- and Y-ranks of the same individual, Spearman's $r = +1.0$. An interchange of any neighboring pair of Y-ranks (i.e., one remove from perfect agreement) produces $r = +0.9$. Starting with perfect disagreement, we find that $r = -1.0$, and backing down one step (one neighboring-rank interchange) we find $r = -0.9$.

Random Frequencies of Spearman's r. In finding out how often the purely random arrangement of Y-ranks in relation to X-ranks would produce the various values of Spearman's r, we make no assumptions about Gaussian distributions, straightness of regression lines, equality of SD's, and so forth. As with differences between sums of ranks in Chapter XIV, we start with a small sample (here $N = 3$) and display all possible arrangements of Y-ranks. Then we increase the sample size by one individual at a time until we find that some information derived from the Gaussian distribution will give us the same verdict about rarity (at 5 per cent and 1 per cent levels of significance) as the exact distribution gives us.

For example, with $N = 3$ the ranks

$$
\begin{array}{cccc}
X & 1 & 2 & 3 \\
Y & 1 & 2 & 3
\end{array}
$$

provide six possible arrangements of the Y's. The frequencies (F) of the r's are as follows:

$$
\begin{array}{ccccc}
r & +1 & +0.5 & -0.5 & -1 \\
F & 1 & 2 & 2 & 1
\end{array}
$$

We note the symmetrical distribution, with the beginning of a peak.

For any particular sample size, $N^3 - N$ is constant, and the "6" in the formula is constant for all sample sizes. Therefore the important thing to find for each N is the distribution of the sums of (D^2). For sample sizes through $N = 8$, these are shown by Kendall (1952), and from those figures the Spearman coefficients were calculated in order to show the 10 per cent, 5 per cent and 1 per cent cut-off points in the usual form:

Sample Size (N)	Random Frequency of Spearman's r (P in Both Tails Combined)		
	0.10—	0.05—	0.01—
4	1.000	————	————
5	0.900	1.000	————
6	0.829	0.886	1.000
7	0.714	0.786	0.929
8	0.643	0.738	0.881

Using this table, if our sample contains 8 individuals and Spearman's r is +0.738 or —0.738, or is numerically greater in either direction, we can say that the coefficient is "significantly" different from zero at the 5 per cent level. That is, of the total possible arrangements of Y-ranks 1, 2, . . . 8, in relation to the X-ranks, less than 2.5 per cent would produce r values of 0.738 or greater in the positive direction, and the same number would occur at —0.738 and beyond.

Fortunately, although somewhat surprisingly, with samples containing more than 8 individuals we can use Table VI in Fisher and Yates' *Tables* — the table that shows P values derived from t-tests applied to Pearson's product-moment correlation coefficient (we have to enter the table, as for Pearson's r, with n = sample size minus 2). Even with N = 8, Fisher and Yates' table would lead astray only those workers who use cut-off points too literally. That is, at a very early stage a Gaussian-derived method can be substituted for the exact distribution of Spearman's r.

Justification of Rank-order Correlations. The justification for rank-order methods in seeking for concomitant variation between measured variables is essentially the same as in analysis of single variables (Chapter XIV). Ease and speed are, of course, not sufficient arguments if those methods fail to give us required information about the measurements as such, e.g., the gradient of a line. But unless we need such information a rank-order (nonparametric) method has the advantage that it keeps us much closer than do parametric methods to card-shuffling phenomena, and the nearer we keep to that the safer we are.

It should be noted also that the product-moment correlation coefficient, by itself, tells us little more than a rank-order coefficient — evidence of the existence of a relationship, its direction (plus or minus) and some idea of whether it is strong or weak. Moreover, even if the X's and Y's are truly (artificially) Gaussian in frequency distribution, we do not lose much power by using Spearman's coefficient instead of Pearson's. If a sample of 90 individuals provides a certain power when the product-moment correlation is used, we have merely to increase it by about 10 individuals to obtain the same power with Spearman's rank-order method. When, as is common, we do not know how non-Gaussian our distributions may be, the more logical technique and in some instances the more powerful, is rank-order correlation. We must remember, however, that it does not protect us against our own foolish interpretations, any more than does Pearson's r.

More details of technique, including the treatment of tied ranks (due to multiple occurrences of the same X-measurement or Y-measurement), can be found in many elementary statistics books, especially those in the behavioral sciences. For more advanced discussion of Spearman's methods and others, reference should be made to the writings of Kendall (1948, 1952).

CHAPTER XVI

SUPPLEMENTARY NOTES
ON TECHNIQUES AND
FURTHER STUDY

1. THE STANDARD DEVIATION (STANDARD ERROR) OF BINOMIAL DISTRIBUTIONS

The Formula

Chapter XI mentions the binomial standard deviation and its curious formula $\sqrt{Npq}$. For many of us a little simple arithmetic suffices to justify the formula, and we are then willing to accept from mathematical statisticians the statement that it is true for any binomial distribution.

Let us suppose that we have an indefinitely large population containing 30 per cent X's and 70 per cent not-X's, and that we propose to take from it random samples of 2. The binomial expression that shows the distribution that we would approach by continued sampling is $(p + q)^2$, where $p = 0.3$ and $q = 0.7$. By the time we had taken a thousand samples we would have a distribution that would be very close to the following:

No. of X's in Sample	Frequency (F)
0	490
1	420
2	90
Total	1000

Let us treat the numbers of X's as if they were measurements. To find the mean we take $(0 \times 490) + (1 \times 420) + (2 \times 90) = 600$, and then we divide by the total number of samples and obtain 0.6 X per sample of 2, i.e., 30 per cent X's as in the population.

To find the standard deviation we proceed as follows:

No. of X's in Sample	Deviation from Mean (D)	D²	Frequency (F)	D² × F
0	−0.6	0.36	490	176.40
1	+0.4	0.16	420	67.20
2	+1.4	1.96	90	176.40
		Total	1000	420.00

Dividing the total sum of squares by the total number of samples, we have 0.42, and SD $= \sqrt{0.42}$.

Using the formula instead of the step-by-step method, we obtain exactly the same result. $\sqrt{Npq} = \sqrt{2 \times 0.3 \times 0.7} = \sqrt{0.42} = 0.648$ X's per sample of 2 individuals.

Alternative Forms. Two other forms of the binomial SD are often met. When the population frequency is expressed as a *proportion* (with 1 as denominator) SD is expressed in the same way. Thus, 0.6 X's per sample of 2, with SD $= 0.648$, is converted into a proportion by dividing by the sample size, and we have the proportion of X's $= 0.3$ with SD $= 0.324$. The formula in this case $= \sqrt{Npq}/N = \sqrt{Npq/N^2} = \sqrt{pq/N} = \sqrt{0.3 \times 0.7/2} = \sqrt{0.105} = 0.324$.

Similarly, we can work entirely in *percentages*. The SD obtained by the step-by-step method is 0.648 X's per sample of 2 individuals $= 32.4$ per cent X's. To find this by formula we write:
$SD(\%) = \sqrt{p\%(1 - p\%/N)} = \sqrt{30 \times 70/N} = \sqrt{1050} = 32.4$ per cent X's.

Uses of the Binomial SD

The use of $\sqrt{Npq}$ in relation to estimates of limits of population frequencies is discussed in Chapter XI. Readers will probably see it used also in the comparison of two binomial samples, instead of the fourfold contingency test by chi-square. The procedure is rather like that of the t-test in the comparison of two samples of measurements. A binomial SD is estimated for each sample and from these SD's the SD of the differences between sample-pairs is estimated. The observed difference is divided by the SD of the sample difference, and if the result is 2 or greater the difference is said to be "significant at the 5 per cent level." With certain modifications, including a form of Yates' correction, this SD test is exactly equivalent to the fourfold contingency chi-square test — the P values from the two tests are identical. There seems, however, to be no particular usefulness in learning two methods of doing the same thing, and chi-square has several advantages, including the fact that it can be used with contingency tables containing any number of cells.

2. ESTIMATION OF LIMITS OF BINOMIAL
POPULATION DIFFERENCES

When we have applied a fourfold contingency test after an experiment such as a drug trial, whether the difference is "significant" or "not significant," it is very desirable to know how large or how small the "real" (population) difference may be, if such a difference exists. Indeed, this information may be much more important than the result of a significance test.

We can, of course, estimate the upper and lower limits (Chapter XI) for each treatment-population separately, but they are apt to give an overestimate of the possible difference. For example, let us suppose that we find from Table I the upper limit of the population percentage of X's in the B-population and the lower limit in the A-population. Treatment B may actually produce a higher percentage of X's than treatment A, but this method of estimating the difference implies that both our samples may have considerably misrepresented their populations — that the B-sample may have been almost in the lower "rare" area of the B-distribution and the A-sample almost in the upper "rare" area of the A-distribution. Such a combined occurrence is unlikely.

What we desire is an estimate of the limits of the *difference* between the percentages of X's in the two populations. The traditional rule for estimating these limits is as follows:

Find the percentage of X's in the A-sample and estimate from it the corresponding standard deviation (by the percentage form of $\sqrt{Npq}$). Do likewise for the B-sample. From these SD's find the SD of differences, as shown in Chapter XIV for measurement data, and write: Observed difference $\pm$ 2 SD of differences.

The result is supposed to be an estimate of the upper and lower limits of the population difference, with a 2.5 per cent risk of overestimation and a 2.5 per cent risk of underestimation. However, it involves using each sample percentage as if it were a population percentage in estimating the SD's, and it involves marking off 2 SD (or 1.96 SD) as if the differences formed a Gaussian distribution. The larger the samples and the nearer the percentages to 50 per cent, the safer are these approximations, but the method can lead us far astray in small-sample work and with percentages that are far from 50. A more fundamental approach is illustrated in the following example:

20 A's contain 5 X's (25 per cent)
20 B's contain 10 X's (50 per cent)

The difference, 25 percentage points, is not significant at the 5 per cent level (Table III). Would differences as small as this be rare if the A- and B-populations contained respectively 15 and 60 per cent X's? We could answer this question by a sampling experiment, starting with two barrels of disks, one containing 15 per cent X's and the other 60 per cent X's. We would take a random sample of 20 disks from each barrel, find the B-A difference in percentages of X, replace the disks and take more sample-pairs, perhaps up to a thousand. We could equate "rare" to less than 5 per cent of sample-pairs in the tails of the distribution, and thereby decide whether the observed sample difference (25 per cent) was compatible, on that standard, with the postulated population percentages.

Instead of actual sampling we could, of course, find the frequency distributions of many thousand such differences from binomial distributions that have been published, but even this method would be too laborious for regular use. It was employed, however, in testing the short-cut method that will now be shown.

Population A. Percentage of X's = 15. SD for random samples of 20 individuals = $\sqrt{15 \times 85/20} = \sqrt{1275/20} = \sqrt{63.75}$.

Population B. Percentage of X's = 60. SD for random samples of 20 individuals = $\sqrt{60 \times 40/20} = \sqrt{120}$.

SD of differences = $\sqrt{63.75 + 120} = \sqrt{183.75} = 13.555$ per cent X's.

Population difference (B − A) = 60 − 15 = 45 per cent X's.

In a Gaussian distribution of differences the lower 5 per cent cut-off point is found by using the expression: Mean minus 1.645 SD. In this instance we have $45 - 1.645 \times 13.555 = 45 - 22.3 = 22.7$ per cent X's. The observed difference (25 per cent) is therefore not below the cut-off point. So far as we can tell from the observed sample difference, we can accept the possibility that the true population values A and B were respectively 15 per cent and 60 per cent X's (a difference of 45 percentage points).

As an exercise the reader could show that the observed sample difference was not compatible with population values of 15 per cent X's in A and 70 per cent X's in B (lower cut-off point for differences = +33.6 per cent X's). With 15 per cent X's in the A-population the boundary between acceptable and unacceptable (compatible and incompatible) values for the B-population would lie between 60 and 70 per cent X's, but nearer the former. For greater precision, we could try values such as 62 per cent.

Tests of this method that I have made by using actual binomial distributions have satisfied me that it is reliable with N values (equal in the two samples) from 10 to 200, and with population values ranging from 5 to 95 per cent X's. This is another example of the usefulness of the Gaussian distribution; but, as always, it had to be thoroughly tested. Tests of the method with unequal samples have not been made in this laboratory.

3. SEQUENTIAL DESIGNS

A general description of sequential designs is given under Q VI – 18. I do not propose here to offer detailed instructions for setting up the boundaries by which an investigator will know whether to stop or continue an experiment; nor will I attempt to probe into the mysterious mathematics that produces the equations for the boundaries. However, having been involved in clinical trials in which sequential designs were used, I have the impression that they offer an even greater temptation to automatic uncomprehending use by research workers than do methods like the t-test. To cross a boundary in a graph seems to be even more definite than to obtain a t-test verdict that P is between 0.05 and 0.01. What we have to ask is: "What does crossing a boundary really tell us?" For many of us, the best way to obtain an answer is by experimentation, and three series of experiments are described here.

Purpose and General Plan

Let us suppose that two treatments, A and B, have been randomly assigned to different members of an indefinitely large population, and that we compare a randomly picked A-treated patient with a randomly picked B-treated patient. If the A and B patients show no difference in outcome (i.e., if they form a "tied pair") we cannot use them for the treatment comparison; but if the A-treated patient has done better than the B-treated patient we count the pair as an "A-preference." Let us suppose that by continuing this process of comparison we would find that among the population of untied pairs 85 per cent were A-preferences and 15 per cent were B-preferences. The Greek letter θ (theta) is used as a general symbol for the proportion of preferences, and for specific values the subscripts 1 and 0 are attached. In this instance we have $\theta_1 = 0.85$ and $\theta_0 = 0.15$.

Let us suppose that if such proportions existed in the population (or would be created if we treated large enough numbers of patients) we would wish to have a very good prospect of detecting an A-B difference in a clinical trial. By "detecting" we mean, as usual, finding a difference that would rarely be found if there were no difference between the effects of A and B, or if half the population were A-preferences and half were B-preferences. By "rare" we mean a difference that we would pronounce "significant at the 5 per cent level" — we set our maximum Type I error at 5 per cent. By "a very good prospect" we mean that 95 per cent of our experiments conducted under these conditions would produce a "significant" difference in the right direction (A preferred to B) — a power of 95 per cent, i.e., a Type II error of 0.05.

In order to find the figures required for setting up a sequential design that will meet our requirements, we turn to Armitage's *Sequential Medical Trials* at Table 3.7 — Restricted Designs for a Series of Preferences. We choose a "restricted" or "closed" design because we do not wish to wander on indefinitely without reaching a verdict. The information obtained from Armitage's table is presented in a somewhat expanded form in our

Table 10. It shows that we are bound to reach a verdict by the 27th preference (untied pair) at the latest.

This table itself can be used in a sequential trial, but the reader can draw for himself a typical sequential graph by setting the values of n (number of preferences, i.e., untied pairs) along a horizontal line (X-axis) at the middle of the graph paper and then inserting the four sets of y-values (two positive and two negative). He will thus produce four boundary lines: uppermost, upper middle, lower middle, and lowermost.

Table 10. Sequential Design for Comparison of Treatments A and B — Population Percentages of Preferences: A, 85; B, 15

(From Armitage's Table 3.7)

n = number of preferences (untied pairs).
y = number of A-preferences minus number of B-preferences.
Type I error = 0.05. Power = 0.95.

n	Uppermost Boundary (Minimum Positive y for Verdict in Favor of A)	Middle Boundaries (Maximum y for "No Signif. Diff.") Upper	Lower	Lowermost Boundary (Minimum Negative y for Verdict in Favor of B)
6	—	—	—	—
7	+7	—	—	−7
11	+9	—	—	−9
14	+10	—	—	−10
16	—	0	0	—
17	+11	+1	−1	−11
18	—	+2	−2	—
19	—	+3	−3	—
20	+12	+4	−4	−12
21	—	+5	−5	—
22	—	+6	−6	—
23	—	+7	−7	—
24	+14	+8	−8	−14
25	—	+9	−9	—
26	+14	+10	−10	−14
27	+13	+11	−11	−13

Experiment Series 1

In a series of experiments with the figures in Table 10, random numbers were taken as a population in which each two-digit number represented a preference for A or for B. The numbers 01 through 85 represented A-preferences and 86 through 00 represented B-preferences. (The two digits in each number should not be confused with the individual patients in a pair.) The first experiment was started at an unselected point in the table of random numbers, and the numbers were taken in vertical order as they came. After the first experiment, the second one was started at the next number below the last one used in the first experiment. The result of the first experiment was as follows:

| Preference | | A — B | Preference | | A — B |
No.(n)	In Favor of	(y)	No.(n)	In Favor of	(y)
1	A	+1	10	A	+4
2	A	+2	11	A	+5
3	B	+1	12	A	+6
4	A	+2	13	A	+7
5	A	+3	14	A	+8
6	A	+4	15	A	+9
7	B	+3	16	A	+10
8	A	+4	17	A	+11
9	B	+3			

If the reader has drawn a graph of the boundaries from Table 10 he can now draw in the zigzag line (y = +1, +2, +1, and so on) representing this first experiment. No boundary was reached until the 17th preference was obtained, and then y became +11, which is the point on the uppermost boundary at n = 17 — a verdict in favor of A.

One hundred such experiments were performed, of which 97 terminated by reaching the uppermost boundary. In no experiment was the lowermost boundary reached, but in 3 experiments a middle boundary was reached, and the verdict was "No significant A-B difference" — Experiment No. 6, n = 18, y = +2; Experiment No. 19, n = 23, y = +7; Experiment No. 77, n = 21, y = +5. That is, 97 of the 100 experiments were "successful" — the Type II error was only 3 per cent.

Experiment Series 2

To demonstrate the Type I error, another series of 100 experiments was conducted, in which the population contained equal numbers of A- and B-preferences, represented respectively by odd and even random digits. (Symbolically, $\theta_1 = \theta_0 = 0.5$.) Ninety-five of the experiments terminated by reaching one or the other of the middle boundaries and thus gave verdicts of "Difference not significant at the 5 per cent level." In 4 of the experiments the uppermost boundary was reached — a verdict in favor of A "significant at the 5 per cent level." One experiment terminated at the lowermost boundary — a verdict in favor of B. The total Type I error was therefore exactly 5 per cent.

Experiment Series 3

Just as in a fixed-sample-size experiment, a "nonsignificant" difference in a sequential experiment does not mean "no real difference." If we set out to catch a big difference we often miss a smaller one. To illustrate this, 100 experiments were performed in which there were in the population 65 per cent A-preferences (random numbers 01 through 65) and 35 per cent B-preferences (random numbers 66 through 00). The figures in Table 10, designed for a population containing 85 per cent A-preferences, were again used.

Seventy of the 100 experiments terminated by reaching one of the middle boundaries — a verdict of "No significant A-B difference." Thirty experiments terminated at the uppermost boundary — a verdict in favor of A.

This series of experiments illustrates what happens when we set up a design that will give us strong assurance of detecting evidence of a difference of a certain magnitude (here 85 per cent A-preferences) if it is present, and then, unknown to us, the actual difference, although very real, is smaller (here 65 per cent A-preferences). In many of the experiments we are not able to detect any "significant" difference. The same thing happens, of course, when we use Table V in determining sample sizes in a fixed-sample-size experiment.

If we wished to have very good assurance (95 per cent power) of detecting an A-B difference when the population contained only 65 per cent A-preferences (and stipulated the Type I error of 5 per cent), we would need to use another set of boundaries (from Armitage's Table 3.5), and the experiment might require as many as 191 preferences (untied pairs) before it gave a verdict.

Experiment Series 3 shows also that, having set up boundaries to insure detection of a certain magnitude of difference, the verdict "significant" does not tell us that the true value is the one that we used in setting up the boundaries. A population containing only 65 per cent A-preferences produced 30 verdicts in favor of A in 100 experiments that were designed to detect an A-B difference in a population that contained 85 per cent A-preferences.

Required Sample Sizes

The three series of experiments provide some information in answer to a very important question: How much do we save by using a sequential design instead of a fixed-sample-size design? Each series of experiments was rather small, but the results with regard to the Type I and Type II errors agreed with the specifications which determined the boundary lines. That is, the series were not aberrant, and presumably we can accept them as fairly typical regarding the numbers of preferences required to reach a verdict.

If a population contained 85 per cent A-preferences and 15 per cent B-preferences and we used, instead of the sequential design, the equivalent nonsequential (fixed-sample-size) design, we would require, for the same Type I error and the same power as in our experiments, 20 preferences (Armitage, Table 3.1) — that is, in a series of 100 experiments we would need 2000 untied pairs. In the three sequential series (each containing 100 experiments) the total numbers of preferences required to reach a verdict were as follows:

Series 1 (Population % A-preferences: 85): 1258
Series 2 (Population % A-preferences: 50): 1846
Series 3 (Population % A-preferences: 65): 1974

In Series 1, in which the population of preferences was as stipulated in the design, there was required only two thirds of the number of preferences that would have been required for the corresponding nonsequential design. In the other two series, in which the population percentages of preferences were less than the 85 per cent for which the boundaries were chosen, the benefit of the sequential design seems rather small. Instead of 20 untied pairs in the nonsequential design, the average number per experiment was 18.46 in Series 2 and 19.74 in Series 3.

These comparisons seem to have an important practical application. The population estimates of treatment differences (percentages of preferences, differences in improvement rates, and so on) on which we have to plan an experiment are often mere guesses, and the figures from these experiments suggest that if we guess too high, and set up the boundaries accordingly, we will be little better off than if we used fixed sample sizes.

It is interesting also to compare the stages at which verdicts were reached in the three series of experiments (100 in each series).

Series	Verdict Reached At 7th Pref.	(Numbers of Expts.) At or Before 11th Pref.	At or Before 20th Pref.	Verdict Not Reached Until 27th Pref.
1	33	59	93	—
2	2	2	76	1
3	3	8	56	10

In Series 1, in which the population of preferences was as stipulated in the design, many of the experiments were terminated quickly, instead of having to continue to the 20th preference as in the nonsequential design. When the preferences for A and B in the population were equal (Series 2) short experiments were rare, and only about three quarters of the total 100 verdicts had been reached before the 21st preference.

In Series 3, in which the population contained 65 per cent A-preferences, there were few quick decisions, less than 60 per cent of the verdicts were reached until after the 20th preference had been examined, and the maximum number, 27 preferences, was required in 10 experiments (7 of them ended with a verdict in favor of A, 3 of them with a "not significant" verdict). It was observed that the excess of A-preferences (65 per cent as against 35 per cent) repeatedly pushed the line of dots (A-B values) toward the uppermost boundary, but often the force was not quite strong enough, and the next observation (a B-preference) pulled the line of dots down again. This seemed to be the reason why verdicts were delayed more in this series than in Series 2, in which there was, on the average, an equal drive toward the uppermost and lowermost boundaries, and the line of dots had a greater opportunity of hitting one of the middle ("nonsignificance") boundaries.

Tied Pairs

The sample sizes discussed so far have been numbers of preferences, i.e., untied pairs; but if tied pairs occur they increase the total number of individuals required, just as they do in a nonsequential matched-pairs experiment. We must always expect tied pairs when we classify subjects binomially (e.g., success, failure; improved, not improved). From any population percentages of S's and F's we can calculate the proportions of tied and untied pairs. Let the population proportions be as follows:

	S's	F's
A-treated	75 per cent (0.75)	25 per cent (0.25)
B-treated	35 per cent (0.35)	65 per cent (0.65)

Then the proportions of the four types of pairs are:

A	B	Proportion	Preference
S	S	$0.75 \times 0.35 = 0.2625$	Neither
S	F	$0.75 \times 0.65 = 0.4875$	A
F	S	$0.25 \times 0.35 = 0.0875$	B
F	F	$0.25 \times 0.65 = 0.1625$	Neither
		Total 1.0000	

Therefore, of the total pairs 0.4250 will be tied and 0.5750 will be untied. Per 100 untied pairs, i.e., preferences that we could use in determining the superiority of A, there will be 74 tied pairs, which we could not use for that purpose. To obtain 20 preferences, we would need on the average a total of $20 + 15 = 35$ pairs.

In order to find the population percentages of A- and B-preferences from the above percentages of S's and F's we take the untied pairs, which comprise 0.5750 of the total pairs. The A-preferences constitute 0.4875 of the total pairs. Then $0.4875/0.5750 = 0.848$, or approximately 0.85. This is the proportion of A-preferences for which Table 10 was designed.

Advantages of Measurements

If we use some form of measurement in assessing the change exhibited by each individual under treatment we are much less likely to meet tied pairs than we are after a binomial type of assessment. This does not imply that we must use a sequential test of the measurements themselves. "Sequential t-tests" have been invented, but in the application of them to much of our small-scale medical research data they introduce, if anything, more problems and uncertainties than do the t-tests that are applied to samples of predetermined size.

In a clinical trial it may be possible, without precise measurement, to rank the degree of change in a certain manifestation of disease, a higher rank meaning more improvement. Then if the A-treated patient in a pair has a higher rank than the B-treated patient the pair counts as an A-preference. This method makes for greater sensitivity, which is reflected in a reduction of the number of tied pairs. The same result can be achieved if it is clinically rational to combine the assessments of several manifestations of the disease. If there are five different manifestations and a patient has improved in four of them he obtains a score of 4. If he is an A-treated patient and his B-treated fellow has a score of 3 or less, the pair is counted as an A-preference. For discussion of this and related topics, the article by Street should be consulted.

Population Estimates in Planning Sequential Experiments

In the planning of a two-sample fixed-sample-size experiment, e.g., by the use of Table V, it is customary to think of the percentages (e.g., S's and F's) in the total populations A and B. In the planning of experiments, either sequential or nonsequential, that involve pairs, the population percentages of preferences are used, and we are concerned with the subpopulation which shows preferences. It should be noted that the percentages of preferences do not give a direct clue to the population percentages of S's and F's, but it was shown above that we can start with these latter values and calculate the percentages of preferences.

By the same method it can be shown that a great variety of population percentages of S's and F's will give, exactly or approximately, the same proportion of preferences — 85 per cent A-preferences and 15 per cent B-preferences. Here are two examples:

Population	S (per cent)	F (per cent)
A	65	35
B	25	75
A	50	50
B	15	85

Bias and Sample Size

The small samples used in sequential experiments are mentioned in the discussion of bias in relation to sample size (Chapter VIII). We can now add an item to that discussion. In the three series of sequential experiments described in this section the members of each pair were selected at random independently of each other, because they were picked from a random numbers table. This is not what we do in sequential clinical trials. If we do not use purposely matched pairs we take the first A-treated patient and pair him with the first B-treated patient, the second A with the second B, and so on.

Let us visualize 100 patients (50 pairs, each showing an A- or a B-preference) whom we would use in a fixed-sample-size experiment. Instead, we perform a sequential experiment and obtain a verdict at the 10th pair. If the 50 pairs are in random order with respect to the behavior of the disease and reaction to treatment, the first 10 pairs will be a random sample of the total; but the randomness of the order is often questionable. Therefore an experiment that terminates early may differ in its verdict from a sequential experiment that terminates later, or from a fixed-sample-size experiment which would use all 50 pairs. Hence the safety of generalization may depend on where a sequential experiment terminates.

Admittedly, generalization from the total 50 pairs to a larger group of patients, at the same place or elsewhere, would always be accompanied by an element of doubt; but here we are doubtful about generalization to patients who would have actually been in the experiment if it had not produced an early verdict. This is one more reason why, in spite of the advantages of the sequential design, we ought to be aware of its limitations.

References

For details of sequential experiment techniques, examples and bibliography, Armitage's book *Sequential Medical Trials* is a standard reference. The work of Bross should also be consulted.

4. SAMPLE SIZES REQUIRED FROM BINOMIAL POPULATIONS

The principles of sample size estimation in Chapter VIII and the discussion of binomial populations in Chapter XI can be applied to Tables I and II in order to answer a question such as the following: If in a certain population of patients 85 per cent would do better on treatment A than on treatment B, and 15 per cent would do better on B than on A, how large a random sample, fixed before the experiment, would we need in order to have strong assurance of demonstrating that treatment A was superior to B in not less than 50 per cent of the population?

By "demonstration" we imply the discovery of a difference from the 50:50 ratio that would be found in less than 5 per cent of random samples if that ratio were the actual ratio in the population (a Type I error of 5 per cent). By "strong assurance" we imply that at least 95 per cent of experiments, with the stipulated population (85 per cent A-preferences) and sample size, would be successful in demonstrating a difference from the 50:50 ratio (a power of at least 0.95).

For the 50 per cent we could substitute 60 per cent or any other percentage less than 85, and for individual patients we could substitute untied pairs as in Section 3 (Sequential Designs). In fact, we can treat thus any units (individuals, pairs or groups) labeled "X", and "not-X." In order to utilize Tables I and II we label those with the lower percentage (the B-preferences) "X" — that is, the population contains 15 per cent X's and 85 per cent not-X's.

First, we must make allowance for possible bad luck. Our sample might contain an unusually high proportion of X's — it might come from the upper tail of a distribution of random samples from the 15 per cent B-preference frequency distribution. Now if we work with Tables I and II from the inside outward, we see that we can begin with a population percentage and find what would be the composition of "rare" random samples — the samples that would occupy the 2.5 per cent tails.

For instance, looking for lower-limit population percentages of 15, we find one at X = 5 and N = 12. This means that if the population percentage of X's were 15, samples of 12 containing 5 or more X's would be rare by our definition. In about 97.5 per cent of our experiments we would be luckier than that, but for safety we allow for that degree of bad luck. If, however, we obtained such a sample of 12 containing 5 X's we would be forced to admit that the actual population percentage of X's might be nearly 72 (the upper limit shown in Table I), and this is far above the 50:50 ratio that we desire.

If we next pass down the table, always looking for a lower limit of 15 per cent X's, we find one at X = 7 and N = 20. The upper limit is now 59 per cent X's. Therefore we are going in the right direction; and when we reach X = 9 and N = 30 we find what we need, for the limits are 15;49. With a population percentage of 15 and samples of 30 we would rarely find a sample containing as many as 9 X's, but even if we met one we would say that the population was unlikely to contain as many as 50 per cent X's. This is equivalent to saying that the percentage is "significantly" lower than 50 per cent, and the Type I error — the risk of rejecting 50 per cent X's if in fact that were the true value — would be less than 2.5 per cent.

If we had even worse luck than we have allowed for, i.e., if we took a sample of 30 and found 10 or more X's in it, we would wrongly accept from Table I the possibility that there might be more than 50 per cent X's in the population (e.g., 53 per cent at X = 10 and N = 30); but such values would be met in less than 2.5 per cent of samples from a population containing 15 per cent X's (85 per cent A-preferences). That is, in more than 97.5 per cent of samples we would rightly conclude that more than 50 per cent of the population were A-preferences — more than 97.5 per cent of experiments conducted under these conditions would be "successful."

It may be noticed that the sample size N = 30, estimated as necessary here, is large compared with size N = 20 specified in Section 3 as necessary in a nonsequential (fixed-sample-size) experiment when a population contains 85 per cent A-preferences and 15 per cent B-preferences. One reason is that, in order to utilize Table I, we have worked with a lower Type I error and a higher power than was adopted in Section 3.

5. BOOKS FOR FURTHER STUDY

Although one aim of this book is to give guidance in the selection and judicious use of analytical techniques, it is rather risky for anyone to pass, without personal guidance, from an introductory text to a book of techniques. However, if investigational designs are kept simple it is surprising how much can be accomplished by the simplest of the techniques discussed in previous chapters, provided that we learn to *think* statistically. This learning never ends, for statistics, applied to the real world, is more an art than a science. One of the best ways of improving our skill in the art is to see how others practice it. For that purpose four recent books can be recommended:

Medical Surveys and Clinical Trials, edited by Witts — a title that has been mentioned more than once in preceding chapters.

Controlled Clinical Trials, issued by the Council for International Organizations of Medical Sciences — papers presented by British investigators to their European colleagues in Vienna in 1959.

The Clinical Evaluation of New Drugs, edited by Waife and Shapiro — a book by American investigators.

It is noteworthy that the majority of the contributors to these three books are not professional statisticians, but clinical and other medical workers who think and act statistically. This is an example of what must happen universally if statistics is to penetrate research without doing harm.

Statistical Methods in Clinical and Preventive Medicine, in which Sir Austin Bradford Hill has reissued papers that were published between 1948 and 1960 — his own articles and lectures, and also reports of work in which he played a major role. They include accounts of drug trials, field trials of vaccines, and medical surveys.

To a small-scale clinical investigator these four titles may seem to lie outside his main field, but the principles displayed in these books, and even many details of method, will give him insight and guidance. Even laboratory workers would benefit by dipping into them. To laboratory workers there can be recommended also Finney's *Experimental Design and Its Statistical Basis,* and *An Introduction to Scientific Research* by a professor of chemistry, E. B. Wilson.

For many years a standard book on computational techniques in the biologic sciences has been Snedecor's *Statistical Methods Applied to Experiments in Agriculture and Biology.* This is concerned largely with "parametric" methods (analysis of variance, regression, and the like). For display of available "nonparametric" methods, reference can be made to Siegel's *Nonparametric Statistics for the Behavioral Sciences.* It should be mentioned, however, that mathematical statisticians who specialize in these methods have criticized some of the statements in that book. Therefore probably the best advice to a research worker who is looking for an appropriate nonparametric technique, is that he select one or two that appear suitable to his needs and then consult a mathematical statistician regarding details of their application and interpretation.

REFERENCES

Arkin, H., and Colton, R. R.: Tables for Statisticians. New York, Barnes and Noble, Inc., 1950 – 1959.

Armitage, P.: Sequential Medical Trials. Oxford, Blackwell; Springfield, Illinois, Charles C Thomas, Publisher, 1960.

Auble, D.: Extended Tables for the Mann-Whitney Statistic. Indiana University Institute of Educational Research, 1953.

Barr, M. L., Bertram, L. F., and Lindsay, H. A.: The morphology of the nerve cell nucleus, according to sex. Anat. Rec. 107:283, 1950.

Belk, W. P., and Sunderman, F. W.: A survey of the accuracy of chemical analyses in clinical laboratories. Am. J. Clin. Path. 17:853, 1947.

Berkson, J.: Limitations of the application of fourfold table analysis to hospital data. Biometrics Bull. 2(3):47, 1946.

Berkson, J.: The statistical study of association between smoking and lung cancer. Proc. Staff Meet. Mayo Clin. 30:319, 1955.

Berkson, J.: Smoking and lung cancer: another view. Lancet 1:807, 1962.

Berkson, J., Magath, T. B., and Hurn, M.: The error of estimate of the blood cell count as made with the hemocytometer. Am. J. Physiol. 128:309, 1940.

Biggs, R., and MacMillan, R. L.: The errors of some haematological methods as they are used in a routine laboratory. J. Clin. Path. 1:269, 1948. The error of the red cell count. Ibid. 288.

Birkelo, C. C., Chamberlain, W. F., and others: Tuberculosis case finding. A comparison of the effectiveness of various roentgenographic and photofluorographic methods. J.A.M.A. 133:359, 1947.

Boyd, E.: The experimental error inherent in measuring the growing human body. Am. J. Phys. Anthrop. 13:389, 1929.

Boynton, P. L., and Herbert, K. G.: Correlational analyses of the influence of basal chronological age on I Q relationships to specified anthropometric measurements. Human Biol. 14:527, 1942.

Bross, I.: Sequential medical plans. Biometrics 8:188, 1952.

Chance, M. R. A.: In Symposium on Humane Technique in the Laboratory. Brit. Med. J. 1:1177, 1957.

Cochrane, A. L.: Discussion of A. Stewart's paper on "Occupational and domiciliary factors in pulmonary tuberculosis." In Medical Research Council: The Application of Scientific Methods to Industrial and Service Medicine. London, H. M. Stationery Office, 1951, p. 36.

Cochrane, A. L., Chapman, P. J., and Oldham, P. D.: Observers' errors in taking medical histories. Lancet 1:1007, 1951.

Comstock, G. W., and Kendrick, M. A.: Blood pressure and the weather. Am. Heart J. 53:825, 1957.

Corner, B. D.: Death at birth. Brit. Med. J. 1:242, 1949.

Corner, G. W.: The Hormones in Human Reproduction. Princeton, Princeton University Press, 1943.

Council for International Organizations of Medical Sciences: Controlled Clinical Trials. Oxford, Blackwell; Springfield, Illinois, Charles C Thomas, 1960.

Crabtree, C.: Sex differences in the structure of Bowman's capsule in the mouse. Science 91:299, 1940.

Daniels, M.: Clinical evaluation of chemotherapy in tuberculosis. Brit. Med. Bull. 7(4):320, 1951.

Densen, P. M., Padget, P., and others: Studies in cardiovascular syphilis. II.

353

Methodologic problems in the evaluation of therapy. Am. J. Syph. 36:64, 1952.

Doll, R.: Occupational factors in peptic ulcer. In Medical Research Council: The Application of Scientific Methods to Industrial and Service Medicine. London, H. M. Stationery Office, 1951, p. 16.

Dublin, L. I.: Longevity in retrospect and in prospect. In Cowdry, E. V. (Editor): Problems of Ageing: Biological and Medical Aspects. Baltimore, Williams and Wilkins, 1942.

Dublin, L. I., and Marks, H. H.: The build of women and its relation to their mortality. New York Assn. of Life Insurance Medical Directors of America, 1938. Mortality of women according to build — experience on substandard issues. Ibid. 1939.

Editorial: Questionaries in clinical trials. Brit. Med. J. 1:1366, 1954.

Erhardt, C. L., and Weiner, L.: Changes in mortality statistics through the use of the New International Statistical Classification. Am. J. Pub. Health 40: 6, 1950.

Finney, D. J.: Experimental Design and Its Statistical Basis. Chicago, University of Chicago Press, 1955.

Fisher, R. A.: Statistical Methods for Research Workers. Edinburgh and London, Oliver and Boyd; New York, Hafner Publishing Co., Inc., 1925 – 1954.

Fisher, R. A.: The Design of Experiments. Edinburgh and London, Oliver and Boyd; New York, Hafner Publishing Co., Inc., 1935 – 1951.

Fisher, R. A., and Yates, F.: Statistical Tables for Biological, Agricultural and Medical Research. Edinburgh and London, Oliver and Boyd; New York, Hafner Publishing Co., Inc., 1938 – 1957.

Fix, E., and Hodges, J. L.: Significance probabilities of the Wilcoxon test. Ann. Math. Stat. 26:301, 1955.

Flagle, C. D.: Operations research in the health services. Operations Research 10:591, 1962.

Florey, M. E., MacVine, J. S., and Bigby, M. A. M.: Treatment of breast abscesses with penicillin. Brit. Med. J. 2: 845, 1946.

Glaser, E. M.: A further note on errors in the use of questionnaires. Clin. Sci. 13:475, 1954.

Gray, H.: Weight-height-age tables for American adults and children. In Piersol and Bortz: Cyclopedia Med., Surg., and Specialties. Vol. 15, p. 1052. Philadelphia, F. A. Davis Co., 1940.

Greenwood, M. (1935) quoted in Editorial: Vaccination against smallpox. Brit. Med. J. 2:311, 1962.

Greenwood, M.: Medical statistics from Graunt to Farr (concluded). Biometrika 33:1, 1943.

Greenwood, M.: Mr. Shaw on doctors. Brit. Med. J. 2:570, 1944.

Haldane, J. B. S.: The use of chi-square as a test of homogeneity in a $(n \times 2)$-fold table when expectations are small. Biometrika 33:234, 1945.

Harvard University Computation Laboratory Staff: Tables of the Cumulative Binomial Probability Distribution. Cambridge, Mass., Harvard University Press, 1955.

Herrera, L.: Bias in the allocation of treatments by random numbers. Science 122:828, 1955.

Herrera, L.: The precision of percentiles in establishing normal limits in medicine. J. Lab. & Clin. Med. 52:34, 1958.

Hill, A. B.: Principles of Medical Statistics. London, The Lancet, 1945. (Ed. 7 – London and New York, Oxford University Press, 1961.)

Hill, A. B. (1951 a): General principles of field surveys. In Medical Research Council: The Application of Scientific Methods to Industrial and Service Medicine. London, H. M. Stationery Office, 1951, p. 7.

Hill, A. B. (1951 b): The clinical trial. Brit. Med. Bull. 7(4):278, 1951.

Hill, A. B.: The clinical trial. New England J. Med. 247:113, 1952.

Hill, A. B.: Observation and experiment. New England J. Med. 248:995, 1953.

Hill, A. B.: Snow — an appreciation. Proc. Roy. Soc. Med. 48:1008, 1955.

Hill, A. B.: Statistical Methods in Clinical and Preventive Medicine. London and New York, Oxford University Press, 1962.

Hogben, L.: Chance and Choice by Cardpack and Chessboard. An introduction to Probability in Practice by Visual Aids. Vol. 1. New York, Chanticleer Press, 1950.

Jamieson, R. A.: Perforated peptic ulcer. Short-term variations in frequency. Brit. Med. J. 2:289, 1947.

Jellinek, E. M.: Clinical tests on effectiveness of analgesic drugs. Biometrics Bull. 2(5):87, 1946.

Johnson, A. H.: The Wit and Wisdom of Alfred North Whitehead. Boston, Beacon Press, 1947.

Kelly, H. J., Souders, H. J., and others: Daily decreases in the body total and stem lengths of normal children. Human Biol. 15:65, 1943.

Kendall, M. G.: Rank Correlation Methods. London, Griffin, 1948.

Kendall, M. G.: The Advanced Theory of Statistics. London, Griffin; New York, Hafner Publishing Co., Inc., Vol. 1, 1952.

Kendall, M. G., and Babington-Smith, B.: Second paper on random sampling numbers. J. Roy. Stat. Soc. Supp. 6:51, 1939.

Kendall, M. G., and Babington-Smith, B.: Tables of Random Sampling Numbers. Tracts for Computers No. XXIV. Cambridge University Press, 1946.

Lieberman, G. J., and Owen, D. B.: Tables of the Hypergeometric Probability Distribution. Stanford, California, Stanford University Press, 1961.

Mackintosh, J. M.: Snow — the man and his times. Proc. Roy. Soc. Med. 48: 1004, 1955.

Mainland, D.: The Treatment of Clinical and Laboratory Data. An Introduction to Statistical Ideas and Methods for Medical and Dental Workers. Edinburgh and London, Oliver and Boyd, 1938.

Mainland, D.: Anatomy as a Basis for Medical and Dental Practice. New York, Hoeber, 1945.

Mainland, D.: Statistical methods in medical research. I. Qualitative statistics (enumeration data). Canad. J. Res., E, 26:1, 1948.

Mainland, D.: The risk of fallacious conclusions from autopsy data on the incidence of diseases, with applications to heart disease. Am. Heart J. 45:644, 1953.

Mainland, D.: Some undesirable effects of laboratory tradition. In Steele, M. J. (Editor): Methods in Medical Research. Chicago, The Year Book Publishers, Vol. 6, 1954, p. 172.

Mainland, D. (1955 a): Use of case records in the study of therapy and other features in chronic disease. I. Planning the survey. Ann. Rheum. Dis. 14:337, 1955.

Mainland, D. (1955 b): An experimental statistician looks at anthropometry. Ann. N. Y. Acad. Sci. 63:474, 1955.

Mainland, D.: Measurement of bone density. Ann. Rheum. Dis. 15:115, 1956.

Mainland, D.: A study of age differences in the X-ray density of the adult human calcaneus — variation and sources of bias. J. Gerontol. 12:53, 1957.

Mainland, D.: The use and misuse of statistics in medical publications. Clin. Pharm. & Therap. 1:411, 1960.

Mainland, D.: Experiences in the development of multiclinic trials. J. New Drugs 1:197, 1961.

Mainland, D., Herrera, L., and Sutcliffe, M. I.: Statistical Tables for Use with Binomial Samples — Contingency Tests, Confidence Limits, and Sample Size Estimates. New York University College of Medicine Department of Medical Statistics, 1956.

Mainland, D., and Murray, I. M.: Tables for use in fourfold contingency tests. Science 116:591, 1952.

Mainland, D., and Sutcliffe, M. I.: Statistical methods in medical research. II. Sample sizes in experiments involving all-or-none responses. Canad. J. Med. Sci. 31:406, 1953.

Mainland, D., and Sutcliffe, M. I.: Hydroxychloroquine sulfate in rheumatoid arthritis, a six month double-blind trial. Bull. Rheum. Dis. 13:287, 1962.

Masserman, Jules H.: Behavior and Neurosis. Chicago, University of Chicago Press, 1943.

Medical Research Council: Streptomycin treatment of pulmonary tuberculosis. Brit. Med. J. 2:769, 1948.

Medical Research Council of Great Britain and American Heart Association: Treatment of acute rheumatic fever in children. A co-operative clinical trial of ACTH, cortisone and aspirin. Circulation 11:343, 1955; Brit. Med. J. 1:555, 1955.

Moroney, M. J.: Facts from Figures. Harmondsworth, Middlesex, Penguin Books, 1951.

Mustard, H. S.: Summary of Vital Statistics, 1948. Department of Health, City of New York, 1948.

Neyman, J.: Statistics — servant of all sciences. Science 122:401, 1955.

Ogilvie, H.: The use of experience. Brit. Med. J. 2:663, 1949.

Osgood, E. E.: Hemoglobin, color index, saturation index and volume index standards: Redetermination based on the findings in one hundred and thirty-seven healthy young men. Arch. Int. Med. 37:685, 1926.

Patterson, W. G.: Review of "Proceedings of the First International Congress on Medical Records." Brit. Med. J. 2:140, 1954.

Rand Corporation: A Million Random Digits with 100,000 Normal Deviates. Glencoe, Illinois, The Free Press, 1955.

Reed, L. J., and Love, A. G.: Biometric studies on U. S. army officers — somatological norms, correlations, and changes with age. Human Biol. 4:509, 1932. Biometric studies on U. S. army officers — somatological norms in disease. Ibid. 5:61, 1933.

Roethlisberger, F. J., and Dickson, W. J.: Management and the Worker. An Account of a Research Program Conducted by the Western Electric Company, Hawthorne Works, Chicago. Cambridge, Mass., Harvard University Press, 1946.

Ruegamer, W. R., and others: Growth, food utilization, and thyroid activity in the albino rat as a function of extra handling. Science 120:184, 1954.

Sartwell, P. E., and Merrell, M.: Influence of the dynamic character of chronic disease on the interpretation of morbidity rates. Am. J. Pub. Health 42:579, 1952.

Schilling, V.: The Blood Picture and Its Clinical Significance. St. Louis, The C. V. Mosby Co., 1929.

Siegel, S.: Nonparametric Statistics for the Behavioral Sciences. New York, McGraw-Hill Book Co., Inc., 1956.

Snedecor, G. W.: Statistical Methods Applied to Experiments in Agriculture and Biology. Ames, Iowa State College Press, 1946. (Ed. 5, 1956.)

Steggerda, M.: Anthropometry of the living: a study on checking of techniques. Anthropological Briefs, New York, No. 2:7, 1942.

Street, E.: A modification of the standard sequential test for the relative effectiveness of two therapies. Clin. Pharm. & Therap. 3:246, 1962.

Stuart, H. C., and Meredith, H. V.: Use of body measurements in the school health program. Am. J. Pub. Health 36:1365, 1946.

Sunderman, F. W., and Boerner, F.: Normal Values in Clinical Medicine. Philadelphia, W. B. Saunders Company, 1949.

Tukey, J. W.: The simplest signed-rank tests. Memorandum 17 (mimeographed). Princeton University Statistical Research Group, 1949.

Universities Federation for Animal Welfare: Handbook on the Care and Management of Laboratory Animals. London, UFAW, 1957.

Vanzant, F. R., Alvarez, W. C., and others: The normal range of gastric acidity from youth to old age. An analysis of 3,746 records. Arch. Int. Med. 49:345, 1932.

Waife, S. O., and Shapiro, A. P. (Editors): The Clinical Evaluation of New Drugs. New York, Hoeber, 1959.

White, C.: The use of ranks in a test of significance for comparing two treatments. Biometrics 8:33, 1952.

Whiteley, M. A., and Pearson, K.: Data for the problem of evolution in man. I. A first study of the variability and correlation of the hand. Proc. Roy. Soc. London 65:126, 1900.

Wilcoxon, F.: Some Rapid Approximate Statistical Procedures. New York, American Cyanamid Company, 1949.

Wilson, E. B.: An Introduction to Scientific Research. New York, McGraw-Hill Book Co., Inc., 1952.

Witts, L. J. (Editor): Medical Surveys and Clinical Trials. Some Methods and Applications of Group Research in Medicine. London and New York, Oxford University Press, 1959.

Woodham-Smith, C.: Florence Nightingale, 1820 – 1910. New York and London, McGraw-Hill Book Co., Inc., 1951, pp. 203 – 204.

World Health Organization: Epidemiological and vital statistics report. 3(4): 104, 1950.

Yule, G. U., and Kendall, M. G.: An Introduction to the Theory of Statistics. London, Griffin, 1949.

APPENDIX

Table I. Limits of Binomial Population Percentages of X's Estimated from Random Samples — No. of X's in Sample: 0–50; Sample Sizes: 1–100

Maximum risks of overestimating lower limit and of underestimating upper limit = 2.5 per cent. X = No. of X's in sample. Bold-faced figures are sample sizes. Lower and upper limits are separated by semicolons. For explanation and method of use, see Chapter XI.

X = 0	**1** 0; 97. 5	**2** 0; 84	**3** 0; 71	**4** 0; 60	**5** 0; 52
	6 0; 46	**7** 0; 41	**8** 0; 37	**9** 0; 34	**10** 0; 31
	12 0; 26	**14** 0; 23	**16** 0; 21	**18** 0; 19	**20** 0; 17
	25 0; 14	**30** 0; 12	**35** 0; 10	**40** 0; 8. 8	**50** 0; 7. 1
	60 0; 6. 0	**70** 0; 5. 1	**80** 0; 4. 5	**90** 0; 4. 0	**100** 0; 3. 62

X = 1	**2** 1. 3; 98. 74	**3** 0. 84; 91	**4** 0. 63; 81	**5** 0. 51; 72	**6** 0. 42; 64
	7 0. 36; 58	**8** 0. 32; 53	**9** 0. 28; 48	**10** 0. 25; 44. 5	**12** 0. 21; 38. 5
	14 0. 18; 34	**16** 0. 16; 30	**18** 0. 14; 27	**20** 0. 13; 25	**22** 0. 12; 23
	25 0. 10; 20	**30** 0. 08; 17	**35** 0. 07; 15	**40** 0. 06; 13	**50** 0. 05; 11
	60 0. 04; 9. 0	**70** 0. 04; 7. 7	**80** 0. 03; 6. 8	**90** 0. 03; 6. 0	**100** 0.025; 5.45

X = 2	**4** 6. 8; 93	**5** 5. 3; 85	**6** 4. 3; 78	**7** 3. 7; 71	**8** 3. 2; 65
	9 2. 8; 60	**10** 2. 5; 56	**11** 2. 3; 52	**12** 2. 1; 48	**14** 1. 8; 43
	16 1. 6; 38	**18** 1. 4; 35	**20** 1. 2; 32	**22** 1. 1; 29	**24** 1. 0; 27
	26 0. 95; 25	**28** 0. 88; 24	**30** 0. 82; 22	**35** 0. 70; 19	**40** 0. 61; 17
	50 0. 49; 14	**60** 0. 41; 12	**70** 0. 35; 10	**80** 0. 30; 9	**90** 0. 27; 8
	100 0. 24; 7. 04				

X = 3	**6** 12; 88	**7** 9. 9; 82	**8** 8. 5; 75. 5	**9** 7. 5; 70	**10** 6. 7; 65
	12 5. 5; 57	**14** 4. 7; 51	**16** 4. 0; 46	**18** 3. 6; 41	**20** 3. 2; 38
	22 2. 9; 35	**24** 2. 7; 32	**26** 2. 4; 30	**28** 2. 3; 28	**30** 2. 1; 27
	35 1. 8; 23	**40** 1. 6; 20	**45** 1. 4; 18	**50** 1. 3; 17	**60** 1. 0; 14
	70 0. 89; 12	**80** 0. 78; 11	**90** 0. 69; 9	**100** 0. 62; 8. 53	

X = 4	**8** 16; 84	**9** 14; 79	**10** 12; 74	**11** 11; 69	**12** 9. 9; 65
	14 8. 4; 58	**16** 7. 3; 52	**18** 6. 4; 48	**20** 5. 8; 44	**22** 5. 2; 40
	24 4. 8; 37	**26** 4. 4; 35	**28** 4. 0; 33	**30** 3. 8; 31	**32** 3. 5; 29
	35 3. 2; 27	**40** 2. 8; 24	**45** 2. 5; 21	**50** 2. 2; 19	**60** 1. 9; 16
	70 1. 6; 14	**80** 1. 4; 12	**90** 1. 2; 11	**100** 1. 10; 9. 93	

X = 5	**10** 19; 81	**11** 17; 77	**12** 15; 72	**14** 13; 65	**16** 11; 59
	18 9. 7; 53	**20** 8. 7; 49	**22** 7. 8; 45	**24** 7. 1; 42	**26** 6. 6; 39
	28 6. 1; 37	**30** 5. 6; 35	**32** 5. 3; 33	**35** 4. 8; 30	**40** 4. 2; 27
	45 3. 7; 24	**50** 3. 3; 22	**60** 2. 8; 18	**70** 2. 4; 16	**80** 2. 1; 14
	90 1. 8; 12. 5	**100** 1. 64; 11. 29			

X = 6	**12** 21; 79	**13** 19; 75	**14** 18; 71	**15** 16; 68	**16** 15; 65
	18 13; 59	**20** 12; 54	**22** 11; 50	**24** 9. 8; 47	**26** 9. 0; 44
	28 8. 3; 41	**30** 7. 7; 39	**32** 7. 2; 36	**35** 6. 6; 34	**37** 6. 2; 32
	40 5. 7; 30	**45** 5. 1; 27	**50** 4. 5; 24	**60** 3. 8; 20. 5	**70** 3. 2; 18
	80 2. 8; 16	**90** 2. 5; 14	**100** 2. 24; 12. 60		

X = 7	**14** 23; 77	**15** 21; 73	**16** 20; 70	**18** 17; 64	**20** 15; 59
	22 14; 55	**24** 13; 51	**26** 12; 48	**28** 11; 45	**30** 9. 9; 42
	32 9. 3; 40	**34** 8. 7; 38	**37** 8. 0; 35	**40** 7. 3; 33	**42** 7. 0; 31
	45 6. 5; 29	**50** 5. 8; 27	**55** 5. 3; 24	**60** 4. 8; 23	**65** 4. 4; 21
	70 4. 1; 20	**80** 3. 6; 17	**90** 3. 2; 15	**100** 2. 86; 13. 90	

Table I *(Continued)*

X = 8	16 25; 75	17 23; 72	18 22; 69	19 20; 66. 5	20 19; 64
	22 17; 59	24 16; 55	26 14; 52	28 13; 49	30 12; 46
	32 11; 43	35 10; 40	37 9. 8; 38	40 9. 0; 36	42 8. 6; 34
	45 8. 0; 32	50 7. 2; 29	55 6. 5; 27	60 5. 9; 25	65 5. 5; 23
	70 5. 1; 21	80 4. 4; 19	90 3. 9; 17	100 3. 51; 15. 16	

X = 9	18 26; 74	19 24; 71	20 23; 68	22 21; 64	24 19; 59
	26 17; 56	28 16; 52	30 15; 49	32 14; 47	34 13; 44
	37 12; 41	40 11; 38	42 10; 37	45 9. 6; 35	47 9. 2; 33
	50 8. 6; 31	55 7. 8; 29	60 7. 1; 27	65 6. 5; 25	70 6. 1; 23
	80 5. 3; 20	90 4. 7; 18	100 4. 20; 16. 40		

X = 10	20 27; 73	21 26; 70	22 24; 68	24 22; 63	26 20; 59
	28 19; 56	30 17; 53	32 16; 50	34 15; 47	37 14; 44
	40 13; 41	42 12; 39	45 11; 37	47 11; 36	50 10; 34
	55 9. 1; 31	60 8. 3; 29	65 7. 6; 26	70 7. 1; 25	80 6. 2; 22
	90 5. 5; 19	100 4. 90; 17. 62			

X = 11	22 28; 72	24 26; 67	26 23; 63	28 21; 59	30 20; 56
	32 19; 53	34 17; 51	36 16; 48	38 15; 46	40 15; 44
	42 14; 42	45 13; 40	47 12; 38	50 12; 36	55 10; 33
	60 9. 5; 30	65 8. 8; 28	70 8. 1; 26	80 7. 1; 23	90 6. 3; 21
	100 5. 62; 18. 83				

X = 12	24 29; 71	25 28; 69	26 27; 67	28 24; 63	30 23; 59
	32 21; 56	34 20; 53. 5	36 19; 51	38 18; 49	40 17; 47
	42 16; 45	45 15; 42	47 14; 40	50 13; 38	55 12; 35
	60 11; 32	65 9. 9; 30	70 9. 2; 28	80 8. 0; 25	90 7. 1; 22
	100 6. 36; 20. 02				

X = 13	26 30; 70	27 29; 68	28 28; 66	29 26; 64	30 25; 63
	32 24; 59	34 22; 56	36 21; 54	38 20; 51	40 19; 49
	42 18; 47	45 16; 44	47 16; 43	50 15; 40	55 13; 37
	60 12; 34	65 11; 32	70 10; 30	75 9. 6; 28	80 9. 0; 26
	90 7. 9; 23	100 7. 11; 21. 20			

X = 14	28 31; 69	30 28; 66	32 26; 62	34 25; 59	36 23; 57
	38 22; 54	40 21; 52	42 20; 50	45 18; 47	47 17; 45
	50 16; 42	55 15; 39	60 13; 36	65 12; 33	70 11; 31
	75 11; 29	80 9. 9; 28	90 8. 8; 25	100 7. 87; 22. 37	

X = 15	30 31; 69	32 29; 65	34 27; 62	36 26; 59	38 24; 57
	40 23; 54	42 22; 52	44 21; 50	46 20; 48	48 19; 46
	50 18; 45	55 16; 41	60 15; 38	65 14; 35	70 13; 33
	75 12; 31	80 11; 29	85 10; 27	90 10; 26	100 8. 645; 23. 53

X = 16	32 32; 68	34 30; 65	36 28; 62	38 26; 59	40 25; 57
	42 23; 54	44 22; 52	46 21; 50	48 20; 48	50 20; 47
	55 18; 43	60 16; 40	65 15; 37	70 14; 34	75 13; 32
	80 12; 30	90 11; 27	100 9. 45; 24. 66		

X = 17	34 32; 68	36 30; 65	38 29; 61	40 27; 59	42 26; 57
	44 24; 55	46 23; 52	48 22; 51	50 21; 49	55 19; 45
	60 17; 41	65 16; 39	70 15; 36	75 14; 34	80 13; 32
	85 12; 30	90 11; 28	100 10. 25; 25. 79		

X = 18	36 33; 67	38 31; 64	40 29; 62	42 28; 59	44 26; 57
	46 25; 55	48 24; 53	50 23; 51	55 21; 47	60 19; 43
	65 17; 40	70 16; 38	75 15; 35	80 14; 33	85 13; 31
	90 12; 30	100 11. 06; 26. 92			

Table I (Continued)

```
X = 19   38 33;67      40 32;64      42 30;61      44 28;59      46 27;57
         48 26;55      50 25;53      55 22;49      60 20;45      65 19;42
         70 17;39      75 16;37      80 15;35      85 14;33      90 13;31
        100 11.86;28.06

X = 20   40 34;66      42 32;64      44 30;61      46 29;59      48 28;57
         50 26;55      55 24;50      60 22;47      65 20;43      70 18;41
         75 17;38      80 16;36      85 15;34      90 14;32     100 12.66;29.19

X = 21   42 34;66      44 32;63      46 31;61      48 29;59      50 28;57
         55 25;52      60 23;48      65 21;45      70 20;42      75 18;40
         80 17;37      85 16;35      90 15;33     100 13.51;30.28

X = 22   44 35;65      46 33;63      48 31;61      50 30;59      55 27;54
         60 25;50      65 23;47      70 21;44      75 19;41      80 18;39
         85 17;36      90 16;35      95 15;33     100 14.35;31.37

X = 23   46 35;65      48 33;63      50 32;61      55 29;56      60 26;52
         65 24;48      70 22;45      75 20;42      80 19;40      85 18;38
         90 17;36      95 16;34     100 15.19;32.47

X = 24   48 35;65      50 34;63      55 30;58      60 28;53      65 25;50
         70 23;47      75 22;44      80 20;41      85 19;39      90 18;37
         95 17;35     100 16.03;33.56

X = 25   50 36;64      55 32;59      60 29;55      65 27;51      70 25;48
         75 23;45      80 21;43      85 20;40      90 19;38      95 18;36
        100 16.88;34.66

X = 26   52 36;64      55 34;61      60 31;57      65 28;53      70 26;50
         75 24;47      80 22;44      85 21;42      90 20;39      95 19;37
        100 17.75;35.72

X = 27   54 36;64      55 35;63      60 32;58      65 29;54      70 27;51
         75 25;48      80 24;45      85 22;43      90 21.41      95 20;39
        100 18.62;36.79

X = 28   56 36;64      60 34;60      65 31;56      70 28;52      75 26;49
         80 25;46      85 23;44      90 22;42      95 21;40     100 19.50;37.85

X = 29   58 37;63      60 35;62      65 32;57      70 30;54      75 28;51
         80 26;48      85 24;45      90 23;43      95 21;41     100 20.37;38.92

X = 30   60 37;63      65 34;59      70 31;55      75 29;52      80 27;49
         85 25;46      90 24;44      95 22;42     100 21.24;39.98

X = 31   62 37;63      65 35;60      70 32;57      75 30;53      80 28;50
         85 26;48      90 25;45      95 23;43     100 22.14;41.02

X = 32   64 37;63      65 37;62      70 34;58      75 31;55      80 29;52
         85 27;49      90 26;46      95 24;44     100 23.04;42.06

X = 33   66 37;63      70 35;59      75 33;56      80 30;53      85 28;50
         90 27;47      95 25;45     100 23.93;43.10

X = 34   68 38;62      70 36;61      75 34;57      80 32;54      85 30:51
         90 28;49      95 26;46     100 24.83;44.15

X = 35   70 38;62      75 35;59      80 33;55      85 31;52      90 29;50
         95 27;47     100 25.73;45.19
```

Table I (*Continued*)

X = 36	**72** 38; 62	**75** 36; 60	**80** 34; 57	**85** 32; 54	**90** 30; 51
	95 28; 48	**100** 26. 65; 46. 20			
X = 37	**74** 38; 62	**75** 38; 61	**80** 35; 58	**85** 33; 55	**90** 31; 52
	95 29; 49	**100** 27. 57; 47. 22			
X = 38	**76** 38; 62	**80** 36; 59	**85** 34; 56	**90** 32; 53	**95** 30; 51
	100 28. 49; 48. 24				
X = 39	**78** 38; 62	**80** 37; 60	**85** 35; 57	**90** 33; 54	**95** 31; 52
	100 29. 41; 49. 26				
X = 40	**80** 39; 61	**85** 36; 58	**90** 34; 55	**95** 32; 53	**100** 30. 33; 50. 28
X = 41	**82** 39; 61	**85** 37; 59	**90** 35; 56	**95** 33; 54	**100** 31. 27; 51. 28
X = 42	**84** 39; 61	**85** 38; 60	**90** 36; 57	**95** 34; 55	**100** 32. 21; 52. 28
X = 43	**86** 39; 61	**90** 37; 59	**95** 35; 56	**100** 33. 15; 53. 27	
X = 44	**88** 39; 61	**90** 38; 60	**95** 36; 57	**100** 34. 09; 54. 27	
X = 45	**90** 39; 61	**95** 37; 58	**100** 35. 03; 55. 27		
X = 46	**92** 39; 61	**95** 38; 59	**100** 35. 99; 56. 25		
X = 47	**94** 40; 60	**95** 39; 60	**100** 36. 95; 57. 23		
X = 48	**96** 40; 60	**100** 37. 91; 58. 21			
X = 49	**98** 40; 60	**100** 38. 87; 59. 19			
X = 50	**100** 39. 83; 60. 17				

Table II. Limits of Binomial Population Percentages of X's Estimated from Random Samples — Percentage of X's in Sample: 50–1; Sample Sizes: 100–1000

Maximum risks of overestimating lower limit and of underestimating upper limit = 2.5 per cent. X per cent = percentage of X's in sample. N = total number of individuals in sample. Lower and upper limits are separated by semicolons. For explanation and method of use, see Chapter XI.

X%	N=100	N=120	N=150	N=200	N=300	N=400	N=500	N=1000	X%
50	40;60	41;59	42;58	43;57	44;56	45;55	46;54	47;53	50
49	39;59	40;58	41;57	42;56	43;55	44;54	45;53	46;52	49
48	38;58	39;57	40;56	41;55	42;54	43;53	44;52	45;51	48
47	37;57	38;56	39;55	40;54	41;53	42;52	43;51	44;50	47
46	36;56	37;55	38;54	39;53	40;52	41;51	42;50	43;49	46
45	35;55	36;54	37;53	38;52	39;51	40;50	41;49	42;48	45
44	34;54	35;53	36;52	37;51	38;50	39;49	40;48	41;47	44
43	33;53	34;52	35;51	36;50	37;49	38;48	39;47	40;46	43
42	32;52	33;51	34;50	35;49	36;48	37;47	38;46	39;45	42
41	31;51	32;50	33;49	34;48	35;47	36;46	37;45	38;44	41
40	30;50	31;49	32;48	33;47	34;46	35;45	36;44	37;43	40
39	29;49	30;48	31;47	32;46	33;45	34;44	35;43	36;42	39
38	28;48	29;47	30;46	31;45	32;44	33;43	34;42	35;41	38
37	28;47	28;46	29;45	30;44	32;43	32;42	33;41	34;40	37
36	27;46	27;45	28;44	29;43	31;42	31;41	32;40	33;39	36
35	26;45	27;44	27;43	28;42	30;41	30;40	31;39	32;38	35
34	25;44	26;43	26;42	27;41	29;40	29;39	30;38	31;37	34
33	24;43	25;42	26;41	27;40	28;39	28;38	29;37	30;36	33
32	23;42	24;41	25;40	26;39	27;38	27;37	28;36	29;35	32
31	22;41	23;40	24;39	25;38	26;37	26;36	27;35	28;34	31
30	21;40	22;39	23;38	24;37	25;36	26;35	26;34	27;33	30
29	20;39	21;38	22;37	23;36	24;34	25;34	25;33	26;32	29
28	20;38	20;37	21;36	22;35	23;33	24;33	24;32	25;31	28
27	19;37	19;36	20;35	21;34	22;32	23;32	23;31	24;30	27
26	18;36	18;35	19;34	20;33	21;31	22;31	22;30	23;29	26
25	17.35	18;34	18;33	19;32	20;30	21;30	21;29	22;28	25
24	16;34	17;33	17;32	18;31	19;29	20;28	20;28	21;27	24
23	15;32	16;32	17;31	17;29	18;28	19;27	19;27	20;26	23
22	14;31	15;30	16;29	16;28	17;27	18;26	18;26	19;25	22
21	14;30	14;29	15;28	16;27	17;26	17;25	18;25	19;24	21
20	13;29	13;28	14;27	15;26	16;25	16;24	17;24	18;23	20
19	12;28	12;27	13;26	14;25	15;24	15;23	16;23	17;22	19
18	11;27	12;26	12;25	13;24	14;23	14;22	15;22	16;21	18
17	10;26	11;25	11;24	12;23	13;22	13;21	14;21	15;19	17
16	9;25	10;24	11;23	11;22	12;21	13;20	13;20	14;18	16
15	8.6;24	9.1;23	9.7;22	10;21	11;20	12;19	12;18	13;17	15
14	7.9;22	8.4;22	8.9;21	9.5;20	10;18	11.18	11;17	12;16	14
13	7.1;21	7.6;20	8.1;19	8.7;18	9.4;17	9.9;17	10;16	11;15	13
12	6.4;20	6.8;19	7.3;18	7.9;17	8.6;16	9.0;16	9.3;15	10;14	12
11	5.6;19	6.0;18	6.5;17	7.0;16	7.7;15	8.1;14	8.4;14	9.1;13	11
X%	N=100	N=120	N=150	N=200	N=300	N=400	N=500	N=1000	X%

Table II (Continued)

X%	N=100	N=120	N=150	N=200	N=300	N=400	N=500	N=1000	X%
10	4.9;18	5.3;17	5.7;16	6.2;15	6.8;14	7.2;13	7.5;13	8.2;12	10
9			5.0;15	5.5;14	6.0;13	6.4;12	6.7;12	7.3;11	9
8			4.2;14	4.7;13	5.2;12	5.6;11	5.8;11	6.4;9.8	8
7			3.6;12	3.9;11	4.4;10	4.8;9.9	5.0;9.6	5.5;8.7	7
6			2.8;11	3.1;10	3.6;9.3	3.9;8.8	4.1;8.4	4.6;7.6	6
5			2.1;9.8	2.4;9.0	2.8;8.1	3.1;7.6	3.3;7.3	3.7;6.5	5
4					2.1;6.9	2.4;6.4	2.5;6.0	2.9;5.4	4
3					1.4;5.6	1.6;5.2	1.8;4.8	2.1;4.2	3
2						0.9;3.9	1.0;3.6	1.3;3.0	2
1						0.3;2.5	0.3;2.3	0.5;1.8	1
X%	N=100	N=120	N=150	N=200	N=300	N=400	N=500	N=1000	X%

Table III. Minimum Contrasts Required in Fourfold Contingency Tables to Insure a Type I Error of Not More Than 5 Per Cent (2.5 Per Cent in Each Tail)

N = number of individuals in each sample. For explanation and method of use, see Chapter XII.

N	No. of X's in Sample(1) / No. of X's in Sample(2)										
4	0/4	1/—									
5	0/4	1/5	2/—								
6	0/5	1/6	2/—								
7	0/5	1/6	2/7	3/—							
8	0/5	1/6	2/7	3/8	4/—						
9	0/5	1/6	2/8	3/8	4/9						
10	0/5	1/7	2/8	3/9	4/10	5/10					
11	0/5	1/7	2/8	3/9	4/10	5/11					
12	0/5	1/7	2/8	3/9	4/10	5/11	6/12				
13	0/5	1/7	2/8	3/9	4/10	5/11	6/12				
14	0/5	1/7	2/8	3/10	4/11	5/12	6/12	7/13			
15	0/5	1/7	2/9	3/10	4/11	5/12	6/13	7/14			
16	0/5	1/7	2/9	3/10	4/11	5/12	6/13	7/14	8/15		
17	0/5	1/7	2/9	3/10	4/11	5/12	6/13	7/14	8/15		
18	0/5	1/7	2/9	3/10	4/11	5/12	6/13	7/14	8/15	9/16	
19	0/5	1/7	2/9	3/10	4/11	5/12	6/14	7/14	8/15	9/16	
20	0/5	1/7	2/9	3/10	4/11	5/13	6/14	7/15	8/16	9/16	10/17
30	0/6	1/8	2/9	3/11	4/12	5/13	6/15	7/16	8/17	9/18	10/19
		15/24									
40	0/6	1/8	2/9	3/11	4/12	5/14	6/15	7/16	8/18	9/19	10/20
		20/30									
50	0/6	1/8	2/10	3/11	4/13	5/14	6/15	7/17	8/18	9/19	10/20
		11/22	25/36								
60	0/6	1/8	2/10	3/11	4/13	5/14	6/16	7/17	8/18	9/20	10/21
		11/22	12/23	13/24	14/26	30/42					
70	0/6	1/8	2/10	3/11	4/13	5/14	6/16	7/17	8/18	9/20	10/21
		11/22	12/23	13/25	18/30	19/32	20/33	35/48			
80	0/6	1/8	2/10	3/11	4/13	5/14	6/16	7/17	8/19	9/20	10/21
		11/22	12/24	13/25	14/26	15/27	16/29	23/36	24/38	40/54	

Table III (Continued)

N	No. of X's in Sample(1) / No. of X's in Sample(2)
90	0/6 1/8 2/10 3/11 4/13 5/14 6/16 7/17 8/19 9/20 10/21 11/23 12/24 13/25 14/26 15/28 20/33 21/35 31/45 32/47 44/59 45/59
100	0/6 1/8 2/10 3/11 4/13 5/15 6/16 7/17 8/19 9/20 10/21 11/23 12/24 13/25 14/27 18/31 19/33 25/39 26/41 50/65
150	0/6 1/8 2/10 3/12 4/13 5/15 6/16 7/18 8/19 9/20 10/22 11/23 12/24 13/26 14/27 15/28 16/30 19/33 20/35 25/40 26/42 32/48 33/50 41/58 42/60 75/93
200	0/6 1/8 2/10 3/12 4/13 5/15 6/16 7/18 8/19 9/21 10/22 11/23 12/25 13/26 14/27 15/29 18/32 19/34 22/37 23/39 27/43 28/45 33/50 34/52 41/59 42/61 51/70 52/72 65/85 66/87 100/121

Table IV. Minimum Contrasts Required in Fourfold Contingency Tables to Insure a Type I Error of Not More Than 1 Per Cent (0.5 Per Cent in Each Tail)

N = number of individuals in each sample. For explanation and method of use, see Chapter XII.

N	No. of X's in Sample(1) / No. of X's in Sample(2)
5	0/5 1/—
6	0/6 1/—
7	0/6 1/7 2/—
8	0/6 1/8 2/8 3/—
9	0/6 1/8 2/9 3/9 4/—
10	0/7 1/8 2/9 3/10 4/—
11	0/7 1/8 2/9 3/10 4/11 5/—
12	0/7 1/8 2/10 3/11 4/11 5/12 6/—
13	0/7 1/9 5/13 6/13
14	0/7 1/9 6/14 7/14
15	0/7 1/9 7/15
16	0/7 1/9 2/10 3/12 4/13 5/14 6/14 8/16
17	0/7 1/9 2/11 7/16 8/16
18	0/7 1/9 2/11 8/17 9/17
19	0/7 1/9 2/11 9/18
20	0/7 1/9 2/11 4/13 5/15 6/16 7/16 10/19
30	0/8 1/10 2/12 3/13 4/15 10/21 15/26
40	0/8 1/10 2/12 3/14 4/15 5/17 8/20 9/22 19/32 20/32
50	0/8 1/10 2/12 3/14 4/15 5/17 6/18 7/20 9/22 10/24 25/39
60	0/8 1/10 2/12 3/14 4/16 5/17 6/19 8/21 9/23 11/25 12/27 19/34 20/36 24/40 25/41 26/41 30/45
70	0/8 1/10 2/12 3/14 4/16 5/17 6/19 7/20 8/22 10/24 11/26 14/29 15/31 21/37 22/39 32/49 33/49 34/50 35/51
80	0/8 1/10 2/12 3/14 4/16 5/18 6/19 7/21 9/23 10/25 12/27 13/29 16/32 17/34 24/41 25/43 38/56 39/56 40/57
90	0/8 1/10 2/12 3/14 4/16 5/18 6/19 7/21 8/22 9/24 11/26 12/28 15/31 16/33 19/36 20/38 28/46 29/48 43/62 44/62 45/63

Table IV *(Continued)*

N	No. of X's in Sample(1) / No. of X's in Sample(2)									
100	0/8	1/10	2/13	3/14	4/16	5/18	6/19	7/21	8/22	9/24	10/25
	11/27	14/30	15/32	18/35	19/37	23/41	24/43	33/52	34/54	47/67
	48/67	50/69
150	0/8	1/11	2/13	3/15	4/16	5/18	6/20	7/21	8/23	9/24	10/26
	11/27	12/29	14/31	15/33	17/35	18/37	21/40	22/42	26/46	27/48
	31/52	32/54	39/61	40/63	51/74	52/76	75/99
200	0/8	1/11	2/13	3/15	4/16	5/18	6/20	7/21	8/23	9/24	10/26
	11/27	12/29	13/30	14/32	16/34	17/36	19/38	20/40	23/43	24/45
	26/47	27/49	31/53	32/55	36/59	37/61	43/67	44/69	51/76	52/78
	63/89	64/91	100/127

Table V. Percentages of Successful Experiments (%S) in Relation to Sample Sizes and to Percentages of X's in Populations A and B

N = number of individuals in each of two samples. For explanation and method of use, see Chapter VIII.

A: 1%, B: 5%

N	% S
5	0.0
10	0.0
15	0.0
20	0.2
30	0.3
50	2.4
70	7.6
100	19.4

A: 1%, B: 10%

N	% S
5	0.0
10	0.1
15	1.1
20	3.6
30	5.6
50	27.2
70	51.5
100	76.9

A: 1%, B: 15%

N	% S
5	0.2
10	0.9
15	5.4
20	14.3
30	23.1
50	63.7
70	86.1
100	97.3

A: 1%, B: 25%

N	% S
5	1.5
10	7.1
15	27.7
20	51.5
30	71.0
50	96.5
70	99.7
100	100.0

A: 1%, B: 33%

N	% S
5	4.2
10	18.8
15	52.9
20	77.5
30	92.0
50	99.8
70	100.0

A: 1%, B: 50%

N	% S
5	18.0
10	57.9
15	90.3
20	98.1
30	99.9
50	100.0

A: 1%, B: 67%

N	% S
5	45.1
10	89.1
15	99.3
20	100.0

A: 1%, B: 75%

N	% S
5	61.3
10	96.0
15	99.9
20	100.0

A: 1%, B: 85%

N	% S
5	81.6
10	99.3
15	100.0

A: 1%, B: 90%

N	% S
5	90.2
10	99.8
15	100.0

A: 1%, B: 95%

N	% S
5	96.7
10	100.0

A: 1%, B: 99%

N	% S
5	99.6
10	100.0

A: 5%, B: 10%

N	% S
5	0.0
10	0.1
15	0.6
20	1.7
30	1.9
50	6.3
70	11.4
100	19.0

A: 5%, B: 15%

N	% S
5	0.2
10	0.6
15	3.0
20	7.0
30	9.3
50	24.3
70	40.7
100	58.6

A: 5%, B: 25%

N	% S
5	1.2
10	4.8
15	16.6
20	29.9
30	43.6
50	74.8
70	90.8
100	98.1

A: 5%, B: 33%

N	% S
5	3.5
10	13.0
15	34.7
20	53.3
30	73.1
50	94.8
70	99.2
100	100.0

A: 5%, B: 50%

N	% S
5	15.1
10	43.1
15	73.6
20	89.4
30	98.2
50	100.0

A: 5%, B: 67%

N	% S
5	38.9
10	75.8
15	94.8
20	99.3
30	100.0

A: 5%, B: 75%

N	% S
5	53.8
10	87.3
15	98.4
20	99.9
30	100.0

A: 5%, B: 85%

N	% S
5	73.7
10	96.4
15	99.9
20	100.0

A: 5%, B: 90%

N	% S
5	83.1
10	98.7
15	100.0

A: 5%, B: 95%

N	% S
5	91.4
10	99.7
15	100.0

A: 5%, B: 99%

N	% S
5	96.7
10	100.0

A: 10%, B: 15%

N	% S
5	0.1
10	0.4
15	1.4
20	2.7
30	2.9
50	5.9
70	9.6
100	13.8

A: 10%, B: 25%

N	% S
5	1.0
10	2.9
15	8.5
20	14.4
30	21.3
50	41.0
70	58.5
100	76.2

Table V (Continued)

Column 1

N	% S
A: 10%, B: 33%	
5	2.7
10	8.0
15	19.6
20	31.1
30	47.6
50	75.7
70	90.1
100	97.6
A: 10%, B: 50%	
5	12.1
10	29.5
15	53.6
20	74.2
30	91.4
50	99.4
70	100.0
A: 10%, B: 67%	
5	32.0
10	60.9
15	85.5
20	96.5
30	99.7
50	100.0
A: 10%, B: 75%	
5	45.1
10	75.9
15	94.4
20	99.2
30	100.0
A: 10%, B: 85%	
5	63.9
10	90.9
15	99.1
20	99.9
30	100.0
A: 10%, B: 90%	
5	73.6
10	95.8
15	99.8
20	100.0
A: 10%, B: 95%	
5	83.1
10	98.7
15	100.0
A: 10%, B: 99%	
5	90.2
10	99.8
15	100.0
A: 15%, B: 25%	
5	0.7

Column 2

N	% S
10	1.7
15	4.2
20	6.6
30	9.2
50	17.1
70	25.3
100	35.9
A: 15%, B: 33%	
5	2.1
10	4.8
15	10.6
20	17.2
30	27.1
50	48.2
70	65.4
100	81.6
A: 15%, B: 50%	
5	9.5
10	19.9
15	37.1
20	57.3
30	77.7
50	95.8
70	99.4
100	100.0
A: 15%, B: 67%	
5	26.0
10	48.0
15	73.8
20	90.0
30	98.4
50	100.0
A: 15%, B: 75%	
5	37.4
10	64.2
15	87.7
20	96.6
30	99.8
50	100.0
A: 15%, B: 85%	
5	54.4
10	83.3
15	97.2
20	99.6
30	100.0
A: 15%, B: 90%	
5	63.9
10	90.9
15	99.1
20	99.9
30	100.0
A: 15%, B: 95%	
5	73.7
10	96.4

Column 3

N	% S
15	99.9
20	100.0
A: 15%, B: 99%	
5	81.6
10	99.3
15	100.0
A: 25%, B: 33%	
5	1.2
10	1.6
15	2.8
20	4.5
30	6.1
50	10.0
70	14.0
100	19.3
A: 25%, B: 50%	
5	5.7
10	8.6
15	15.7
20	26.9
30	41.3
50	67.5
70	83.1
100	94.5
A: 25%, B: 67%	
5	16.4
10	27.6
15	48.3
20	66.1
30	87.9
50	98.8
70	99.9
100	100.0
A: 25%, B: 75%	
5	24.4
10	42.1
15	67.6
20	83.4
30	97.0
50	99.9
70	100.0
A: 25%, B: 85%	
5	37.4
10	64.2
15	87.7
20	96.6
30	99.8
50	100.0
A: 25%, B: 90%	
5	45.1
10	75.9
15	94.4
20	99.2
30	100.0

Column 4

N	% S
A: 25%, B: 95%	
5	53.8
10	87.3
15	98.4
20	99.9
30	100.0
A: 25%, B: 99%	
5	61.3
10	96.0
15	99.9
20	100.0
A: 33%, B: 50%	
5	3.6
10	4.1
15	7.1
20	11.6
30	18.7
50	34.3
70	46.4
100	64.4
A: 33%, B: 67%	
5	10.8
10	16.4
15	30.1
20	43.8
30	68.4
50	91.5
70	97.8
100	99.8
A: 33%, B: 75%	
5	16.4
10	27.6
15	48.3
20	66.1
30	87.9
50	98.8
70	99.9
100	100.0
A: 33%, B: 85%	
5	26.0
10	48.0
15	73.8
20	90.0
30	98.4
50	100.0
A: 33%, B: 90%	
5	32.0
10	60.9
15	85.5
20	96.5
30	99.7
50	100.0

Table V (Continued)

N	% S
A: 33%, B: 95%	
5	38.9
10	75.8
15	94.8
20	99.3
30	100.0
A: 33%, B: 99%	
5	45.1
10	89.1
15	99.3
20	100.0
A: 50%, B: 67%	
5	3.6
10	4.1
15	7.1
20	11.6
30	18.7
50	34.3
70	46.4
100	64.4
A: 50%, B: 75%	
5	5.7
10	8.6
15	15.7
20	26.9
30	41.3
50	67.5
70	83.1
100	94.5
A: 50%, B: 85%	
5	9.5
10	19.9
15	37.1
20	57.3
30	77.7
50	95.8
70	99.4
100	100.0
A: 50%, B: 90%	
5	12.1
10	29.5
15	53.6
20	74.2
30	91.4
50	99.4
70	100.0
A: 50%, B: 95%	
5	15.1
10	43.1
15	73.6
20	89.4
30	98.2
50	100.0

N	% S
A: 50%, B: 99%	
5	18.0
10	57.9
15	90.3
20	98.1
30	99.9
50	100.0
A: 67%, B: 75%	
5	1.2
10	1.6
15	2.8
20	4.5
30	6.1
50	10.0
70	14.0
100	19.3
A: 67%, B: 85%	
5	2.1
10	4.8
15	10.6
20	17.2
30	27.1
50	48.2
70	65.4
100	81.6
A: 67%, B: 90%	
5	2.7
10	8.0
15	19.6
20	31.1
30	47.6
50	75.7
70	90.1
100	97.6
A: 67%, B: 95%	
5	3.5
10	13.0
15	34.7
20	53.3
30	73.1
50	94.8
70	99.2
100	100.0
A: 67%, B: 99%	
5	4.2
10	18.8
15	52.9
20	77.5
30	92.0
50	99.8
70	100.0

N	% S
A: 75%, B: 85%	
5	0.7
10	1.7
15	4.2
20	6.6
30	9.2
50	17.1
70	25.3
100	35.9
A: 75%, B: 90%	
5	1.0
10	2.9
15	8.5
20	14.4
30	21.3
50	41.0
70	58.5
100	76.2
A: 75%, B: 95%	
5	1.2
10	4.8
15	16.6
20	29.9
30	43.6
50	74.8
70	90.8
100	98.1
A: 75%, B: 99%	
5	1.5
10	7.1
15	27.7
20	51.5
30	71.0
50	96.5
70	99.7
100	100.0
A: 85%, B: 90%	
5	0.1
10	0.4
15	1.4
20	2.7
30	2.9
50	5.9
70	9.6
100	13.8
A: 85%, B: 95%	
5	0.2
10	0.6
15	3.0
20	7.0
30	9.3
50	24.3
70	40.7
100	58.6

N	% S
A: 85%, B: 99%	
5	0.2
10	0.9
15	5.4
20	14.3
30	23.1
50	63.7
70	86.1
100	97.3
A: 90%, B: 95%	
5	0.0
10	0.1
15	0.6
20	1.7
30	1.9
50	6.3
70	11.4
100	19.0
A: 90%, B: 99%	
5	0.0
10	0.1
15	1.1
20	3.6
30	5.6
50	27.2
70	51.5
100	76.9
A: 95%, B: 99%	
5	0.0
10	0.0
15	0.0
20	0.2
30	0.3
50	2.4
70	7.6
100	19.4

Table VI. Signed-ranks Test (Wilcoxon)

(Prepared by M.I. Sutcliffe)

N = number of pairs. P = probability (randomization frequency) in both tails combined. Minimum algebraic sums of ranks required to insure that P is not greater than the specified values. For explanation and method of use, see Chapter XIV.

N	P (Both Tails) 0.10−	0.05−	0.01−	N	P (Both Tails) 0.10−	0.05−	0.01−
5	15	—	—	25	125	147	189
6	17	21	—	26	131	155	201
7	22	24	—	27	140	164	212
8	26	30	36	28	146	174	224
9	29	35	43	29	155	183	235
10	35	39	49	30	163	191	247
11	40	46	56	31	170	202	260
12	44	52	64	32	178	210	272
13	49	57	73	33	187	221	285
14	55	63	81	34	195	231	299
15	60	70	90	35	204	240	312
16	66	78	98	36	212	250	324
17	71	85	107	37	221	261	339
18	77	91	117	38	229	271	353
19	84	98	126	39	238	282	366
20	90	106	136	40	248	292	380
21	97	115	147				
22	103	123	157				
23	110	130	168				
24	118	138	178				

Table VII. The Gaussian Distribution — Frequency of Random Samples Lying Beyond Specified Multiples of the Standard Deviation Measured Above and Below the Mean

(Based on R.A. Fisher's Table of the Normal Distribution)

P = probability (relative frequency in random sampling).

Multiple of SD	P (Both Tails)	P (One Tail)
0.063	0.95	0.475
0.126	0.90	0.45
0.253	0.80	0.40
0.385	0.70	0.35
0.524	0.60	0.30
0.674	0.50	0.25
0.842	0.40	0.20
1.036	0.30	0.15
1.282	0.20	0.10
1.645	0.10	0.05
1.960	0.05	0.025
2.326	0.02	0.01
2.576	0.01	0.005
3.291	0.001	0.0005

Table VIII. Two-sample Ranks Test (Wilcoxon-White)

(Prepared by M. I. Sutcliffe)

N_1 and N_2 = sample sizes, N_1 not greater than N_2. P = probability (randomization frequency) in both tails combined. Extreme (minimum; maximum) sums of ranks in N_1 required to insure that P is not greater than the specified values. For explanation and method of use, see Chapter XIV.

N_1	N_2	P (Both Tails) 0.10−	0.05−	0.01−	N_1	N_2	P (Both Tails) 0.10−	0.05−	0.01−
2	4	--	--	--	4	16	24;60	21;63	15;69
	5	3;13	--	--		17	25;63	21;67	16;72
	6	3;15	--	--		18	26;66	22;70	16;76
	7	3;17	--	--					
	8	4;18	3;19	--		19	27;69	23;73	17;79
						20	28;72	24;76	18;82
	9	4;20	3;21	--					
	10	4;22	3;23	--	5	5	19;36	17;38	15;40
	11	4;24	3;25	--		6	20;40	18;42	16;44
	12	5;25	4;26	--		7	21;44	20;45	16;49
	13	5;27	4;28	--		8	23;47	21;49	17;53
						9	24;51	22;53	18;57
	14	6;28	4;30	--					
	15	6;30	4;32	--		10	26;54	23;57	19;61
	16	6;32	4;34	--		11	27;58	24;61	20;65
	17	6;34	5;35	--		12	28;62	26;64	21;69
	18	7;35	5;37	--		13	30;65	27;68	22;73
						14	31;69	28;72	22;78
	19	7;37	5;39	3;41					
	20	7;39	5;41	3;43		15	33;72	29;76	23;82
3	3	6;15	--	--		16	34;76	30;80	24;86
	4	6;18	--	--		17	35;80	32;83	25;90
	5	7;20	6;21	--		18	37;83	33;87	26;94
	6	8;22	7;23	--		19	38;87	34;91	27;98
	7	8;25	7;26	--					
						20	40;90	35;95	28;102
	8	9;27	8;28	--	6	6	28;50	26;52	23;55
	9	10;29	8;31	6;33		7	29;55	27;57	24;60
	10	10;32	9;33	6;36		8	31;59	29;61	25;65
	11	11;34	9;36	6;39		9	33;63	31;65	26;70
	12	11;37	10;38	7;41		10	35;67	32;70	27;75
	13	12;39	10;41	7;44		11	37;71	34;74	28;80
	14	13;41	11;43	7;47		12	38;76	35;79	30;84
	15	13;44	11;46	8;49		13	40;80	37;83	31;89
	16	14;46	12;48	8;52		14	42;84	38;88	32;94
	17	15;48	12;51	8;55		15	44;88	40;92	33;99
	18	15;51	13;53	8;58		16	46;92	42;96	34;104
	19	16;53	13;56	9;60		17	47;97	43;101	36;108
	20	17;55	14;58	9;63		18	49;101	45;105	37;113
4	4	11;25	10;26	--		19	51;105	46;110	38;118
	5	12;28	11;29	--		20	53;109	48;114	39;123
	6	13;31	12;32	10;34	7	7	39;66	36;69	32;73
	7	14;34	13;35	10;38		8	41;71	38;74	34;78
	8	15;37	14;38	11;41		9	43;76	40;79	35;84
						10	45;81	42;84	37;89
	9	16;40	14;42	11;45		11	47;86	44;89	38;95
	10	17;43	15;45	12;48					
	11	18;46	16;48	12;52		12	49;91	46;94	40;100
	12	19;49	17;51	13;55		13	52;95	48;99	41;106
	13	20;52	18;54	13;59		14	54;100	50;104	43;111
						15	56;105	52;109	44;117
	14	21;55	19;57	14;62		16	58;110	54;114	46;122
	15	22;58	20;60	15;65					

Table VIII (Continued)

N_1	N_2	P (Both Tails)			N_1	N_2	P (Both Tails)		
		0.10—	0.05—	0.01—			0.10—	0.05—	0.01—
7	17	61;114	56;119	47;128	12	12	120;180	115;185	105;195
	18	63;119	58;124	49;133		13	125;187	119;193	109;203
	19	65;124	60;129	50;139		14	129;195	123;201	112;212
	20	67;129	62;134	52;144		15	133;203	127;209	115;221
						16	138;210	131;217	119;229
8	8	51;85	49;87	43;93					
	9	54;90	51;93	45;99		17	142;218	135;225	122;238
	10	56;96	53;99	47;105		18	146;226	139;233	125;247
	11	59;101	55;105	49;111		19	150;234	143;241	129;255
	12	62;106	58;110	51;117		20	155;241	147;249	132;264
	13	64;112	60;116	53;123	13	13	142;209	136;215	125;226
	14	67;117	62;122	54;130		14	147;217	141;223	129;235
	15	69;123	65;127	56;136		15	152;225	145;232	133;244
	16	72;128	67;133	58;142		16	156;234	150;240	136;254
	17	75;133	70;138	60;148		17	161;242	154;249	140;263
	18	77;139	72;144	62;154		18	166;250	158;258	144;272
	19	80;144	74;150	64;160		19	171;258	163;266	147;282
	20	83;149	77;155	66;166		20	175;267	167;275	151;291
9	9	66;105	62;109	56;115	14	14	166;240	160;246	147;259
	10	69;111	65;115	58;122		15	171;249	164;256	151;269
	11	72;117	68;121	61;128		16	176;258	169;265	155;279
	12	75;123	71;127	63;135		17	182;266	172;276	159;289
	13	78;129	73;134	65;142		18	187;275	179;283	163;299
	14	81;135	76;140	67;149		19	192;284	183;293	168;308
	15	84;141	79;146	69;156		20	197;293	188;302	172;318
	16	87;147	82;152	72;162	15	15	192;273	184;281	171;294
	17	90;153	84;159	74;169		16	197;283	190;290	175;305
	18	93;159	87;165	76;176		17	203;292	195;300	180;315
	19	96;165	90;171	78;183		18	208;302	200;310	184;326
	20	99;171	93;177	81;189		19	214;311	205;320	189;336
10	10	82;128	78;132	71;139		20	220;320	210;330	193;347
	11	86;134	81;139	73;147					
	12	89;141	84;146	76;154	16	16	219;309	211;317	196;332
	13	92;148	88;152	79;161		17	225;319	217;327	201;343
	14	96;154	91;159	81;169		18	231;329	222;338	206;354
	15	99;161	94;166	84;176		19	237;339	228;348	210;366
	16	103;167	97;173	86;184		20	243;349	234;358	215;377
	17	106;174	100;180	89;191	17	17	249;346	240;355	223;372
	18	110;180	103;187	92;198		18	255;357	246;366	228;384
	19	113;187	107;193	94;206		19	262;367	252;377	234;395
	20	117;193	110;200	97;213		20	268;378	258;388	239;407
					18	18	280;386	270;396	252;414
11	11	100;153	96;157	87;166		19	287;397	277;407	258;426
	12	104;160	99;165	90;174		20	294;408	283;419	263;439
	13	108;167	103;172	93;182					
	14	112;174	106;180	96;190	19	19	313;428	303;438	283;458
	15	116;181	110;187	99;198		20	320;440	309;451	289;471
	16	120;188	113;195	102;206	20	20	348;472	337;483	315;505
	17	123;196	117;202	105;214					
	18	127;203	121;209	108;222					
	19	131;210	124;217	111;230					
	20	135;217	128;224	114;238					

INDEX